# Bio-Inspired Regenerative Medicine

# Bio-Inspired Regenerative Medicine

Materials, Processes, and Clinical Applications

edited by

**Simone Sprio**
**Anna Tampieri**

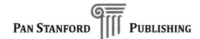

PAN STANFORD PUBLISHING

*Published by*

Pan Stanford Publishing Pte. Ltd.
Penthouse Level, Suntec Tower 3
8 Temasek Boulevard
Singapore 038988

Email: editorial@panstanford.com
Web: www.panstanford.com

**British Library Cataloguing-in-Publication Data**
A catalogue record for this book is available from the British Library.

**Bio-Inspired Regenerative Medicine: Materials, Processes, and Clinical Applications**

Copyright © 2016 Pan Stanford Publishing Pte. Ltd.

*All rights reserved. This book, or parts thereof, may not be reproduced in any form or by any means, electronic or mechanical, including photocopying, recording or any information storage and retrieval system now known or to be invented, without written permission from the publisher.*

For photocopying of material in this volume, please pay a copying fee through the Copyright Clearance Center, Inc., 222 Rosewood Drive, Danvers, MA 01923, USA. In this case permission to photocopy is not required from the publisher.

ISBN 978-981-4669-14-6 (Hardcover)
ISBN 978-981-4669-15-3 (eBook)

Printed in the USA

# Contents

*Preface*                                                                   xiii

**1. Biologically Inspired Nanomaterials and Nanobiomagnetism: A Synergy among New Emerging Concepts in Regenerative Medicine**                1

*Anna Tampieri, Monica Sandri, Silvia Panseri, Alessio Adamiano, Monica Montesi, and Simone Sprio*

| | | |
|---|---|---|
| 1.1 | The New Concept of Bio-Inspiration toward Biomimetics | 2 |
| 1.2 | Bio-Inspired Scaffolds for Regeneration of Bone and Multi-Functional Hard Tissues | 5 |
| 1.3 | Nanobiomagnetism as a New Concept to Boost Tissue Regeneration | 10 |
| 1.4 | Conclusions | 15 |

**2. Biomimetic Nanostructured Platforms for Biologically Inspired Medicine**                21

*Silvia Minardi, Alessandro Parodi, Francesca Taraballi, Bruna Corradetti, Bradley K. Weiner, and Ennio Tasciotti*

| | | | |
|---|---|---|---|
| 2.1 | | Mimicry of the Extracellular Matrix Composition and Its Functions | 22 |
| | 2.1.1 | The Extracellular Matrix: A Modulator of Cell Activity in Tissues | 22 |
| | 2.1.2 | Artificial Extracellular Matrices for Tissue Engineering Applications | 23 |
| | 2.1.3 | Surface Modifications of Biomaterials | 24 |
| | | 2.1.3.1 Integrin adhesion sites | 25 |
| | | 2.1.3.2 Growth factors | 26 |

|  |  | 2.1.3.3 | Glycosamminoglycans and proteoglycans | 27 |

2.1.3.3 Glycosamminoglycans and
proteoglycans ... 27

2.1.3.4 Molecules and artificial ECM:
new players in immune-modulation ... 28

2.2 Biomimicry of the Biochemical Gradients
Occurring in the Regenerative Process ... 30

  2.2.1 Control Over Growth Factor Release ... 31

    2.2.1.1 Polymeric vectors ... 31

    2.2.1.2 Silica-based vectors ... 32

    2.2.1.3 Bioactive coatings to mimic cell
functions ... 33

  2.2.2 Composite Vectors ... 34

## 3. Nano-Apatites with Designed Chemistry and Crystallinity for Bone Regeneration and Nanomedical Applications ... 47

*Michele Iafisco and Daniele Catalucci*

3.1 Introduction ... 48

3.2 Apatite Nanocrystals in Biological Systems ... 49

3.3 Nanocrystalline Apatite ... 58

3.4 Nanocrystalline Apatite for Bone Regeneration
and Nanomedical Applications ... 63

## 4. New Biomimetic Strategies for Regeneration of Load-Bearing Bones ... 85

*Simone Sprio, Andrea Ruffini, Massimiliano Dapporto,
and Anna Tampieri*

4.1 Bone Tissue: Structure, Biomechanics and
Remodelling ... 86

4.2 Main Limitations in Current Approaches for
Regeneration of Load-Bearing Bones ... 89

4.3 Regeneration of Long Segmental Bones:
New Biomorphic Porous Devices ... 94

4.4 Treatment of Osteoporosis-Related Fractures:
New Biomimetic Injectable Devices ... 101

## Contents | vii

**5. New Bio-Inspired Processes for Synthesis and Surface Treatments of Biomaterials**     **119**

*Frank A. Müller*

| | | |
|---|---|---|
| 5.1 | Introduction | 119 |
| 5.2 | Biomimetic Apatite | 120 |
| 5.3 | Literature Survey | 122 |
| 5.4 | In vitro Apatite Formation | 124 |
| | 5.4.1   Simulated Body Fluid | 125 |
| | 5.4.2   Bioactive Surfaces | 127 |
| | 5.4.3   Structure and Properties of Biomimetic Apatite | 129 |
| |      5.4.3.1   Nucleation and crystal growth | 129 |
| |      5.4.3.2   Carbonate substitution | 133 |
| |      5.4.3.3   Growth orientation | 135 |
| 5.5 | Conclusions | 137 |

**6. Fibre-Reinforced, Biphasic Composite Scaffolds with Pore Channels and Embedded Stem Cells Based on Alginate for the Treatment of Osteochondral Defects**     **145**

*F. Despang, C. Halm, K. Schütz, B. Fischer, A. Lode, and M. Gelinsky*

| | | |
|---|---|---|
| 6.1 | Osteochondral Defects and the Tissue Engineering Approach | 145 |
| 6.2 | Scaffolds with Parallel Aligned Pores Generated from the Biopolymer Alginate | 148 |
| | 6.2.1   Biopolymer Alginate and Its Structure Formation Phenomenon of Directed Ionotropic Gelation | 148 |
| | 6.2.2   Influence of Selected Process Parameters on Pore Channel Formation during Ionotropic Gelation | 151 |
| 6.3 | Biphasic Alginate-Based Scaffolds with Channel-Like Pores | 157 |
| | 6.3.1   Components of the Biphasic Scaffolds beyond Alginate | 158 |
| | 6.3.2   Macro- and Microstructure of Alginate Scaffolds Including Fibres | 160 |

| | | | |
|---|---|---|---|
| | 6.3.3 | Mechanical Strengthening by Fibre Reinforcement of Alginate Based Scaffolds | 162 |
| | 6.3.4 | Evaluation of Cytocompatibility | 163 |
| | | 6.3.4.1 Evaluation of cytocompatibility by indirect exposure | 163 |
| | | 6.3.4.2 Generation of cell-laden scaffolds with embedded stem cells and long-term analysis of cell viability | 166 |
| 6.4 | Summary and Outlook | | 170 |

## 7. Hybrid Nanocomposites with Magnetic Activation for Advanced Bone Tissue Engineering          179

*Ugo D'Amora, Teresa Russo, Roberto De Santis, Antonio Gloria, and Luigi Ambrosio*

| | | |
|---|---|---|
| 7.1 | Introduction | 180 |
| 7.2 | Bone Tissue Engineering | 181 |
| 7.3 | Magnetism in Biomedicine: Basic Principles in the Design of Magnetic Scaffolds | 187 |
| 7.4 | Magnetic Scaffolds for Advanced Bone Tissue Engineering | 192 |
| 7.5 | Conclusions and Future Trends | 198 |

## 8. Bio-Inspired Organized Structures Guiding Nerve Regeneration          211

*Rahmat Cholas, Marta Madaghiele, Luca Salvatore, and Alessandro Sannino*

| | | | |
|---|---|---|---|
| 8.1 | Introduction | | 211 |
| | 8.1.1 | Key Aspects of Peripheral Nerve Development, Regeneration, and Structure | 213 |
| 8.2 | Spontaneous Nerve Regeneration | | 216 |
| 8.3 | Surgical Approaches to Neurotmesis | | 217 |
| | 8.3.1 | Direct Repair | 217 |
| | 8.3.2 | Autologous Nerve Graft | 219 |
| | 8.3.3 | Tubulization | 220 |
| 8.4 | Bio-Inspired Design of Nerve Regenerative Templates | | 222 |

|  |  | 8.4.1 | Mimicking Native Nerve ECM Topography | 222 |
|  |  | 8.4.2 | Mimicking Native Nerve ECM Biochemistry | 225 |
|  |  | 8.4.3 | Multi-Faceted Approaches | 228 |
|  | 8.5 | Conclusion | | 230 |

## 9. Biomimetic Scaffolds Integrated with Patterns of Exogenous Growth Factors — **241**

*Silvia Minardi, Francesca Taraballi, Bayan Aghdasi, and Ennio Tasciotti*

| 9.1 | Scaffolds and Bioactive Molecules in Orthopedic Surgery: Potential and Pitfalls | 241 |
| 9.2 | Conventional Fabrication Methods of Scaffold Functionalized with Bioactive Molecules | 243 |
|  | 9.2.1 | Layer-by-Layer Assembly of Growth Factor-Coated Implants | 243 |
|  | 9.2.2 | Electrospun Scaffolds Functionalized with Bioactive Molecules | 244 |
| 9.3 | Mimicry of the Natural Biochemical Gradients | 246 |
|  | 9.3.1 | Functionalization of Scaffolds with Nano- and Microstructured Delivery Systems | 247 |
|  | 9.3.2 | Spatial and Temporal Patterning of Biomimetic Scaffolds and Hydrogels with Multiple Proteins | 250 |

## 10. Heart Failure and MicroRNA-Based Therapy: A Perspective on the Use of Nanocarriers — **259**

*Michele Miragoli, Michael V. G Latronico, Gianluigi Condorelli, and Daniele Catalucci*

| 10.1 | Introduction | 260 |
| 10.2 | The Pathophysiology of Cardiac Hypertrophy and Failure | 261 |
|  | 10.2.1 | Cardiac Ion Channel Remodeling and Arrhythmogenesis | 262 |
| 10.3 | MicroRNA: A Class of Abundant Non-Protein Regulators | 263 |
|  | 10.3.1 | MicroRNA Biogenesis | 264 |

| | | | |
|---|---|---|---|
| | 10.3.2 | Function and Mechanism of Action of MicroRNA | 265 |
| | 10.3.3 | MicroRNA and Cardiac Pathophysiology | 266 |
| | | 10.3.3.1 Cardiac miRNAs: A close-up on miR-1 and miR-133 | 267 |
| | 10.3.4 | MicroRNA-Based Therapies | 269 |
| 10.4 | | Nanoparticles and the Heart | 270 |
| | 10.4.1 | Side A of the Coin: Nanoparticle Cardiotoxicity | 271 |
| | 10.4.2 | Side B of the Coin: The Physicochemical Nature of Nanoparticles | 271 |
| 10.5 | | Nanoparticle-Mediated Delivery of MicroRNA to the Heart: Future Perspectives | 273 |

## 11. Triggering Cell–Biomaterial Interaction: Recent Approaches for Osteochondral Regeneration  283

*Monica Montesi and Silvia Panseri*

| | | |
|---|---|---|
| 11.1 | Introduction | 283 |
| 11.2 | Biomaterial Chemical Features | 285 |
| 11.3 | View within Article | 286 |
| 11.4 | Scaffold Architecture: From Macro- to Molecular Level | 288 |
| 11.5 | Biosignals to Enhance the Cellular Interactions with Biomaterials | 291 |
| 11.6 | Magnetic Remote Control: Innovative Solution for Tissue Regeneration | 293 |

## 12. Biomimetic Materials in Regenerative Medicine: A Clinical Perspective  305

*Maurilio Marcacci, Giuseppe Filardo, Giulia Venieri, Lorenzo Milani, and Elizaveta Kon*

| | | |
|---|---|---|
| 12.1 | Introduction | 306 |
| 12.2 | Smart Biomimetic Materials | 307 |
| 12.3 | Tendons | 308 |
| 12.4 | Ligaments | 309 |
| 12.5 | Menisci | 310 |

| | | |
|---|---|---|
| 12.6 | Osteochondral Defects | 311 |
| 12.7 | Bone | 313 |
| 12.8 | Conclusions | 315 |

## 13. Clinical Aspects in Regeneration of Articular Regions: New Biologically Inspired Multifunctional Scaffolds — 321

*Elizaveta Kon, Giuseppe Filardo, Francesco Tentoni, Andrea Sessa, and Maurilio Marcacci*

| | | |
|---|---|---|
| 13.1 | Introduction | 321 |
| 13.2 | The Osteochondral Strategy | 323 |
| 13.3 | Clinical Results in Osteochondral Regeneration | 325 |
| 13.4 | Conclusions | 330 |

## 14. Biomimetic Materials in Spinal Surgery: A Clinical Perspective — 335

*Giandomenico Logroscino, Giampiero Salonna, and Carlo Ambrogio Logroscino*

| | | |
|---|---|---|
| 14.1 | Introduction | 335 |
| 14.2 | Historical Background and Indications for Spinal Fusion | 336 |
| 14.3 | Biomimetic Bone Substitutes | 341 |
| 14.4 | Tissue Engineering Strategies | 342 |
| | 14.4.1 Smart Materials: Biomimetic Scaffolds | 342 |
| | 14.4.2 "*Doped*" Ceramic Substitutes | 343 |
| | 14.4.3 Bioactivity of Ceramic Materials | 345 |
| | 14.4.4 Fiber-Reinforced Ceramic Materials | 346 |
| | 14.4.5 Control of the Material Resorption Velocity | 346 |
| 14.5 | Current Research: Future Prospects | 347 |
| 14.6 | Cell-Based and Gene Therapy | 347 |
| 14.7 | Factor-Based Therapy | 348 |
| | 14.7.1 Demineralized Bone Matrix | 348 |
| | 14.7.2 Platelet-Rich Plasma | 349 |
| | 14.7.3 Bone Morphogenetic Proteins | 349 |
| 14.8 | Conclusion | 349 |

xii | Contents

**15. Bioartificial Endocrine Organs: At the Cutting Edge of Translational Research in Endocrinology** 357

*Roberto Toni, Elena Bassi, Fulvio Barbaro, Nicoletta Zini, Alessandra Zamparelli, Marco Alfieri, Davide Dallatana, Salvatore Mosca, Claudia della Casa, Cecilia Gnocchi, Giuseppe Lippi, Giulia Spaletta, Elena Bassoli, Lucia Denti, Andrea Gatto, Francesca Ricci, Pier Luigi Tazzari, Annapaola Parrilli, Milena Fini, Monica Sandri, Simone Sprio, and Anna Tampieri*

15.1 Introduction 358

    15.1.1 Basic Principles for ex situ Growth and Differentiation of Endocrine Cells to Engineer Complex, 3D Organomorphic Bioconstructs 358

    15.1.2 Lessons from Embryonic Development for an ex situ Developmental Bioengineering of Endocrine Organs: The Organomorphic Principle 361

    15.1.3 Current Results on ex situ Bioengineering of Bioartificial Endocrine Organs 365

15.2 The New Concept of the Organomorphic Scaffold-Bioreactor Unit for Endocrine Organ Bioengineering 366

    15.2.1 Design of a Thyromorphic, Scaffold-Bioreactor Unit for ex situ Bioengineering, and Its Application to Patient-Tailored Bioconstructs 368

    15.2.2 Studies on the Role of the Native Stroma in Addressing the Morphogenesis of the Embryonic Human Thyroid Gland 373

    15.2.3 Studies on the Growth and Differentiation of Adult Rat Thyroid Cells in 3D Culture Systems 374

    15.2.4 Studies on the ex situ Bioengineering of the Rat Anterior Pituitary Gland, Adrenal Cortex, Thymus and Cerebral Neocortex 376

15.3 Conclusions 378

*Index* 389

# Preface

The field of regenerative medicine is today a melting pot of interdisciplinary competences spanning from materials science, biology and medicine. Indeed, only strong interdisciplinary approaches can successfully face the challenge to establish new regenerative therapies significantly improving the life quality of millions of people worldwide.

As biomaterials play a major role in this field, material scientists are being increasingly pushed to develop advanced constructs mimicking the extracellular matrix in a tissue-specific fashion. In this respect, the driving concept is *biomimetics*, pinning on both a close reproduction of the physico-chemical, morphological, and mechanical features of the host tissues, and on smart functionalization, aiming to provide the biomaterials with ability of smart response to specific physiological conditions and, possibly, of boosting the regenerative cascade.

With this in mind, the book was conceived and developed to capture broad interest among young chemists, physicists, engineers, and biologists acting in biomaterials development. After an introduction describing the most recent trends in regenerative medicine, each of the following chapters is dedicated to specific topics and application fields, so that they are stand-alone contributions that can be consulted independently.

We thank Pan Stanford Publishing for having invited us to edit such a book and all the authors for having accepted to contribute to it. We hope that the book may provide the readers with a good overview of the recent advances in this important field and possibly be a source of inspiration for new research.

**Simone Sprio**
**Anna Tampieri**
Faenza, February 2016

# Chapter 1

# Biologically Inspired Nanomaterials and Nanobiomagnetism: A Synergy among New Emerging Concepts in Regenerative Medicine

Anna Tampieri, Monica Sandri, Silvia Panseri, Alessio Adamiano, Monica Montesi, and Simone Sprio

*Institute of Science and Technology for Ceramics,*
*National Research Council of Italy, ISTEC-CNR,*
*Via Granarolo 64, 48018 Faenza, Italy*

anna.tampieri@istec.cnr.it

Materials science is today experiencing a paradigmatic change in the development of new smart devices for biomedical applications. Indeed there is a strong demand for new solutions able to face and solve degenerative and highly invalidating diseases that involve a steadily increasing number of people, also due to the progressive ageing of the population. In particular, the regeneration of hard tissues (i.e. bone, cartilage, tooth) is one of the most demanding issues in medicine and requires smart devices showing high mimicry of the host tissues and able to instruct and address progenitor cells to the regeneration of new functional tissue. This chapter highlights the emerging concepts of bio-inspiration, by which natural processes can be reproduced in lab and

*Bio-Inspired Regenerative Medicine: Materials, Processes, and Clinical Applications*
Edited by Simone Sprio and Anna Tampieri
Copyright © 2016 Pan Stanford Publishing Pte. Ltd.
ISBN 978-981-4669-14-6 (Hardcover), 978-981-4669-15-3 (eBook)
www.panstanford.com

addressed to the synthesis of scaffolds mimicking complex multi-functional tissues. Besides, nanobiomagnetism is presented as a new strategy to develop *on demand* bio-devices that can be activated and controlled by non-invasive remote signaling. These new concepts promise to be among the most relevant drivers for the development of new generation smart biomedical devices with high regenerative performance in the next decade.

## 1.1 The New Concept of Bio-Inspiration toward Biomimetics

During the last few years, "bio-nanocomposite" has become a common term to designate those nanocomposites involving a naturally occurring polymer (biopolymer) in combination with an inorganic phase, and showing at least one dimension on the nanometer scale. Similar to conventional nanocomposites, which involve synthetic polymers, these bio-hybrid materials (i.e. organic/inorganic structures with complex interaction at the molecular scale) exhibit improved structural and functional properties of great interest for different applications spanning from optical, magnetic, and electrochemical to biological ones. In particular, bio-nanocomposites show the remarkable advantage of exhibiting biocompatibility, biodegradability and, in some cases, complex tissue-like features that provide them with functional properties given by the interaction between the organic and inorganic components. This kind of interaction has been recently described as *binary cooperative complementary phenomena* [1] i.e. the coexistence of two entirely opposite physical statuses such as positive/negative, hydrophobic/hydrophilic, hard/soft, optically dense/loose matter. Once the distance between the two nanoscopic components is comparable to the characteristic length of some physical interactions, the cooperation between these complementary building blocks become dominant and endows the macroscopic materials with novel and superior properties.

The inspiration for the design and development of bio-nanocomposites takes place from living organisms that are able to produce natural nanocomposites showing an amazing hierarchical arrangement of their organic and inorganic components from the nanoscale to the macroscopic scale (Fig. 1.1). Nacre in pearls and shells, ivory, bones, ligaments, enamel and dentine, as well as woods, plants, insects and shells are fine examples of bio-nanocomposites found in Nature.

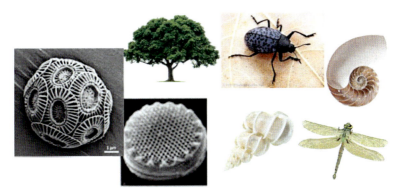

**Figure 1.1** Examples of natural structures with hierarchically organized morphology.

Biological materials science focuses on the structure–function–property–processing paradigm, which is a common theme in materials science, however synthesis and growth of natural materials is quite different from the procedures of fabrication of synthetic materials. Almost all biological systems follow some fundamental design principles [2]: (i) *self-assembly*; (ii) *fitting form to function*, since biological systems grow, self-repair, and evolve as needed to survive and to actuate superior functions; (iii) *hierarchical structures*: Efficiency and multi-functionality are organized over a range of scale levels (nanoscale to macroscale).

Differently, synthetic ceramics and composites imply harsh synthesis and fabrication procedures to be built as 3D constructs, but often right these processes are responsible for bioactivity loss and degradation of most of the other biological performances. On the other hand, biomimetic processes mimicking the natural phenomena of organization-assembling and nucleation enable the development of 3D structures with high level of functional ability using mild synthesis conditions [3, 4].

Biomineralization, responsible for the natural bone and tooth formation, is an example of natural process generating bio-nanocomposite endowed with superior biological and mechanical performance. It was recently reproduced and merged in a single process at the lab level to develop biomimetic bone and osteochondral scaffolds [5, 6].

During the past decade, in the orthopedic field, the well-established approach for curing diseased bone parts, based on replacement with inert substitutes, has progressively given way to new regenerative approaches, based on the use of bioactive and biomimetic devices. Such devices should have the task to trigger the correct cascade of biological events that lead to tissue regeneration, exposing cells to an adequate array of signals. Native extra-cellular matrix contains multiple signals whose presentation follows precise spatial and temporal patterns. In designing scaffolds for bone or osteochondral tissue regeneration, such signals must be reproduced so as to give chemical, physical, structural, and morphological information to cells and compel them to express specific phenotypes.

Bone tissue is one of the most representative examples of natural hybrid nanocomposites: In case of bone loss or bone critical size defects (i.e. a defect that does not heal spontaneously), one of the best approaches to facilitate bone regeneration is through the development of scaffolds. An ideal scaffold guiding tissue regeneration should not only maintain, induce, and restore biological functions, but also have adequate properties with respect to degradation, cell binding, cellular uptake, non-immunogenicity, mechanical strength, and flexibility. The key technical aspects that have to be met by a scaffold can be summarized as the *4Fs*: *form*, *function*, *fixation*, and *formation* [7].

An adequate *form* enables adaptation of the scaffold to the bone defect cavities for a suitable filling. *Function* is the load-bearing property of the scaffolds in compliance with biomechanical demands in specific anatomic sites. An adequate *fixation* of the scaffold provide an adequate interface and interconnection with the surrounding bone, preventing or at least diminishing motion between scaffold and bone and thereby avoid non-union. *Formation* means that bone scaffolds should promote new bone formation. In this respect, the essential characteristics of regenerative bone scaffolds are biocompatibility, which includes appropriate degradation profile without host tissue responses such as inflammation or fibrous encapsulation of the implant; osteoconductivity, i.e. the ability to serve as a template for bone cells, thus guiding bone formation along the scaffold surfaces (i.e. outside and inside the scaffold pores) by supporting cells to adhere and proliferate; bioactivity that enables the scaffold to form chemical bonds with the surrounding host bone; osteoinductivity, i.e. ability to induce bone formation as postulated for nanohydroxyapatite [8].

Among the several different approaches in developing scaffold for regenerative medicine, a great consensus is now consolidating around the concept of "*biomimetics.*" Such a definition indicates the ability of a synthetic material to closely reproduce chemical composition, physical properties, and 3D architecture of native tissues. The idea embodied in such a concept is that the physicochemical and morphological features of the scaffold, once implanted, are, by themselves, signals able to stimulate cell chemotaxis and colonization by autologous cells. In this way, the human body can be seen as a natural bioreactor able to guide proper tissue regeneration starting from a biomimetic scaffold without addition of cells or other biological factors simply recalling autologous cells and preserving the physiologic equilibrium.

In the case of bone tissue, the reproduction of its complex structure, made of elements characterized by a defined chemistry and with a morphology hierarchically organized from the macroscopic down to the molecular scale, can be obtained by reproducing the conditions for activating several intrinsic control mechanisms: chemical, structural, and morphological mechanisms that control the hybrid nanocomposites' final characteristics.

By these mechanisms, the organic template transfers information to the mineral phase at the molecular level that in turn reflect on the upper levels of hierarchy, toward the macroscopic size: (a) The chemical interaction of HA with collagen prevents the crystallization and growth of the mineral phase, which results in a poorly crystalline phase with an apatite-like lattice; (b) the growth of nuclei is controlled by organic matrix and the size and shape of the nuclei are constrained up to few nanometers; (c) the topotactic interaction induce a specific crystal orientation of the mineral phase growing on the collagen fiber; (d) finally, lamellae organize through different hierarchical levels up to the macroscopic bone [9–15].

## 1.2 Bio-Inspired Scaffolds for Regeneration of Bone and Multi-Functional Hard Tissues

Actually chemical factors are crucial in affecting the bioactivity and bioavailability of the biomaterials: In the case of synthetic

HA/Collagen hybrid composites [5], collagen fibers, which act as sites of heterogeneous nucleation, hamper HA crystals growth and crystallization, allowing the entrapment of ions naturally present in the physiological environment (i.e. $Mg^{2+}$, $CO_3^{2-}$, $Na^+$, $K^+$, $SiO_4^{4-}$) into the mineral lattice. In bone mineral, $CO_3^{2-}$ ions mainly substitute phosphate (B type position) and, to a smaller extent, $OH^-$ (A type position) ions [10]. The substitution of $CO_3^{2-}$ ions for $PO_4^{3-}$ ions is the major source of structural disorder in bone mineral, and consequently increases its chemical reactivity (dissolution and thermal decomposition). In particular, B-type carbonation enhances the apatite solubility without altering the surface polar property and the affinity of the osteoblast cells. Besides, $CO_3^{2-}$ ions also exist in non-apatitic domains, mainly located in a hydrated layer surrounding apatite crystals; their amount is high in young bone, thus representing a reservoir of ions that promote the remodeling processes. Among the substituting cations, magnesium is associated with the first stages of bone formation (5 mol%) and decreases with increasing calcification and with ageing of the individual [11]. The presence of magnesium increases the nucleation kinetics of HA on collagen fibers but retards its crystallization, giving rise to small mineral nuclei/particles (<20 nm), thus increasing the bioavailability of the mineral phase. For this reason, the magnesium concentration is higher in cartilage and young bone than in mature tissues. Silicon, as well, is an essential element for healthy skeletal and cartilage growth and development in higher biological organisms [12, 16], and is especially high in the metabolically active state of the cell. Silicon is also known to bind to glycosaminoglycan macromolecules and has been shown to play a role in the formation of cross-links between collagen and proteoglycans [17], thus resulting in the stabilization of bone matrix molecules and preventing their enzymatic degradation. The consequence of chemical substitutions, from the structural point of view, is the formation of a nearly amorphous calcium phosphate with increased solubility at physiological pH and tendency to structural reorganization, which implies ions exchange and movement at the crystal/physiological environment interface. Similarly, spatial factor and structural factor, consisting in the control exerted by the insoluble macromolecules acting as templates for the nucleation of mineral phases, play a crucial role in affecting the bioactivity of the composites. Crystal growth is limited to very few unit cells of the apatite lattice, with values ranging from 30–50 nm long, 15–30 nm wide, and 2–10 nm thick, the high value of specific surface reflects in increased bioactivity [13–15, 18–20].

The apatite platelets develop along the long axis of collagen, so that the apatite crystals grow preferentially along the $c$ axis of the hexagonal apatite lattice. This specific growth direction, induced by the presence of particular functional chemical groups on the surface of the organic template, affects the surface polarity of the final hybrid composites and consequently protein adhesion and cell attachment.

Finally, a morphologic control is activated (morphogenesis) where, on a macroscopic scale, the mineral phase assumes a complex architecture, strictly dependent on the combination of the various above-described phenomena, which hierarchically occur on different dimensional scales in correspondence with the sites of heterogeneous nucleation.

All these control mechanisms, reproducing phenomena occurring in biological processes, synergistically act toward the realization of 3D hybrid composites manifesting complex functions and capacity of remodeling, and specific interaction with cells. The amount and morphology of the porosity in hybrid composite, usually above 80% for bone and osteochondral regeneration, can be directed and customized by freeze drying processes.

The in-lab reproduction of phenomena occurring in biological processes can be considered as a conceptually new approach for nanotechnology and may pave the way for the development of new devices with outstanding properties. On the basis of the recognition of the different requirements to regenerate cartilaginous and bony part, such processes can be directed to graded scaffolds reproducing different histological areas in the osteochondral tissue by simply varying the degree of mineralization and the alignment of collagen fibers [6]. Therefore, hydrogels with designed features can be engineered into three-layered devices reproducing the sub-chondral bone (mineralization = 60–70 wt%), mineralized cartilage (mineralization = 30–40 wt%), and the hyaline cartilage (no mineralization) (Fig. 1.2). In particular, the collagen-like layer, based on collagen and added with hyaluronic acid to create microstructural features improving the hydrophilic behavior of the construct, reproduces some cartilaginous environmental cues such as the formation of a columnar-like structure converging toward the external surface where it forms horizontal flat ribbons, resembling the morphology of the *lamina splendens* [5, 6].

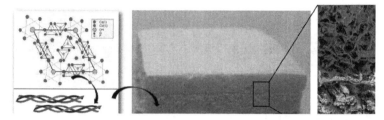

**Figure 1.2** Left: scheme of the crystal structure of hydroxyapatite, heterogeneously nucleating in the gap of collagen molecule; middle: three-layer hybrid composite mimicking osteochondral region; right: SEM image of the different tissue-mimicking morphology of the different layers.

Such composites have demonstrated enhanced cell proliferation with very spread cell morphology (Fig. 1.3), as well as high osteoinductivity and regenerative potential. The HA/collagen graded composites differentially support cartilage and bone tissue formation in the different histological layers, as demonstrated by comparative in vivo study carried out on adult sheep, where HA/collagen graded composites have been implanted on femoral condyles [21]. In particular, histological evaluation showed the formation of new hyaline-like tissue and good integration of scaffolds with host cartilage, with a strong proteoglycan staining and columnar rearrangement of chondrocytes, and an underlying well-ordered sub-chondral trabecular bone.

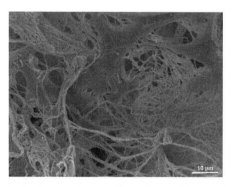

**Figure 1.3** Colonization and spreading of osteoblast cells cultivated on hybrid HA/Collagen scaffold.

In this section, it has been discussed that biologic processes pin on information exchanged at a molecular scale and on boundary conditions exerted by the polymer template and environmental conditions that guide the process toward the establishment of 3D hybrid composites with defined characteristics. This implies that bio-inspired syntheses are flexible processes that can be directed to fabricate specific devices *on demand*. In this respect, hybrid collagen/hydroxyapatite composites can be developed to assume specific 3D morphologies thus mimicking human multifunctional tissues such as periodontal regions. Indeed, human tooth is a complex organ formed by a multifunctional region (i.e. the periodontium, formed by alveolar bone and cementum, linked together by the periodontal ligament) firmly bound to the root, and the dentin, a highly mineralized collagen matrix with tubular organization that is protected by the enamel (see Fig. 1.4).

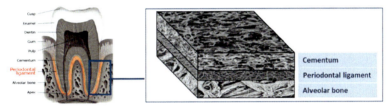

**Figure 1.4**   Scheme of tooth structure (left) and of three-layer constructs designed for regeneration of Periodontium.

All the components of tooth form upon biologic phenomena close to those leading to formation of bone and cartilage [22]. The relevant differences are related to the mineralization extent of the different tissues (i.e. alveolar bone ~70 wt%, cementum ~50 wt%, dentine ~75 wt%, enamel ~98%), the degree of aggregation of collagen fibers and the structural organization. Therefore, bio-inspired in-lab mineralization can be directed to develop new biomimetic scaffolds mimicking the different parts of teeth by varying the concentration of calcium and phosphate ions in respect to collagen thus achieving the desired mineralization extent. Then, oriented channel-like porosity mimicking the tubular organization of dentine can be obtained by ionotropic gelation techniques applied to the as-synthesized hydrogels (see Fig. 1.5).

Hence, preliminary research shows that the application of flexible bio-inspired synthesis techniques can enable the development of new implantable devices for the complete regeneration of dental tissues. This is one of the most demanding clinical needs and a target of high impact in materials science and regenerative medicine.

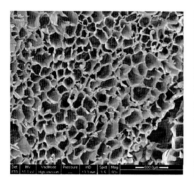
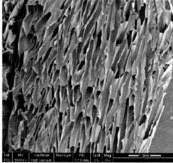

**Figure 1.5** Hybrid porous constructs based on collagen mineralized with hydroxyapatite showing dentin-like oriented tubular porosity.

## 1.3 Nanobiomagnetism as a New Concept to Boost Tissue Regeneration

Since biomimetic scaffolds effectively drive bone tissue regeneration, also providing progressive replacing of the scaffold itself with new healthy tissue (bio-resorption process), the patients' metabolism plays an important role in the regulation of the kinetics and extent of new bone formation. For this reason metabolic diseases, as well as the degenerative condition induced by aging, are a concern and new bone formation and fracture healing are reduced. Causes include a reduced number of recruited osteoblast precursors and the advanced age-related changes occurring in bone matrix. This fact impacts the delicate relationship between bone resorption and bone formation so that imbalance can occur, thus leading to osteopenia and osteoporosis. In consideration of the ever-increasing ageing of the world population, the occurrence of degenerative diseases is expected to steadily rise in the next decades, thus new therapeutic approaches are strongly required to boost tissue regeneration in patients with reduced endogenous regenerative potential. Systemic approaches are now being recognized as scarcely suitable to this purpose, as the patients are exposed to a number of harmful side effects and, indeed, the systemic administration of growth factors has limited efficacy due to the short lifetime. Therefore biomimetic and osteoconductive scaffolds should ensure prolonged and controlled biochemical stimulation that should be delivered *on demand* and in temporo-spatially defined fashion.

In this respect, recent advances in material science suggest that the use of weak magnetic fields is appealing as remote signaling for non-destructive and non-invasive controlling of biomedical devices in vivo. The use of magnetic materials in nanomedicine is thus raising a steadily growing interest, due to the numerous possible applications including cancer therapy by hyperthermia, magnetic resonance imaging and other diagnostic approaches based on the guiding of such particles to specific targeted areas in vivo and their use as nanoprobes. This represents a very interesting and promising tool for new personalized therapies [23–28]. However, the currently used superparamagnetic iron oxide nanoparticles (SPION, i.e. mainly magnetite and maghemite) exhibit long-term toxicity by progressive accumulation in soft tissues and organs such as liver and kidney [29, 30]. Recently, Tampieri et al. developed a new biocompatible and bioresorbable superparamagnetic phase by doping HA with $Fe^{2+}/Fe^{3+}$ ions (FeHA) [31]. This new biomaterial has been developed by selective and dosed substitution of Fe ions in the two specific crystal sites of calcium. Since FeHA exhibit composition very close to the one of mineral bone, it exhibits very good biocompatibility. This was confirmed by in vitro studies revealing that FeHA nanoparticles do not reduce cell viability and at the same time enhance cell proliferation compared to HA particles. This effect was even significantly increased when a magnetic field was applied [32].

Moreover, a pilot animal study of bone repair (a rabbit critical bone defect model) demonstrated the in vivo biocompatibility and biodegradability of FeHA [32].

The achievement of biocompatible nanobiomaterials with magnetic properties opens new perspectives in therapeutics and more specifically in regenerative medicine. In this scenario, it is possible to identify two main paths for the development of new biomedical devices of high socio-economic impact: (1) new biomimetic scaffolds with ability of remote activation and switching; (2) magnetic cells obtained by internalization of new biocompatible magnetic nanophases (Fig. 1.6).

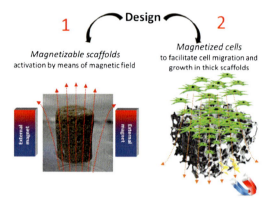

**Figure 1.6**  Scheme of the possible applications of biocompatible/bioactive superparamagnetic phases in regenerative medicine.

Indeed, the development of scaffolds enhancing bone regeneration by remote magnetic activation is now an emerging concept in regenerative medicine [33], since it has been demonstrated that weak magnetic or pulsed electromagnetic fields are effective in promoting bone fracture healing, spinal fusion, and bone ingrowth in animal models [34–38].

Moreover, several works have demonstrated that magnetic scaffolds have a positive effect on osteoinductivity with and without application of external magnetic force. However, the incorporation of magnetic phases into ceramic bone scaffolds is made difficult by the need of consolidating green ceramic bodies by a high temperature treatment that often provokes oxidation of superparamagnetic iron oxides and losing of their properties [32]. In this respect FeHA can also be synthesized by inducing heterogeneous nucleation on Type I collagen that functions as a 3D self-assembling fibrous template, thus reproducing the biomineralization process as already described in Section 1.1 [39]. This method yields biomimetic hybrid scaffolds with mineralization extent that can be tailored from cartilage to bone-like level. The presence of a mineral phase with bone-like features and ability to be activated by remote magnetic signal make this new biomaterial very promising to boost regeneration of extended bone and osteochondral regions, even in patients with reduced endogenous regenerative potential [40–43].

Thanks to its high biocompatibility and safety, FeHA phase can also be used in techniques of tissue engineering to enhance the efficacy of regenerative devices. Indeed, a key limiting factor in the regeneration of extended bone defects is the inability of cells to self-propagate in the inner part of the scaffold and to establish new bone and vascular tissue [44]. Recent progress shows that it is possible to locally guide the migration of magnetic nanoparticles and nanoparticle-labeled cells through the use of an externally applied magnetic field gradient [45]. In this respect FeHA nanoparticles can be easily incorporated into cells by endocytosis, thus obtaining "magnetic cells" without negatively affect cell behavior (e.g. proliferation, morphology, differentiation) (see Fig. 1.7). Through the application of an external magnetic field of low intensity, these cells can be guided within a scaffold, in order to have a faster and more selective seeding for tissue engineering application. Besides, cells can be moved selectively into different anatomic regions so to achieve high cell concentration, thus reducing the cell loss typical of the current cell therapies. The feasibility of safe generation of magnetic cells opens new generation approach in cell therapies and cell homing.

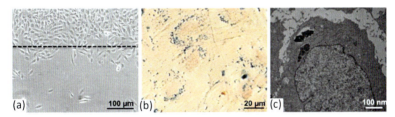

**Figure 1.7** (a) Magnetic cells aligned by a static magnetic field application; (b) FeHA nanoparticles endocytosed by cells stained with Prussian blue; (c) TEM analysis of FeHA nanoparticles uptaken by cells.

The progress in the investigation of magnetism in nanomaterials will lead to advanced functionalization techniques and specific applications for magnetic nanoparticle targeting and magnetic nanomaterials. Along with novel nanomaterials, new multimodality therapeutic and diagnostic materials will emerge, characterized by high sensitivity, specificity, and efficacy.

In this respect, among the new approaches in therapeutics and regenerative medicine, one of the most challenging is the development of smart drug delivery systems with ability to release active molecules *on demand* and under defined temporo-spatial

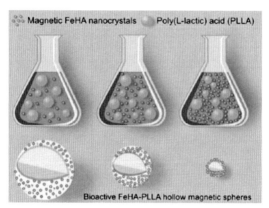

**Figure 1.8** Scheme of functionalization of polylactic acid spheres with superparamagnetic FeHA.

patterns. In this respect, many techniques are being investigated to conjugate bioactive molecules to magnetic nanoparticles [46–51]. Recently, the use of biocompatible magnetic media such as FeHA phase enabled the development of magnetic hybrid inorganic–polymeric composites in the form of hollow micro-nano spheres (Fig. 1.8) [52–54]. These devices may enable multiple functionalization, by taking advantage of the active surface sites of the polymer and the apatite phase; moreover, drugs or bioactive molecules can be loaded in the cavity of the spheres. The chemical-physical features of the spheres such as size, polymer crystallinity, surface charge, and magnetization can be tailored by the amount of FeHA. In this respect they displayed good biocompatibility toward bone marrow mesenchymal stem cells, and the spheres coated with higher amount of FeHA exhibited better cell proliferation than those coated with lower amount. These magnetic materials have potential uses as building blocks for the preparation of scaffolds for hard tissue regeneration as well as carriers of biomolecules for nanomedical applications. In fact, due to the presence of magnetic FeHA nanoparticles these new devices can be remotely activated through alternate magnetic fields. Such a stimulus can be dosed to obtain mild effect (magneto-shaking) or to trigger hyperthermia effect by which spheres can be disrupted thus releasing the bioactive agent [55]. Therefore, further development of this approach may represent a new tool enabling the release of different chemical species under defined patterns thus achieving more advanced and personalized therapies. Besides,

FeHA phase can be used as safe and biocompatible nanoparticles for applications at the frontier of knowledge such as *magnetovaccination* and *magnetofection* that are envisaged for advanced cell and gene therapies [56, 57].

## 1.4 Conclusions

The emerging concept of biomimetics applied to material science is gaining ground as a milestone for the development of new generation devices with smart properties and ability to respond to urgent clinical needs, most of which related to the progressive aging of the population. In particular, inspiration from nature is to be considered as a key paradigm for material scientists, to overcome the limitation of the current processes and products and to provide new nanomaterials with real mimicry of native tissues and ability to establish an active cross-talk with cells.

Besides, the urging need for smart and personalized solutions is pushing scientists toward investigation of the effects of weak magnetic fields on cell metabolism, that may enable switching on/off mechanisms for the on-demand control and activation of biomedical devices. Therefore, further progress in the understanding of fundamental science related to physical, chemical, and biological aspects of living tissues in interaction with magnetic fields will pave the way to identify new approaches in theranostics and regenerative medicine that may significantly improve the life of people worldwide.

### Acknowledgment

The authors would like to acknowledge the EC-funded project SMILEY (GA n. 310637) for the financial support

### References

1. Su, B., Guo, W., and Jiang, L. (2014). Learning from nature: Binary cooperative complementary nanomaterials, *Small*, DOI: 10.1002/smll.201401307.

2. Fratzl, P., and Weinkamer, R. (2007). Nature's hierarchical materials, *Prog. Mater. Sci.*, **52**, pp. 1263–1334.

3. Reis, R. L., and San Román, J., eds. (2005). *Biodegradable systems in Tissue Engineering and Regenerative Medicine*, CRC Press.

4. Kumbar, S. G., Laurencin, C. T., Deng, M., eds. (2014). *Natural and Synthetic Natural Polymers*, Elsevier.

5. Tampieri, A., Celotti, G., Landi, E., Sandri, M., Roveri, N., and Falini, G. (2003). Biologically inspired synthesis of bone like composite: Self-assembled collagen fibers/hydroxyapatite nanocrystals, *J. Biomed. Mater. Res.*, **67A**, pp. 618–625.

6. Tampieri, A., Sandri, M., Landi, E., Pressato, D., Francioli, S., Quarto, R., and Martin, I. (2008). Design of graded biomimetic osteochondral composite scaffolds, *Biomaterials*, **29**(26), pp. 3539–3546.

7. Hollister, S. J., and Murphy, W. L. (2011). Scaffold translation: Barriers between concept and clinic, *Tissue Eng. Part B Rev.*, **17**(6), pp. 459–474.

8. Wagoner Johnson, A. J., and Herschler, B. A. (2011).A review of the mechanical behavior of CaP and CaP/polymer composites for applications in bone replacement and repair, *Acta Biomater.*, **7**(1), pp. 16–30.

9. LeGeros, R. Z. (1991). *Calcium Phosphate in Oral Biology and Medicine*, Karger.

10. Boskey, A. L. (2006). Mineralization, structure and function of bone. In *Dynamics of Bone and Cartilage Metabolism* (Seibel, M. J., Robins, S. P., and Bilezikian, J. P., eds.), Academic Press, pp. 201–212.

11. Bigi, A., Foresti, E., Gregorini, R., Ripamonti, A., Roveri, N., and Shah, J. S. (1992). The role of magnesium on the structure of biological apatite, *Calcif. Tissue Int.*, **50**, pp. 439–444.

12. Matsko, N. B., Žnidaršič, N., Letofsky-Papst, I., Dittrich, M., Grogger, W., Štrus, J., and Hofer, F. (2011). Silicon: The key element in early stages of biocalcification, *J. Struct. Biol.*, **174**, pp. 180–186.

13. Lowenstam, H. A., and Weiner, S. (1989). *On Bio-Mineralization*, Oxford University Press.

14. Robinson, R. A., and Watson, M. L. (1952). Collagen–crystal relationships in bone as seen in the electron microscope, *Anat. Rec.*, **114**, pp. 383–409.

15. Jackson, S. A., Cartwright, A. G., and Lewis, D. (1978). The morphology of bone-mineral crystals, *Calcif. Tissue Res.*, **25**(1), pp. 217–222.

16. Pietak, A. M., Reid, J. W., Stott, M. J., and Sayer, M. (2007). Silicon substitution in the calcium phosphate bioceramics, *Biomaterials*, **28**, pp. 4023–4032.

17. Schwarz, K. (1973). A bound form of Si in glycosaminoglycans and polyuronides, *Proc. Natl. Acad. Sci. U. S. A.*, **70**, pp. 1608–1612.

18. Eppell, S. J., Tong, W. D., Katz, J. L., Kuhn, L., and Glimcher, M. J. (2001). Shape and size of isolated bone mineralites measured using atomic force microscopy, *J. Orthop. Res.*, **19**, pp. 1027–1034.

19. Weiner, S., and Price, P. A. (1986). Disaggregation of bone into crystals, *Calcif. Tissue Int.*, **39**, pp. 365 375.

20. Traub, W., Arad, T., and Weiner, S. (1989). Three-dimensional ordered distribution of crystals in turkey tendon collagen fibers, *Proc. Natl. Acad. Sci.*, **86**, pp. 9822–9826.

21. Kon, E., Delcogliano, M., Filardo, G., Fini, M., Giavaresi, G., Francioli, S., Martin, I., Pressato, D., Arcangeli, E., Quarto, R., Sandri, M., and Marcacci, M. (2010). Orderly osteochondral regeneration in a sheep model using a novel nano-composite multilayered biomaterial, *J. Orthop. Res.*, **28**, pp. 116–124.

22. Linde, A., and Goldberg, M. (1993). Dentinogenesis, *Crit. Rev. Oral Biol. Med.*, **4**(5), pp. 679–728.

23. Meng, J., Xiao, B., Zhang, Y., Liu, J., Xue, H., Lei, J., Kong, H., Huang, Y., Jin, Z., Gu, N., and Xu, H. (2013). Super-paramagnetic responsive nanofibrous scaffolds under static magnetic field enhance osteogenesis for bone repair in vivo, *Sci. Rep.*, **3**, pp. 2655–2662.

24. Panseri, S., Russo, A., Sartori, M., Giavaresi, G., Sandri, M., Fini, M., Maltarello, M. C., Shelyakova, T., Ortolani, A., Visani, A., Dediu, V., Tampieri, A., and Marcacci, M. (2013). Modifying bone scaffold architecture in vivo with permanent magnets to facilitate fixation of magnetic scaffolds, *Bone*, **56**, pp. 432–439.

25. Shan, D., Shi, Y., Duan, S., Wei, Y., Cai, Q., and Yang, X. (2013). Electrospun magnetic poly(L-lactide) (PLLA) nanofibers by incorporating PLLA-stabilized $Fe_3O_4$ nanoparticles, *Mater. Sci. Eng. C*, **33**, pp. 3498–3505.

26. Meng, J., Zhang, Y., Qi, X., Kong, H., Wang, C., Xu, Z., Xie, S., Gu, N., and Xu, H. (2010). Paramagnetic nanofibrous composite films enhance the osteogenic responses of pre-osteoblast cells. *Nanoscale*, **2**, pp. 2565–2569.

27. Hou, R., Zhang, G., Du, G., Zhan, D., Cong, Y., Cheng, Y., and Fu, J. (2013). Magnetic nanohydroxyapatite/PVA composite hydrogels for promoted osteoblast adhesion and proliferation, *Colloids Surf. B*, **103**, pp. 318–325.

28. Mertens, M. E., Hermann, A., Bühren, A., Olde-Damink, L., Möckel, D., Gremse, F., Ehling, J., Kiessling, F., and Lammers, T. (2014). Iron

oxide-labeled collagen scaffolds for non-invasive MR imaging in tissue engineering, *Adv. Funct. Mater.*, **24**, pp. 754–762.

29. Lewinski, N., Colvin, V., and Drezek, R. (2008). Cytotoxicity of nanoparticles, *Small*, **4**, pp. 26–49.

30. Singh, N., Jenking, G. J. S, Asadi, R., and Doak, S. H. (2010). Potential toxicity of superparamagnetic iron oxide nanoparticles (SPION), *Nano Rev.*, **1**, pp. 53–58.

31. Tampieri, A., D'Alessandro, T., Sandri, M., Sprio, S., Landi, E., Bertinetti, L., Panseri, S., Pepponi, G., Goettlicher, J., Bañobre-López, M., and Rivas, J. (2012) Intrinsic magnetism and hyperthermia in bioactive Fe-doped hydroxyapatite, *Acta Biomater.*, **8(2)**, pp. 843–851.

32. Panseri, S., Cunha, C., D'Alessandro, T., Sandri, M., Giavaresi, G., Marcacci, M., Hung, C. T., and Tampieri, A. (2012). Intrinsically super-paramagnetic Fe-hydroxyapatite nanoparticles positively influence osteoblast-like cell behavior, *J. Nanobiotechnol.*, **10**, pp. 32–42.

33. Clavijo-Jordan, V., Kodibagkar, V. D., Beeman, S. C., Hann, B. D., and Bennett, K. M. (2012). Principles and emerging applications of nano magnetic materials in medicine, *WIREs Nanomed. Nanobiotechnol.*, **4**, pp. 345–365.

34. Grace, K. L. R., Revell, W. J., and Brookes, M. (1998). The effects of pulsed electromagnetism on fresh fracture healing: Osteochondral repair in the rat femoral groove, *Orthopedics*, **21**, pp. 297–302.

35. Glazer, P. A., Heilmann, M. R., Lotz, J. C., and Bradford, D. S. (1997). Use of electromagnetic fields in a spinal fusion: A rabbit model, *Spine*, **22**, pp. 2351–2356.

36. Yan, Q. C., Tomita, N., and Ikada, Y. (1998). Effects of static magnetic field on bone formation of rat femurs, *Med. Eng. Phys.*, **20**, pp. 397–402.

37. Assiotis, A., Sachinis, N. P., and Chalidis, B. E. (2012). Pulsed electromagnetic fields for the treatment of tibial delayed unions and nonunions. A prospective clinical study and review of the literature, *J. Orthop. Sur. Res.*, **7**, p. 24.

38. Chalidis, B., Sachinis, N., Assiotis, A., and Maccauro, G. (2011). Stimulation of bone formation and fracture healing with pulsed electromagnetic fields: Biologic responses and clinical implications, *Int. J. Immunopathol. Pharmacol.*, **24**, pp. 17–20.

39. Tampieri, A., Iafisco, M., Sandri, M., Panseri, S., Cunha, C., Sprio, S., Savini, E., Uhlarz, M., and Herrmannsdörfer, T. (2014). Magnetic bio-inspired hybrid nanostructured collagen-hydroxyapatite scaffolds

supporting cell proliferation and tuning regenerative process, *ACS Appl. Mater. Interf.*, **6**(18), pp. 15697–15707.

40. Torbet, J., and Ronziere, M. C. (1984). Magnetic Alignment of collagen during self-assembly, *Biochem. J.*, **219**, pp. 1057–1059.

41. Higashi, T., Yamagishi, A., Takeuchi, T., Kawaguchi, N., Sagawa, S., Onishi, S., and Date, M. (1993). Orientation of erythrocytes in a strong static magnetic field, *Blood*, **82**, pp. 1328–1334.

42. Kotani, H., Kawaguchi, H., Shimoaka, T., Iwasaka, M., Ueno, S., Ozawa, H., Nakamura, K., and Hoshi, K. (2002). Strong static magnetic field stimulates bone formation to a definite orientation in vitro and in vivo, *J. Bone Miner. Res.*, **17**, pp. 1814–1821.

43. Xu, H.-Y., and Gu, N. (2014). Magnetic responsive scaffolds and magnetic fields in bone repair and regeneration, *Front. Mater. Sci.*, **8**, pp. 20–31.

44. Sprio, S., Sandri, M., Iafisco, M., Panseri, S., Filardo, G., Kon, E., Marcacci, M., and Tampieri, A. (2014). Composite biomedical foams for engineering bone tissue. In: *Biomedical Foams for Tissue Engineering Applications* (Netti, P. A., ed.), Woodhead Publishing Limited, Cambridge (UK), pp. 249–280.

45. Ganguly, R., and Puri, I. K. (2010). Microfluidic transport in magnetic MEMS and bioMEMS, *WIREs Nanomed. Nanobiotechnol.*, **2**, pp. 382–399.

46. Veiseh, O., Gunn, J. W., and Zhang, M. Q. (2010). Design and fabrication of magnetic nanoparticles for targeted drug delivery and imaging, *Adv. Drug Deliv. Rev.*, **62**, pp. 284–304.

47. Sperling, R. A., and Parak, W. J. (2010). Surface modification, functionalization and bioconjugation of colloidal inorganic nanoparticles, *Philos. Trans. A Math. Phys. Eng. Sci.*, **368**, pp. 1333–1383.

48. Yiu, H. H., McBain, S. C., Lethbridge, Z. A., Lees, M. R., and Dobson, J. (2010). Preparation and characterization of polyethylenimine-coated $Fe_3O_4$-MCM-48 nanocomposite particles as a novel agent for magnetassisted transfection, *J. Biomed. Mater. Res. A*, **92**, pp. 386–392.

49. Schellenberger, E., Schnorr, J., Reutelingsperger, C., Ungethum, L., Meyer, W., Taupitz, M., and Hamm, B. (2008). Linking proteins with anionic nanoparticles via protamine: Ultrasmall protein-coupled probes for magnetic resonance imaging of apoptosis, *Small*, **4**, pp. 225–230.

50. Yu, M. K., Jeong, Y. Y., Park, J., Park, S., Kim, J. W., Min, J. J., Kim, K., and Jon, S. (2008). Drug-loaded superparamagnetic iron oxide nanoparticles

for combined cancer imaging and therapy in vivo, *Angew. Chem. Int. Ed. Engl.*, **47**, pp. 5362–5365.

51. Dilnawaz, F., Singh, A., Mohanty, C., and Sahoo, S. K. (2010). Dual drug loaded superparamagnetic iron oxide nanoparticles for targeted cancer therapy, *Biomaterials*, **31**, pp. 3694–3706.

52. Bañobre-Lopez, M., Piñeiro-Redondo, Y., De Santis, R., Gloria, A., Ambrosio, L., Tampieri, A., Dediu, V., and Rivas, J. (2011). Poly(caprolactone) based magnetic scaffolds for bone tissue engineering, *J. Appl. Phys.*, **109**, p. 07B313.

53. Gloria, A., Russo, T., D'Amora, U., Zeppetelli, S., D'Alessandro, T., Sandri, M., Bañobre-Lopez, M., Piñeiro-Redondo, Y., Uhlarz, M., Tampieri, A., Rivas, J., Herrmannsdörfer, T., Dediu, V. A., Ambrosio, L., and De Santis, R. (2013). Magnetic poly($\varepsilon$-caprolactone)/iron-doped hydroxyapatite nanocomposite substrates for advanced bone tissue engineering, *J. R. Soc. Interface*, **10**, p. 20120833.

54. Iafisco, M., Sandri, M., Panseri, S., Delgado-Lopez, J. M., Gomez-Morales, J., and Tampieri, A. (2013). Magnetic bioactive and biodegradable hollow Fe-doped hydroxyapatite coated poly(L-lactic) acid micro-nanospheres, *Chem. Mater.*, **25**, pp. 2610–2617.

55. Nappini, S., Bonini, M., Bombelli, F. B., Pineider, F., Sangregorio, C. L., Baglioi, P., and Norden, B. (2011). Controlled drug release under a low frequency magnetic field: Effect of the citrate coating on magnetoliposomes stability, *Soft Matter*, **7**, pp. 1025–1037.

56. Long, C. M., van Laarhoven, H. W., Bulte, J. W., and Levitsky, H. I. (2009). Magnetovaccination as a novel method to assess and quantify dendritic cell tumor antigen capture and delivery to lymph nodes, *Cancer Res.*, **69**, pp. 3180–3187.

57. Scherer, F., Anton, M., Schillinger, U., Henke, J., Bergemann, C., Krüger, A., Gänsbacher, B., and Plank, C. (2002). Magnetofection: Enhancing and targeting gene delivery by magnetic force in vitro and in vivo, *Gene Ther*, **9**(2), pp. 102–109.

## Chapter 2

# Biomimetic Nanostructured Platforms for Biologically Inspired Medicine

**Silvia Minardi,[a,b] Alessandro Parodi,[a] Francesca Taraballi,[a] Bruna Corradetti,[a] Bradley K. Weiner,[a] and Ennio Tasciotti[a]**

[a]*The Houston Methodist Research Institute, Houston, USA*
[b]*Institute of Science and Technology for Ceramics, National Research Council, ISTEC-CNR, Via Granarolo 64, 48018 Faenza (RA), Italy*

sminardi@houstonmethodist.org

It is well recognized that biological processes are a source of inspiration in a wide range of fields, including nanoscience. The shapes of organisms, animal coat patterns, and seashells are becoming more often an inspiring source. Materials scientists have been vastly learning from Nature; for example, structures found on water lilies, on butterfly wings or marine organism's skeleton could find application in the construction of water-repellant materials, photonic structures, or optical fibers [1]. Moreover, biomaterials found in nature not only have very interesting properties but also are inspiring in the way they are made.

Biomimicry is a term used to describe different kinds of therapeutic/biomedical approaches: Mimicking nature form or

*Bio-Inspired Regenerative Medicine: Materials, Processes, and Clinical Applications*
Edited by Simone Sprio and Anna Tampieri
Copyright © 2016 Pan Stanford Publishing Pte. Ltd.
ISBN 978-981-4669-14-6 (Hardcover), 978-981-4669-15-3 (eBook)
www.panstanford.com

function, organization, and biomolecular working mechanism are just a few examples of this new research field [2]. Mimicking nature's form or function can be applied as a paradigm in the tissue engineering applications.

## 2.1 Mimicry of the Extracellular Matrix Composition and Its Functions

The final goal of tissue engineering is to create neo-tissues similar in architecture, function, and compatibility to native human structures [3]. Although this approach is very promising, many challenges have to be addressed to achieve effective tissue regeneration through the reproduction of complex mechanisms of living system [4]. Observation and understanding of the fundamentals operating in native tissue represents the starting point to develop biohybrid artificial substitutes. Inside a tissue, cells of different phenotypes are interconnected by a complex network of macromolecules comprising proteins and polysaccharides secreted by the cells themselves. This natural environment refers to the extracellular matrix (ECM) that has the role of structurally and functionally organizing the overall tissue.

### 2.1.1 The Extracellular Matrix: A Modulator of Cell Activity in Tissues

The ECM serves as a channel for cell–cell communication. It is enriched with a number of cell surface receptors (e.g., integrins, laminin, and syndecans) and structural proteins (e.g., collagens, laminins, fibronectin, vitronectin, and elastin, which allow adhesion, migration, proliferation, and differentiation [5]. Artificial two- and three-dimensional extracellular scaffolds are typically employed by tissue-engineering to reproduce a native functional tissue and thereby improve the recovery of the patient and tissue regeneration [6]. As an artificial environment meant to support different processes in tissue formation, the ECM should ideally (i) provide structural support for cells residing in that tissue to attach, grow, migrate, and respond to signals, (ii) give the tissue its structural and mechanical properties associated with the tissue functions, (iii) provide bioactive cues to the residing cells, (iv) act as a reservoir of growth factors (GF), and (v) provide a degradable environment to allow neovascularization and remodeling in response to developmental, physiological and pathological challenges (e.g., homeostasis and wound healing) [7]. Because of the tight connection between the cytoskeleton and the ECM achieved through cell surface receptors, cells sense and respond to the mechanical properties of their environment by converting mechanical signals into chemical signals [8, 9]. Consequently, the biophysical properties of ECM influence various cell functions, including adhesion and migration. Moreover, the fibrillar structure of matrix components have been demonstrated to alter cell behavior by bringing about adhesion ligand clustering [10]. Structural ECM features, such as fibrils and pores, are often of a size compatible with cellular processes involved in migration, which may influence the strategy by which cells migrate through the ECM [11].

## 2.1.2 Artificial Extracellular Matrices for Tissue Engineering Applications

The principles of biomimicry are based on strict adherence to the proper replication of natural science as a medium for promoting cellular repair. This coupled with control over the chemical and physical cues of the scaffold will provide the proper environment for cells to integrate and proliferate with the surrounding recipient tissue site. Demonstrating control over the platform for cell growth is important to achieving multi-functionality [12]. In order to create an artificial extracellular matrix, a wide range of options exist (natural, synthetic, and hybrid materials).

- *Natural materials* have biological activity and biocompatibility. The degradation products of these kinds of materials are natural metabolic products such as sugars, amino acids, or minerals that reduce the possibility of cytotoxicity and inflammation [13]. They can be grouped into three classes: (i) ceramics and ceramics composites (shells, bones, material with mineral component), (ii) biopolymer and biopolymer composite (ligament and silk), and (iii) cellular materials (feathers, wood, cancellous bone).
- *Biomimetic Synthetic materials* represent biologically multifunctional hydrogel-based structures, synthesized or not under physiological-like conditions [14, 15], that mimic

natural ECMs at the biochemical and biophysical level such as poly(ε-caprolactone) (PCL), poly(lactic-co-glycolic) acid (PGLA), and Polyethylene glycol (PEG).
- *Hybrid materials* are systems composed by at least two distinct classes of material (synthetic and biological), for example, synthetic polymers, and proteins domains. The combination results in new materials that possess novel properties [16].

Although natural biomaterials have proved effective in many basic and clinical applications [17] synthetic materials more effectively control their physical and chemical properties and can be further modified through biochemical means [18].

### 2.1.3 Surface Modifications of Biomaterials

For the successful design of materials to serve as artificial ECMs, knowledge of molecular interactions that occur within the tissues and between the cells and the ECM is required [19–21] (Fig. 2.1).

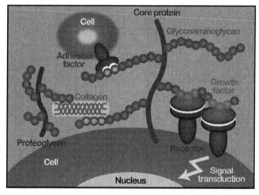

**Figure 2.1** Schematic of the interaction between the extra cellular matrix and cells.

The composition, structure, and manufacturing methods could affect the structural and mechanical properties of the tailored scaffold and the in vivo degradation [22]. Attempts to determine synthetic material surface modifications and to improve the modulation of cell–material interactions have led to the alteration of physicochemical features of biomaterials like chemistry [23] or topography [24–26]. Current methods of biomaterial functionalization include specific surface coatings and the incorporation of bioactive molecules such as adhesion sites, growth factors, anti-inflammatory mediators or drugs, either alone or combined [27, 28]. Biomaterial surface functionalization can be performed either by physical or by wet chemical treatments. Physical modifications include electron-beam or UV-radiation-induced coupling of molecules [6, 7], surface-radical-induced coupling of molecules, and functionalization by non-polymerizing plasma-generated species. Each of these approaches has specific advantages and disadvantages concerning the variability, selectivity, and stability of the obtained functionalization, as well as the question of polymer structure retention or destruction. At present, most functionalization approaches result in surfaces that exhibit a mix of different functional groups [8–12]. It is notable that plasma activation offers a convenient way to alter the surface properties, such as bioactivity and hydrophilicity, or hydrophobicity, while retaining the favorable bulk properties such as biostability, or biodegradability [13, 18].

Taking into account the multifunctional and the nature of biological components, the major challenge into this direction is a chemical one: the need to proceed through bio-orthogonal reactions and under the benign reaction conditions that would preserve and respect the functionality and structure of biological building blocks. In 2001, Sharpless and coworkers [16] introduced the concept of "click chemistry" that successively had an wide impact on the chemical community driving the design of new generation of synthetic biomaterials [29]. These versatile reactions represent a formidable way to engineer hydrogel networks, decorated 2D cell culture surfaces and 3D scaffold. It also provides control over the conformation of the protein or peptide immobilized, thereby maximizing its bioactivity. Finally, the evolution of click-chemistry with the Diels–Alder Click Immobilization is the new era of "reagent-free" click reaction that does not require catalyst, photoinitiator, or radical initiation [30–32].

### 2.1.3.1 Integrin adhesion sites

The knowledge of cell adhesion molecules (CAMs) is already being widely investigated [33]. Integrins are proteins known to be involved in the process of cell adhesion, motility, growth, shape and differentiation [34]. The functionalization of biomaterials with short sequences derived from ECM proteins has been shown to improve cell-specific adhesion and function. The most commonly used peptides are derived from proteins like fibronectin (e.g., RGD, KQAGDV, REDV and PHSRN), laminin (e.g., IKLLI, LRE, LRGDN, PDGSR, IKVAV, LGTIPG, and YIGSR), collagen (e.g., DGEA, GFOGER) and elastin (e.g., VAPG). The most widely used is the arginine-glycine-aspartate (RGD) sequence, a ubiquitous receptor adhesion motif found in most ECM proteins [29]. RGD modified surfaces have been used in a variety of applications such as engineering neuronal tissue [35], improving human embryonic stem cells growth in vitro [29] and increasing the biocompatibility of orthopedic materials [36]. Regarding the integrin domain functionalization some key aspects need to be taken into account. The density and *presentation* of these peptides have been reported to highly affect the overall cellular functions [37, 38] such as cell proliferation, gene expression and differentiation [29]. This effect can be attributed to the variation in adhesion strength between the cells and the substrate. Moreover, spacer sequences (commonly polyethylene glycol) must be long enough, depending of the exposed signal in order) [39] to prevent steric hindrance and to allow for maximal receptor binding, but they must also be short enough to allow for synergistic interactions. The presence of spacers allows for the peptide to present to the cell in a more stable conformation and effectively interact with several receptors [40]. To avoid this limitation, some researchers have explored functionalization using recombinant fragments of native ECM proteins to maintain the native folding of the protein, to retain the same binding motif conformation and orientation and also to inhibit antigenicity.

### 2.1.3.2 Growth factors

Cellular functions are not solely controllable by promoting adhesion and direct interaction with integrins and other cell surface receptors. The induction of a specific growth factor's response is crucial to effectively modulating cell activity. Biodegradable coatings that locally release incorporated growth factors (i.e., Bone Morphogenic Protein-2 (BMP-2), IGF and TGF-$\beta$) have been successfully tested to stimulate fracture healing and to improve biomaterial performance [41]. However, emerging approaches have focused on controlling growth factor release kinetics in order to decrease the effective dose and potential side effects [42]. Sponges [43], hydrogels [44], pastes [45, 46], putties, particulates and various micro- and nanocarriers [44] have been used to successfully deliver growth factors over long timescales. A more sophisticated approach is to exploit the potential of the ECM to regulate the release and functions of growth factors. Artificial ECMs have been developed by functionalizing collagen matrices with glycosamminoglycans (GAGs) and proteoglycans (PGs) [47] to produce a material able to recreate the in vivo environment.

### 2.1.3.3 Glycosamminoglycans and proteoglycans

GAGs are long, unbranched carbohydrate chains consisting of repeating disaccharide units. They are located primarily on the surface of cells or in the ECM. Sugar chains can be modified by sulfate groups as in chondroitin sulfate (CS), heparan sulfate (HS), dermatan sulfate, and keratin sulfate (KS). The only non-sulfated GAG is hyaluronic acid (HA). It is also not attached to a protein core, whereas the sulfated GAGs are linked to serine-rich proteins to form proteoglycans. The glycan matrix of the ECM serves as lubricant and not only provides a reservoir for signaling molecules (growth factors) but also regulates their gradients and mode of action. Components of the ECM (mainly PGs) retain the soluble mediators via electrostatic interactions between the negatively charged sulfate groups of the PGs and the positively charged surface of the signaling molecules [48]. Such interaction has different biological consequences since it affects the local concentration, biological activity, and stabilization of growth factors [49, 50]. Secreted growth factors usually have a short half-life due to the proteolytic degradation that characterizes the extracellular microenvironment. Furthermore, the linkage of growth factors to the ECM protects them from enzymatic cleavage and prevents fast diffusion within the tissue [49]. In addition, growth factor activity may be enhanced by localization within the ECM, allowing interaction with its specific ligands [49]. Conversely, some growth factors (examples) may be inactivated by their adhesion to the ECM and while they can act on their target when released by matrix proteolysis [51], requiring the action of ECM-degrading enzymes expressed by the cells regulated by growth factors and ECM adhesion domains.

### 2.1.3.4 Molecules and artificial ECM: new players in immune-modulation

In tissue engineering, biomaterial implantation is usually accompanied by the injury provoked by the surgical procedure. Tissue or organ injury initiates an inflammatory response to the biomaterial starting with the formation of a provisional matrix [30, 52]. The ability of the immune system to correctly resolve the entire wound healing phases is important in determining the final success of the implanted biomaterials. As such, another crucial role of the ECM is regulating and integrating different and consecutive key processes during the wound healing: hemostasis, inflammation, proliferation, and remodeling of the injured tissue.

During hemostasis, platelets are activated by signals from damaged vascular tissue that induce clot formation. In this phase, there is a formation of a provisional matrix consisting of fibrin and entrapped erythrocytes [52]. Additionally, the secretion of chemokines initiates the recruitment of neutrophils, macrophages, fibroblasts, and resident cells [53]. During the early phases of inflammation, neutrophils are the first cells to be recruited and to arrive at the wound site. They start to phagocyte all the foreign material, bacteria, or dead cells around the wound site while secreting biomolecular cytokines to recruit macrophages. Pro-inflammatory macrophages (M1 phenotype) secrete cytokines and chemokines that promote the further recruitment of other leukocytes to the site of injury [54]. Macrophages then change to a more reparative phenotype (M2 phenotype, also called "alternatively activated") in order to remove apoptotic neutrophils, thus leading to the resolution of the inflammatory phase [53, 55], and, ultimately, to the remodeling phase. The proliferation process involves cellular proliferation, angiogenesis, and new ECM deposition. These are largely mediated via cytokines secreted by macrophages, T lymphocytes, and other cells within the wound site [55]. Finally the remodeling phase is characterized by the degradation and remodeling of the newly deposited ECM, which is mediated by metalloproteinase (MMP) and tissue inhibitor of metalloproteinase (TIMP), This generally results in scar tissue formation or maturation [53–56].

In particular, the foreign body reaction (FBR), composed of macrophages and foreign body giant cells, has been shown to play a critical role in the successful performance of the artificial ECM and mediates the rejection of the implant [30]. For this particular event the biomaterials surface plays the most important role. In fact, in the very early process of implantation, blood/material interactions occur with protein adsorption to the biomaterial surface and development of a blood-based transient provisional matrix that forms on and around the biomaterial. On the contrary, the appropriate functionalization of the biomaterials to be implanted can help in inducing a newly described mechanism that switched macrophages from a detrimental (inflammatory, M1) to a beneficial (regenerative, M2) phenotype [31, 32]. This process, known as "macrophage polarization" can thereby influence macrophages consequent behavior, such as phagocytosis and cytokines secretion. Significant efforts have focused on modifying material properties using various anti-inflammatory polymeric surface coatings to generate more biocompatible implants. The specific features of any synthetic biomaterials are able to tune the formation of giant cells. These multinucleate macrophages can be found at biomaterial surfaces even years following implantation. Recent studies have demonstrated that altering the properties of the bulk materials it is possible to influence the preferential polarization of macrophages [57, 58]. Indeed, natural derived biomaterials elicit a different immune response due to their native structure and surface, as well as the presence of natural ligands that promote constructive tissue remodeling. This anabolic process has been directly linked to the ability of material to polarize macrophage phenotypes [59, 60]. This suggests that biomaterial design strategies able to control the macrophage phenotype may improve the regenerative medicine applications.

A better understanding of the context-specific biological mechanisms, which underlie the macrophage response and macrophage polarization, is essential for the development of biomimetic strategies for appropriate functional tissue remodeling responses.

Different strategies of coatings of anti-inflammatory molecules have been exploited in order to release drugs by passive mechanism [61–63] or by enzymatic secondary reaction [64–66]. As an example of passive mechanism, dexamethasone, a synthetic glucocorticoid hormone, has been used as an anti-inflammatory agent and has been shown to locally reduce the inflammation of the surrounding tissues [67, 68]. Another example of bio-inspired materials can be demonstrated by coating of superoxide dismutase (scavenger enzyme with anti-inflammatory properties) covalently attached to a polyethylene surface to reduce neutrophil recruitment [69]. To achieve the desired in vivo response appropriate coatings need to be designed.

Tunable, immune-modulatory materials may be able to actively direct cell behavior and activity surrounding the implant, thereby encouraging more desirable interactions.

## 2.2 Biomimicry of the Biochemical Gradients Occurring in the Regenerative Process

Several issues affect the therapeutic efficacy of GFs, including their short protein half-life in vivo, side-effects caused by the multiple or high doses administered to reach the desirable concentration in the cell, and possible denaturation of the protein during manipulation, and these should be carefully considered in the design of GF-based therapeutics [70]. Most therapeutic proteins (e.g., GFs, cytokines) that are administered in their native form and without any protection are susceptible to biodegradation, resulting in insufficient amounts of those proteins at the active site, or resulting in the generation of inactive variants [70]. In the search for methods that can overcome these disadvantages, encapsulation of a GF in a delivery system has been demonstrated to be very promising for GF-based therapeutics. This technology, known as localized delivery, is frequently the only feasible strategy if a locally controlled concentration of a GF is necessary, and it has found wide spread use in wound healing and tissue regeneration.

Nanomedicine has been offering numerous innovative possibilities also in this regenerative strategies [71]. However, of the diverse array of particles developed in laboratories, only a few have made their way to the clinic [72]. The ideal carrier for tissue engineering applications should be biocompatible, biodegradable, present a high surface area to accommodate a high amount of molecules and also modifiable to tune the release [70]. Herein, we have been focusing on the advances in molecules and protein release to create temporal and spatial patterns of molecules and GFs to mimic the biochemical gradients of the natural healing process.

## 2.2.1 Control Over Growth Factor Release

The action of GFs is typically concentration dependent [73]. Thus, GFs release has to be precisely controlled. A plethora of nanostructured particulate technologies have been developed, aiming at delivering proteins [74], peptides [75], drugs [76], and genetic materials [77], in a controlled fashion in the site to be regenerated [71, 78, 79].

### 2.2.1.1 Polymeric vectors

Polymeric materials are frequently used to allow controlled, sustained, and localized delivery of proteins. Polymer delivery vehicles allow to control the kinetics and dose of protein release while also protecting the protein from degradation until release [71].

At the end of 1980s it was clear that tissue engineering could benefit of a controlled delivery of GFs and the number and complexity of delivery systems tremendously rose [80]. Several delivery systems prepared from gelatin and collagen were developed as implants [81]. Another material which has been greatly exploited is alginate, to synthesize beads ionically cross-linked [82, 83]. Furthermore, injectable gelatin microspheres were developed by the group of Tabata [84, 85]. In mid-1990s, research further focused on the design of new delivery systems based on biodegradable microspheres. In particular, polylactic acid and poly(lactic-co-glycolic acid) (PLA and PLGA) generated tremendous interest due to their excellent biocompatibility as well as the possibility to tailor their biodegradability by varying composition (lactide/glycolide ratio) [86, 87], molecular weight and chemical structure (i.e., capped and uncapped end-groups) [80]. In particular, FDA approval of PLGA use in humans led to the availability of copolymers characterized by a wide range of in vivo life-times, ranging from 3 weeks to over 1 year [63]. Drug microencapsulation within PLGA copolymers, in form of micro- and nanoparticles, was regarded as a powerful mean to achieve sustained release for long time-frames and, in the case of labile molecules, such as proteins, effectively protect the molecule from in vivo degradation occurring at the administration site. Protein encapsulation in PLGA microspheres is a challenging task due to stability issues occurring during microsphere-processing, shelf-life and protein release [63]. Techniques to entrap protein in PLGA microspheres feature partly competing and partly complementary characteristics [88], and are all joined by the common aim of realizing experimental conditions as mild as possible. Fabrication methods actively used for physical encapsulation of growth factors include solvent casting and particulate leaching, freeze drying, phase separation, melt molding, phase emulsion, in situ polymerization and gas foaming [74]. A key issue is minimizing exposure of factors to harsh conditions during processing in order to protect the activity of the biomolecules [88].

Currently, the synthesis of PLGA follows well established protocols that provide the flexibility of producing PLGA particles with various size, shape, surface chemistry and also nanostructured enclosures [89, 90]. Moreover, PLGA is hydro-soluble, and not immunogenic. Some of this carriers have also the unique ability to co-encapsulate multiple molecules and control the release of each agent in a temporal fashion, or to trigger the release by responding to environmental changes, such as pH, temperature, light, and mechanical stress [5]. However, the preservation of proteins' stability during particles' fabrication still remains a concern.

### 2.2.1.2 Silica-based vectors

A successful approach to preserve protein stability and at the same time allowing for an efficient protein loading has been proposed by De Rosa et al., who tested mesoporous silica (pSi) particles for high loading of proteins, and an agarose coating to further increase protein stability in the carrier [91]. pSi has been widely used for tissue engineering and drug delivery by virtue of its biodegradable and biocompatible nature [92, 93]. For therapeutic delivery, pSi has been administered orally [94], intravenously [95], or injected percutaneously and intraperitonealy in humans for brachytherapy without notable side effects [96]. A wide variety of therapeutic and imaging agents have been successfully loaded into and released from pSi particles including antibiotics [97], hormones [98], proteins [99], liposomes [17] and carbon nanotubes [100], showing the great versatility of this material as a delivery system. As a scaffold, pSi is suitable for directing the growth of neuronal cells [101] and for stimulating mineralization in bone tissue engineering [102, 103]. pSi structure and the idea of using it in nanotechnology applications came mimicking the structure of diatoms shell, which is characterized by a regular structure and high surface area [104, 105]. The size and shape as well as the porosity and pore size of the pSi particles can be engineered and tightly controlled during manufacturing [106], in order to provide a material with constant and uniform physical features at the micro- and nanometer scale and to control degradation time and kinetics as well as biodistribution and bioaccumulation [107, 108].

Additionally, their surface can be functionalized to be linked to scaffold or to control the release kinetics of the payload [91, 109]. Bovine serum albumin (BSA) and BMP-2 were also loaded into pSi particles to examine in vitro release kinetics of the proteins [109]. Furthermore, pSi itself has a regenerative potential: it is osteoinductive (it has the capacity to stimulate primitive stem cells or immature bone cells to grow and mature, forming healthy bone tissue) and also osteoconductive (it can serve as a scaffold on which bone cells can attach and grow so that the bone healing response is lead towards the graft site) [110]. The osteoconductivity of pSi can be controlled by altering the interfacial chemistry and microstructure of the pores. The range of pore size and structure affords the identification of the preferred morphology for osteoblast adhesion, growth, protein matrix synthesis, and mineralization.

Several coating strategies were also developed to avoid the burst release of proteins from the pores and to achieve a sustained and tunable release over the course of weeks [109, 111].

### 2.2.1.3 Bioactive coatings to mimic cell functions

From targeted therapy obtained by modifying the surface of the carriers with antibodies and peptides, a new bio-engineering field is emerging with a focus on isolating, manipulating and treating disease with technology formed in part by biological material. Erythrocyte ghosts represent the first attempts in this direction with promising results [112]. Red blood cells are used as carriers for drugs and biologicals (enzymes, siRNAs, etc.) to develop a 100% personalized, safe and un-expensive approach. Erythrocyte ghosts were shown to be effective in improving payload delivery in many pathological conditions such as vascular treatment, circulating macrophage treatment (e.g., lysosomal storage related disease), infections, ant-inflammatory and anti-cancer agents [113, 114]. Unfortunately the physical or chemical procedure to load red blood cells was shown to create surface damage to cells, which affected circulation time and biocompatibility [115]. However this approach still showed significant advantages over synthetic carriers along parameters such as safety and reproducibility [116]. Leukocytes are another circulating cell phenotype that attracted the attention of researchers for new bio-inspired delivery systems. The Leukolike vector is a hybrid particle formed by a synthetic mesoporous silicon core and a shell derived from the membrane of infiltrating leukocytes [117]. This system was proven to possess high biocompatibility and to delay the unspecific internalization by the cells of the mononuclear system. The surface of these hybrid particles in fact is enriched with many biomarkers related to the tolerance and the self-recognition of the leukocytes [117]. In addition it was shown that the system was provided with active receptors able to target and decrease the barrier function of inflamed vasculature, thereby overcoming all the limitations related to enhanced permeation and retention effect (Fig. 2.2). The system was able to target tumor vasculature of melanoma cancer model in vivo while avoiding internalization of resident macrophages. These technologies represent the most advanced system of the bio-inspired approach, because the pSi utilized to load the payload acquired properties and functions typical of the cell used to coat the particles.

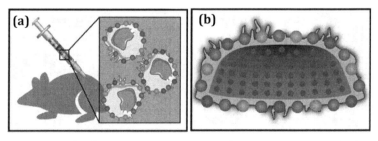

**Figure 2.2** The leukocytes are obtained from a host (a), and their membranes are used to coat mesoporous silicon particles (b).

## 2.2.2 Composite Vectors

The importance of GFs in the regulation of various cell processes, and the need to carefully regulate GF presentation, suggests that sophisticated approaches to their delivery will be crucial to affect desired cellular responses [118]. As discussed above, PLGA has been extensively used for its several advantages. However, PLGA release rates (as well as for pSi) are characterized by an initial burst release that partially hinders the ability to control the timed delivery of payloads [119, 120]. Also, the by-products of PLGA degradation decrease the pH of the surrounding microenvironment resulting in the inherent destabilization or denaturation of the protein payload [121]. In order to address these issues, Fan et al. introduced a composite delivery platform composed of a pSi core encapsulated in a PLGA shell (PLGA-pSi) (Fig. 2.3) [109].

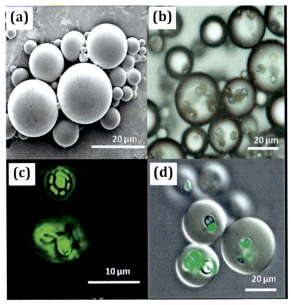

**Figure 2.3** PLGA-pSi characterized by (a) SEM, (b) optical microscope, (c) fluorescence and (d) confocal microscope, with fluorescently labeled pSi particles.

The authors demonstrated that silicon nanoparticles had no immunogenic or toxic effects and that both the PLGA and the pSi component were fully biodegradable [122]. The use of pSi in combination with PLGA enabled the double controlled delivery of molecules, resulting in the extension of the therapeutic window and prevented the acidification of the system during the degradation process resulting in better stabilization of the payload and in a better in vivo therapeutic outcome [109, 123]. Compared with pSi, a larger quantity of biomolecules could be loaded and stored into the PLGA-pSi composite microparticles.

Recently, Bhattacharyya et al. also proposed a PEG-coated mesoporous silica nanoparticles (MSN) with incorporated trypsin inhibitor (a model protein molecule for growth factors) [124]. Due to the goal of incorporating large protein molecules, the pore size of the as-synthesized MSNs was expanded by a hydrothermal treatment prior to payload incorporation. In vitro release from the MSNs without the thin polymer film shows an initial burst followed by continuous release. In the case of polymer-coated MSNs the initial burst release was completely suppressed and approximate zero order release was achieved for 4 weeks.

## References

1. Lopez, P. J., et al., Mimicking biogenic silica nanostructures formation. *Current Nanoscience*, 2005. **1**(1), pp. 73–83.

2. Cramer, M., *Biomimicry: Innovation inspired by nature-Benyus, JM.* 1997, Bowker Magazine Group Cahners Magazine Division 249 W 17th St, New York, NY 10011.

3. Weber, B., et al. *Tissue Engineering on Matrix: Future of Autologous Tissue Replacement.* in *Seminars in Immunopathology.* 2011. Springer.

4. Sreejalekshmi, K. G., and P. D. Nair, Biomimeticity in tissue engineering scaffolds through synthetic peptide modifications— Altering chemistry for enhanced biological response. *Journal of Biomedical Materials Research Part A*, 2011. **96**(2), pp. 477–491.

5. Daley, W. P., S. B. Peters, and M. Larsen, Extracellular matrix dynamics in development and regenerative medicine. *Journal of Cell Science*, 2008. **121**(3), pp. 255–264.

6. Bosman, F. T., and I. Stamenkovic, Preface to extracellular matrix and disease. *The Journal of Pathology*, 2003. **200**(4), pp. 421–422.

7. Kim, B.-S., and D. J. Mooney, Development of biocompatible synthetic extracellular matrices for tissue engineering. *Trends in Biotechnology*, 1998. **16**(5), pp. 224–230.

8. Galbraith, C. G., and M. P. Sheetz, Forces on adhesive contacts affect cell function. *Current Opinion in Cell Biology*, 1998. **10**(5), pp. 566–571.

9. Geiger, B., et al., Transmembrane crosstalk between the extracellular matrix and the cytoskeleton. *Nature Reviews Molecular Cell Biology*, 2001. **2**(11), pp. 793–805.

10. Maheshwari, G., et al., Cell adhesion and motility depend on nanoscale RGD clustering. *Journal of Cell Science*, 2000. **113**(10), pp. 1677–1686.

11. Friedl, P., Prespecification and plasticity: Shifting mechanisms of cell migration. *Current Opinion in Cell Biology*, 2004. **16**(1), pp. 14–23.

12. Hollister, S. J., Scaffold design and manufacturing: From concept to clinic. *Advanced Materials*, 2009. **21**(32–33), pp. 3330–3342.

13. Wegst, U., and M. Ashby, The mechanical efficiency of natural materials. *Philosophical Magazine*, 2004. **84**(21), pp. 2167–2186.

14. Nuttelman, C. R., et al., Macromolecular monomers for the synthesis of hydrogel niches and their application in cell encapsulation and tissue engineering. *Progress in Polymer Science*, 2008. **33**(2), pp. 167–179.

15. Lutolf, M., and J. Hubbell, Synthetic biomaterials as instructive extracellular microenvironments for morphogenesis in tissue engineering. *Nature Biotechnology*, 2005. **23**(1), pp. 47–55.

16. Kopeček, J., and J. Yang, Smart Self-Assembled Hybrid Hydrogel Biomaterials. *Angewandte Chemie International Edition*, 2012. **51**(30), pp. 7396–7417.

17. Ha, T. L. B., and T. M. Quan, *Naturally Derived Biomaterials: Preparation and Application.* 2013.

18. Zhu, J., Bioactive modification of poly (ethylene glycol) hydrogels for tissue engineering. *Biomaterials*, 2010. **31**(17), pp. 4639–4656.

19. Stevens, M. M., and J. H. George, Exploring and engineering the cell surface interface. *Science*, 2005. **310**(5751), pp. 1135–1138.

20. Hynes, R. O., Integrins: Versatility, modulation, and signaling in cell adhesion. *Cell*, 1992. **69**(1), pp. 11–25.

21. Adams, J. C., and F. M. Watt, Regulation of development and differentiation by the extracellular matrix. *Development-Cambridge*, 1993. **117**, pp. 1183–1183.

22. Badylak, S. F., D. O. Freytes, and T. W. Gilbert, Extracellular matrix as a biological scaffold material: Structure and function. *Acta Biomaterialia*, 2009. **5**(1), pp. 1–13.

23. Scotchford, C. A., et al., Protein adsorption and human osteoblast-like cell attachment and growth on alkylthiol on gold self-assembled monolayers. *Journal of Biomedical Materials Research*, 2002. **59**(1), pp. 84–99.

24. Chen, S., et al., Characterization of topographical effects on macrophage behavior in a foreign body response model. *Biomaterials*, 2010. **31**(13), pp. 3479–3491.

25. Dalby, M., et al., In vitro reaction of endothelial cells to polymer demixed nanotopography. *Biomaterials*, 2002. **23**(14), pp. 2945–2954.

26. Schulte, V. A., et al., Surface topography induces fibroblast adhesion on intrinsically nonadhesive poly (ethylene glycol) substrates. *Biomacromolecules*, 2009. **10**(10), pp. 2795–2801.

27. Franz, S., et al., Immune responses to implants—A review of the implications for the design of immunomodulatory biomaterials. *Biomaterials*, 2011. **32**(28), pp. 6692–6709.

28. Boontheekul, T., and D. J. Mooney, Protein-based signaling systems in tissue engineering. *Current Opinion in Biotechnology*, 2003. **14**(5), pp. 559–565.

29. Rahmany, M. B., and M. Van Dyke, Biomimetic approaches to modulate cellular adhesion in biomaterials: A review. *Acta Biomaterialia*, 2012. **9**(3), pp. 5431–5437.

30. Anderson, J. M., Biological responses to materials. *Annual Review of Materials Research*, 2001. **31**(1), pp. 81–110.

31. Collier, T., and J. Anderson, Protein and surface effects on monocyte and macrophage adhesion, maturation, and survival. *Journal of Biomedical Materials Research*, 2002. **60**(3), pp. 487–496.

32. Shen, M., et al., Effects of adsorbed proteins and surface chemistry on foreign body giant cell formation, tumor necrosis factor alpha release and procoagulant activity of monocytes. *Journal of Biomedical Materials Research Part A*, 2004. **70**(4), pp. 533–541.

33. Hynes, R. O., and Q. Zhao, The evolution of cell adhesion. *The Journal of Cell Biology*, 2000. **150**(2), pp. F89–F96.

34. Siebers, M., et al., Integrins as linker proteins between osteoblasts and bone replacing materials. A critical review. *Biomaterials*, 2005. **26**(2), pp. 137–146.

35. Subramanian, A., U. M. Krishnan, and S. Sethuraman, Development of biomaterial scaffold for nerve tissue engineering: Biomaterial mediated neural regeneration. *Journal of Biomedical Science*, 2009. **16**(1), p. 108.

36. Navarro, M., et al., Biomaterials in orthopaedics. *Journal of the Royal Society Interface*, 2008. **5**(27), pp. 1137–1158.

37. Massia, S., and J. Hubbell, Human endothelial cell interactions with surface-coupled adhesion peptides on a nonadhesive glass substrate and two polymeric biomaterials. *Journal of Biomedical Materials Research*, 1991. **25**(2), pp. 223–242.

38. Roberts, C., et al., Using mixed self-assembled monolayers presenting RGD and (EG) 3OH groups to characterize long-term attachment of bovine capillary endothelial cells to surfaces. *Journal of the American Chemical Society*, 1998. **120**(26), pp. 6548–6555.

39. Schmidt, D. R., and W. J. Kao, Monocyte activation in response to polyethylene glycol hydrogels grafted with RGD and PHSRN separated by interpositional spacers of various lengths. *Journal of Biomedical Materials Research Part A*, 2007. **83**(3), pp. 617–625.

40. Taraballi, F., et al., Glycine-spacers influence functional motifs exposure and self-assembling propensity of functionalized substrates tailored for neural stem cell cultures. *Frontiers in Neuroengineering*, 2010. 3 doi. 10.3389/neuro.16.001.2010.

41. Schmidmaier, G., et al., Collective review: Bioactive implants coated with poly(D,L-lactide) and growth factors IGF-I, TGF-$\beta$1, or BMP-2 for stimulation of fracture healing. *Journal of Long-Term Effects of Medical Implants*, 2006. **16**(1), pp. 61–69.

42. Suárez-González, D., et al., Controllable mineral coatings on PCL scaffolds as carriers for growth factor release. *Biomaterials*, 2012. **33**(2), pp. 713–721.

43. Takahashi, Y., M. Yamamoto, and Y. Tabata, Enhanced osteoinduction by controlled release of bone morphogenetic protein-2 from biodegradable sponge composed of gelatin and *$\beta$*-tricalcium phosphate. *Biomaterials*, 2005. **26**(23), pp. 4856–4865.

44. Yamamoto, M., Y. Takahashi, and Y. Tabata, Controlled release by biodegradable hydrogels enhances the ectopic bone formation of bone morphogenetic protein. *Biomaterials*, 2003. **24**(24), pp. 4375–4383.

45. Kempen, D. H., et al., Retention of in vitro and in vivo BMP-2 bioactivities in sustained delivery vehicles for bone tissue engineering. *Biomaterials*, 2008. **29**(22), pp. 3245–3252.

46. Li, R., et al., rhBMP-2 injected in a calcium phosphate paste ($\alpha$-BSM) accelerates healing in the rabbit ulnar osteotomy model. *Journal of Orthopaedic Research*, 2003. **21**(6), pp. 997–1004.

47. Rammelt, S., et al., Coating of titanium implants with collagen, RGD peptide and chondroitin sulfate. *Biomaterials*, 2006. **27**(32), pp. 5561–5571.

48. Kreuger, J., et al., Interactions between heparan sulfate and proteins: the concept of specificity. *The Journal of Cell Biology*, 2006. **174**(3), pp. 323–327.

49. Schultz, G. S., and A. Wysocki, Interactions between extracellular matrix and growth factors in wound healing. *Wound Repair and Regeneration*, 2009. **17**(2), pp. 153–162.

50. Rosso, F., et al., From cell–ECM interactions to tissue engineering. *Journal of Cellular Physiology*, 2004. **199**(2), pp. 174–180.

51. Hynes, R. O., *The extracellular matrix: not just pretty fibrils.* Science, 2009. **326**(5957), pp. 1216–1219.

52. Clark, R. A., Fibrin and wound healing. *Annals of the New York Academy of Sciences*, 2001. **936**(1), pp. 355–367.

53. Werner, S., and R. Grose, Regulation of wound healing by growth factors and cytokines. *Physiological Reviews*, 2003. **83**(3), pp. 835–870.

54. Barrientos, S., et al., Growth factors and cytokines in wound healing. *Wound Repair and Regeneration*, 2008. **16**(5), pp. 585–601.

55. Adamson, R., Role of macrophages in normal wound healing: An overview. *Journal of Wound Care*, 2009. **18**(8), pp. 349–351.

56. Mantovani, A., et al., The chemokine system in diverse forms of macrophage activation and polarization. *Trends in Immunology*, 2004. **25**(12), pp. 677–686.

57. Brown, B. N., et al., Macrophage phenotype as a predictor of constructive remodeling following the implantation of biologically derived surgical mesh materials. *Acta Biomaterialia*, 2012. **8**(3), pp. 978–987.

58. Bota, P., et al., Biomaterial topography alters healing in vivo and monocyte/macrophage activation in vitro. *Journal of Biomedical Materials Research Part A*, 2010. **95**(2), pp. 649–657.

59. Badylak, S. F., et al., Macrophage phenotype as a determinant of biologic scaffold remodeling. *Tissue Engineering Part A*, 2008. **14**(11), pp. 1835–1842.

60. Brown, B. N., et al., Macrophage phenotype and remodeling outcomes in response to biologic scaffolds with and without a cellular component. *Biomaterials*, 2009. **30**(8), pp. 1482–1491.

61. Benkirane-Jessel, N., et al., Control of monocyte morphology on and response to model surfaces for implants equipped with anti-inflammatory agent. *Advanced Materials*, 2004. **16**(17), pp. 1507–1511.

62. Schultz, P., et al., Polyelectrolyte multilayers functionalized by a synthetic analogue of an anti-inflammatory peptide, *α*-MSH, for coating a tracheal prosthesis. *Biomaterials*, 2005. **26**(15), pp. 2621–2630.

63. Anderson, J. M., and M. S. Shive, Biodegradation and biocompatibility of PLA and PLGA microspheres. *Advanced Drug Delivery Reviews*, 1997. **28**(1), pp. 5–24.

64. Lutolf, M. P., et al., Cell-responsive synthetic hydrogels. *Advanced Materials*, 2003. **15**(11), pp. 888–892.

65. Zisch, A. H., et al., Cell-demanded release of VEGF from synthetic, biointeractive cell ingrowth matrices for vascularized tissue growth. *The FASEB Journal*, 2003. **17**(15), pp. 2260–2262.

66. Bae, M., et al., Metalloprotease-specific poly (ethylene glycol) methyl ether-peptide-doxorubicin conjugate for targeting anticancer drug delivery based on angiogenesis. *Drugs Under Experimental and Clinical Research*, 2003. **29**(1), pp. 15–24.

67. Norton, L., et al., Vascular endothelial growth factor and dexamethasone release from nonfouling sensor coatings affect the foreign body response. *Journal of Biomedical Materials Research Part A*, 2007. **81**(4), pp. 858–869.

68. Patil, S. D., F. Papadmitrakopoulos, and D. J. Burgess, Concurrent delivery of dexamethasone and VEGF for localized inflammation control and angiogenesis. *Journal of Controlled Release*, 2007. **117**(1), pp. 68–79.

69. Udipi, K., et al., Modification of inflammatory response to implanted biomedical materials in vivo by surface bound superoxide dismutase mimics. *Journal of Biomedical Materials Research*, 2000. **51**(4), pp. 549–560.

70. Balasubramanian, V., et al., Protein delivery: From conventional drug delivery carriers to polymeric nanoreactors. *Expert Opinion on Drug Delivery*, 2010. **7**(1), pp. 63–78.

71. Shi, J., et al., Nanotechnology in drug delivery and tissue engineering: From discovery to applications. *Nano Letters*, 2010. **10**(9), pp. 3223–3230.

72. Peer, D., et al., Nanocarriers as an emerging platform for cancer therapy. *Nature Nanotechnology*, 2007. **2**(12), pp. 751–760.

73. Tayalia, P., and D. J. Mooney, Controlled growth factor delivery for tissue engineering. *Advanced Materials*, 2009. **21**(32–33), pp. 3269–3285.

74. Lee, K., E. A. Silva, and D. J. Mooney, Growth factor delivery-based tissue engineering: General approaches and a review of recent developments. *Journal of The Royal Society Interface*, 2011. **8**(55), pp. 153–170.

75. Amidi, M., et al., Chitosan-based delivery systems for protein therapeutics and antigens. *Advanced Drug Delivery Reviews*, 2010. **62**(1), pp. 59–82.

76. Ranade, V. V., and J. B. Cannon, *Drug Delivery Systems*. 2011, CRC press.

77. Srinivas, R., S. Samanta, and A. Chaudhuri, Cationic amphiphiles: Promising carriers of genetic materials in gene therapy. *Chemical Society Reviews*, 2009. **38**(12), pp. 3326–3338.

78. Grattoni, A., et al., Nanotechnologies and regenerative medical approaches for space and terrestrial medicine. *Aviation, Space, and Environmental Medicine*, 2012. **83**(11), pp. 1025–1036.

79. Malmsten, M., Inorganic nanomaterials as delivery systems for proteins, peptides, DNA, and siRNA. *Current Opinion in Colloid & Interface Science*, 2013. **18**(5), pp. 468–480.

80. Quaglia, F., Bioinspired tissue engineering: The great promise of protein delivery technologies. *International Journal of Pharmaceutics*, 2008. **364**(2), pp. 281–297.

81. Buckley, A., et al., Sustained release of epidermal growth factor accelerates wound repair. *Proceedings of the National Academy of Sciences*, 1985. **82**(21), pp. 7340–7344.

82. Downs, E. C., et al., Calcium alginate beads as a slow-release system for delivering angiogenic molecules in vivo and in vitro. *Journal of Cellular Physiology*, 1992. **152**(2), pp. 422–429.

83. Lee, K. Y., et al., Controlled growth factor release from synthetic extracellular matrices. *Nature*, 2000. **408**(6815), pp. 998–1000.

84. Tabata, Y. and Y. Ikada, Vascularization effect of basic fibroblast growth factor released from gelatin hydrogels with different biodegradabilities. *Biomaterials*, 1999. **20**(22), pp. 2169–2175.

85. Tabata, Y., et al., Neovascularization effect of biodegradable gelatin microspheres incorporating basic fibroblast growth factor. *Journal of Biomaterials Science, Polymer Edition*, 1999. **10**(1), pp. 79–94.

86. Borselli, C., et al., Bioactivation of collagen matrices through sustained VEGF release from PLGA microspheres. *Journal of Biomedical Materials Research Part A*, 2010. **92A**(1), pp. 94–102.

87. Ungaro, F., et al., Microsphere-integrated collagen scaffolds for tissue engineering: Effect of microsphere formulation and scaffold properties on protein release kinetics. *Journal of Controlled Release*, 2006. **113**(2), pp. 128–136.

88. Freitas, S., H. P. Merkle, and B. Gander, Microencapsulation by solvent extraction/evaporation: Reviewing the state of the art of microsphere preparation process technology. *Journal of Controlled Release*, 2005. **102**(2), pp. 313–332.

89. Cheng, J., et al., Formulation of functionalized PLGA–PEG nanoparticles for in vivo targeted drug delivery. *Biomaterials*, 2007. **28**(5), pp. 869–876.

90. Müller, M., et al., Surface modification of PLGA microspheres. *Journal of Biomedical Materials Research Part A*, 2003. **66A**(1), pp. 55–61.

91. De Rosa, E., et al., Agarose surface coating influences intracellular accumulation and enhances payload stability of a nano-delivery system. *Pharmaceutical Research*, 2011. **28**(7), pp. 1520–1530.

92. Martinez, J. O., et al., Evaluation of cell function upon nanovector internalization. *Small*, 2012. **9**(9–10), pp. 1696–1702.

93. Canham, L. T., Bioactive silicon structure fabrication through nanoetching techniques. *Advanced Materials*, 1995. **7**, pp. 1033–1037.

94. Canham, L. T., Nanoscale semiconducting silicon as a nutritional food additive. *Nanotechnology*, 2007. **18**, pp. 185704.

95. Martin, F. J., et al., Acute toxicity of intravenously administered microfabricated silicon dioxide drug delivery particles in mice: Preliminary findings. *Drugs in R&D*, 2005. **6**(2), pp. 71–81.

96. Anthony Soon-Whatt, G., et al., A novel approach to brachytherapy in hepatocellular carcinoma using a phosphorous32 (32P) brachytherapy delivery device—a first-in-man study. *International Journal of Radiation Oncology, Biology, Physics*, 2007. **67**(3), pp. 786–792.

97. Murphy, M. B., et al., A multifunctional nanostructured platform for localized sustained release of analgesics and antibiotics. *European Journal of Pain Supplements*, 2011. **5**(S2), pp. 423–432.

98. Foraker, A. B., et al., Microfabricated porous silicon particles enhance paracellular delivery of insulin across intestinal caco-2 cell monolayers. *Pharmaceutical Research*, 2003. **20**(1), pp. 110–116.

99. Prestidge, C. A., et al., Loading and release of a model protein from porous silicon powders. *Physica Status Solidi (a)*, 2007. **204**(10), pp. 3361–3366.

100. Tasciotti, E., et al., Mesoporous silicon particles as a multistage delivery system for imaging and therapeutic applications. *Natue Nanotechnology*, 2008. **3**(3), pp. 151–157.

101. Mayne, A. H., et al., Biologically interfaced porous silicon devices. *Physica Status Solidi (a)*, 2000. **182**(1), pp. 505–513.

102. Whitehead, M. A., et al., High-porosity poly($\varepsilon$-caprolactone)/ mesoporous silicon scaffolds: Calcium phosphate deposition and biological response to bone precursor cells. *Tissue Engineering Part A*, 2008. **14**(1), pp. 195–206.

103. Whitehead, M. A., et al., Accelerated calcification in electrically conductive polymer composites comprised of poly(epsilon-caprolactone), polyaniline, and bioactive mesoporous silicon. *Journal of Biomedical Materials Research Part A*, 2007. **83A**(1), pp. 225–234.

104. Losic, D., J. G. Mitchell, and N. H. Voelcker, Diatomaceous lessons in nanotechnology and advanced materials. *Advanced Materials*, 2009. **21**(29), pp. 2947–2958.

105. Vrieling, E. G., et al., Diatom silicon biomineralization as an inspirational source of new approaches to silica production. *Journal of Biotechnology*, 1999. **70**(1–3), pp. 39–51.

106. Decuzzi, P., et al., Size and shape effects in the biodistribution of intravascularly injected particles. *Journal of Controlled Release*, 2010. **141**(3), pp. 320–327.

107. Chiappini, C., et al., Tailored porous silicon microparticles: Fabrication and properties. *ChemPhysChem*, 2010. **11**(5), pp. 1029–1035.

108. Martinez, J. O., et al., Short and long term, in vitro and in vivo correlations of cellular and tissue responses to mesoporous silicon nanovectors. *Small*, 2013. **9**(9–10), pp. 1722–1733.

109. Fan, D., et al., Mesoporous silicon-PLGA composite microspheres for the double controlled release of biomolecules for orthopedic tissue engineering. *Advanced Functional Materials*, 2012. **22**(2), pp. 282–293.

110. Sun, W., et al., Porous silicon as a cell interface for bone tissue engineering. *Physica Status Solidi (a)*, 2007. **204**(5), pp. 1429–1433.

111. De Rosa, E., et al., Agarose surface coating influences intracellular accumulation and enhances payload stability of a nano-delivery system. *Pharmaceutical Research*, 2011. **28**(7), pp. 1520–1530.

112. Hu, C. M. J., R. H. Fang, and L. Zhang, Erythrocyte-inspired delivery systems. *Advanced Healthcare Materials*, 2012. **1**(5), pp. 537–547.

113. Kolesnikova, T. A., A. G. Skirtach, and H. Möhwald, Red blood cells and polyelectrolyte multilayer capsules: Natural carriers versus polymer-based drug delivery vehicles. *Expert Opinion on Drug Delivery*, 2013. **10**(1), pp. 47–58.

114. Abolmaali, S. S., A. M. Tamaddon, and R. Dinarvand, A review of therapeutic challenges and achievements of methotrexate delivery systems for treatment of cancer and rheumatoid arthritis. *Cancer Chemotherapy and Pharmacology*, 2013, pp. 1–16.

115. Magnani, M., F. Pierigè, and L. Rossi, Erythrocytes as a novel delivery vehicle for biologics: From enzymes to nucleic acid-based therapeutics. *Therapeutic Delivery*, 2012. **3**(3), pp. 405–414.

116. Gutiérrez Millán, C., et al., Cell-based drug-delivery platforms. *Therapeutic Delivery*, 2012. **3**(1), pp. 25–41.

117. Parodi, A., et al., Synthetic nanoparticles functionalized with biomimetic leukocyte membranes possess cell-like functions. *Nature Nanotechnology*, 2012. **8**, pp. 61–68.

118. Shi, J., et al., Nanotechnology in drug delivery and tissue engineering: From discovery to applications. *Nano Letters*, 2010. **10**(9), pp. 3223–3230.

119. Habraken, W. J. E. M., et al., PLGA microsphere/calcium phosphate cement composites for tissue engineering: In vitro release and degradation characteristics. *Journal of Biomaterials Science, Polymer Edition*, 2008. **19**(9), pp. 1171–1188.

120. Allison, S. D., Analysis of initial burst in PLGA microparticles. *Expert Opinion on Drug Delivery*, 2008. **5**(6), pp. 615–628.

121. van de Weert, M., W. E. Hennink, and W. Jiskoot, Protein instability in poly(lactic-co-glycolic acid) microparticles. *Pharmaceutical Research*, 2000. **17**(10), pp. 1159–1167.

122. Park, J.-H., et al., Biodegradable luminescent porous silicon nanoparticles for in vivo applications. *Natue Materials*, 2009. **8**(4), pp. 331–336.

123. Murphy, M., et al., Multi-composite bioactive osteogenic sponges featuring mesenchymal stem cells, platelet-rich plasma, nanoporous silicon enclosures, and peptide amphiphiles for rapid bone regeneration. *Journal of Functional Biomaterials*, 2011. **2**(2), pp. 39–66.

124. Bhattacharyya, S., H. Wang, and P. Ducheyne, Polymer-coated mesoporous silica nanoparticles for the controlled release of macromolecules. *Acta Biomaterialia*, 2012. **8**(9), pp. 3429–3435.

# Chapter 3

# Nano-Apatites with Designed Chemistry and Crystallinity for Bone Regeneration and Nanomedical Applications

**Michele Iafisco[a] and Daniele Catalucci[b]**

[a]*Institute of Science and Technology for Ceramics (ISTEC),
National Research Council of Italy (CNR),
Via Granarolo 64, Faenza (RA), 48018, Italy*
[b]*Institute of Genetic and Biomedical Research (IRGB),
National Research Council (CNR) and Humanitas Clinical and Research Center,
Via Manzoni, 113, Rozzano (MI), 20089, Italy*
michele.iafisco@istec.cnr.it

Apatite nanocrystals constitute the inorganic part of mammalian hard tissues and an increasing interest in the preparation of synthetic equivalents able to precisely mimic the morphological and physical-chemical features of biological apatite is emerging. These compounds exhibit many differences in comparison to stoichiometric hydroyapatite ceramics, such as non-stoichiometric composition, nanometric size, plate-shape morphology and hydrate layer on the crystal surface. This chapter is intended to give the reader an overview on the occurrence of apatites in human tissues, their peculiar physical-chemical and biological properties, the main synthetic strategies and their applications in bone tissue regeneration and in nanomedicine.

---

*Bio-Inspired Regenerative Medicine: Materials, Processes, and Clinical Applications*
Edited by Simone Sprio and Anna Tampieri
Copyright © 2016 Pan Stanford Publishing Pte. Ltd.
ISBN 978-981-4669-14-6 (Hardcover), 978-981-4669-15-3 (eBook)
www.panstanford.com

## 3.1 Introduction

Calcium phosphates (CaPs) are very attractive compounds in many scientific fields such as geology, paleontology, chemistry, material science, biology and medicine [1]. Geologically, CaPs are found in different regions mostly as deposits of apatites (belong to igneous rocks), mainly as phosphorites (called phosphate rock or rock phosphate), which is a non-detrital sedimentary rock containing high amounts of phosphate or fluorapatite ($Ca_5(PO_4)_3F$) (Fig. 3.1) [2].

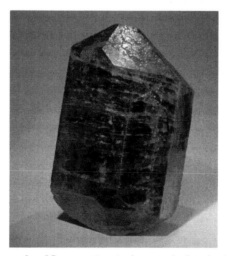

**Figure 3.1** Example of fluorapatite single crystal of geological origin.

In biological systems, CaPs are the main constituent of normal (bone, dentine, fish scales, horns of different animals) and pathological (e.g., dental and urinary calculi, tendon mineralization, calcification of blood vessels) calcifications [1]. Except for small portions of the inner ear, all hard tissues of the human body are made of CaPs. Structurally, with the exception of enamel, which has a high degree of crystallinity, they occur mainly in the form of ionic substituted (mainly by F, Na, Mg, and carbonate) nanocrystalline apatites [3].

In the last years, different synthetic approaches have been developed to prepare synthetic "biomimetic analogs" via soft and green chemistry [4]. In fact, the ability to modulate structure and morphology of apatites opens several possibilities in medical sciences. Besides their excellent properties as biomaterial, one of the most interesting characteristics of nanocrystalline apatites is their surface reactivity and capability to bind a wide variety of biomolecules due to their high surface area to volume ratio and different available ionic sites on the surface [5]. Surface properties as well as other structural and chemical properties such as dimensions and morphology, can be exploited and tailored by materials scientists to obtain nanostructured and apatite based bioactive biomaterials, in particular, in view of drug delivery and tissue engineering applications [6]. The present chapter outlines the recent progress in the preparation of multifunctional nanocrystalline apatites with tailored properties and their applications as biomedical material. The chapter is structured in three sections. In Section 3.1 biologically related CaPs in bones, teeth and pathological calcifications are depicted. Section 3.2 is devoted to the description of the peculiar properties of nanocrystalline apatite, their differences in comparison with stoichiometric hydroxyapatite and the some of the latest published works regarding their preparation with tailored surfaces properties. Section 3.3 deals with some examples of the most important applications of apatite nanocrystals related to materials for treatment bone disease and with the most novelty and fascinating applications of apatites nanoparticles in the field of nanomedicine such as bio-imaging and drug delivery.

## 3.2   Apatite Nanocrystals in Biological Systems

In biological systems, CaPs are the main constituent of normal (bone, dentine, fish scales, horns of different animals) and pathological (e.g., dental and urinary calculi, tendon mineralization, calcification of blood vessels) calcifications [4]. Except for small portions of the inner ear, which are made of calcium carbonate, all hard tissues of the human body are made of CaPs. Structurally, with the exception of enamel, they occur in the form of poorly crystallized non-stoichiometric carbonate-substituted apatite nanocrystals [3]. In this section, details about the principal characteristics of the structure and the mineral phases of bones, teeth, and pathological calcifications will be given.

Bones are the major mineralized tissues of the human body, and their function is (i) to move, support and protect organs of the body; (ii) produce red and white blood cells and (iii) store minerals [7]. Bone is composed of about 65 wt.% of mineral phase (nanosized crystals of apatite), 25 wt.% of organic phase (basically type-I collagen, non-collagenous proteins (NCPs) and minor organic molecules such as citrate) and 10 wt.% of water. Bone is a dynamic tissue that is constantly reshaped by osteoblasts that build bone and osteoclasts that resorb it [8]. Bones appear in a variety of shapes and have a complex internal and external structure. Essentially, they are lightweight, yet strong and hard, in addition to satisfying their many other functions. The structure of bones differs greatly among the different locations in the skeleton reflecting the fine-tuning and the adaptation of the structure to function [9]. However, all have in common the basic building block, which primarily comprises collagen type I fibrous matrix mineralized with carbonated-apatite nanocrystals [10]. Bone is a hierarchically structured hybrid material that has continually fascinated scientists due to its particular structure and unique mechanical properties and remodeling ability [11]. To well understand the intricate bone architecture, several hierarchical models have been proposed in the past. The most known is the model proposed by Weiner and Wagner describing seven hierarchical levels that range from the nano- to the macro-scale (Fig. 3.2) [12].

The first level consists of the single molecular components: (i) type I collagen fibrils, (ii) carbonated apatite nanocrystals, (iii) water, and (iv) non-collagenous bone proteins. There are more than 200 non-collagenous proteins (NCPs) and among them, osteonectin, osteocalcin, bone morphogenetic proteins, bone proteoglycan, and bone sialoprotein are the probably the most important and studied [8].

The main function of collagen is the integrity and mechanical reinforcement of soft and hard connective tissue [13]. Type I collagen, as the major organic component of bone, is made up of three polypeptide strands called alpha peptides forming a triple helical assembly with approximately 300 nm long and 1.5 nm in diameter [14]. The trimeric polypeptidic molecule consisting of two $\alpha 1$ and one $\alpha 2$ peptide chains that comprise a repeating glycine (Gly)–X–Y triplet, in which X and Y can be a residue but are usually proline (Pro) and hydroxyproline (Hyp), respectively [15].

Apatite Nanocrystals in Biological Systems | 51

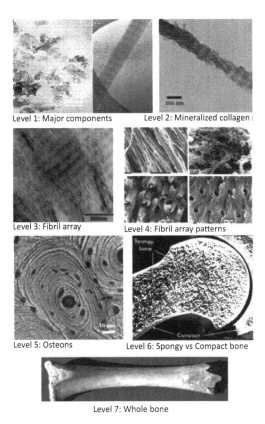

**Figure 3.2** The seven hierarchical levels of bone according to the model proposed by Weiner and Wagner.

The triple helical collagen molecules self-assemble with their long axes in parallel into a staggered arrangement in which each molecule is shifted with respect to its neighboring molecules forming characteristic D-periodic cross-striated pattern (where $D = 67$ nm is the characteristic axial periodicity of collagen) (Fig. 3.3) [16–18].

The typical 67 nm period of cross-striation pattern of collagen assembly can be observed by transmission electron microscope (TEM), atomic force microscope (AFM), and X-ray diffraction (XRD) analyses [18, 19]. The most widely accepted model for packing of collagen molecules is that five triple helices align hexagonally in cross section and longitudinally with approximately a quarter of the molecular length of staggered arrangement to form the five stranded microfibrils. The diameter of the collagen fibrils in the five-stranded packing model should be about 4 nm according to 1.5 nm of diameter of single collagen molecule, which has been verified by TEM examination of native collagen fibrils [20]. The collagen microfibrils are then assembled into collage fibrils of about 35–500 nm in diameter that are further combined, oriented and laid up to form ordered structures with particular morphologies for tissues [17].

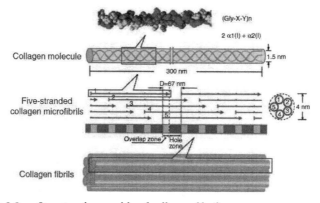

**Figure 3.3** Structural assembly of collagen fibrils.

The second level is formed by the mineralized collagen fibrils (Fig. 3.4). In the mineralized collagen fibrils, tiny plate-shaped crystallites of carbonated apatite with hexagonal symmetry are organized into parallel arrays with their $c$-axes co-aligned with the long axes of the collagen fibril [21]. The first-formed minerals nucleate initially in the "hole" zones of assembled collagen fibrils with continuous growth, and then penetrate into the overlap regions of the fibrils. There are more mineral crystals in the gap than in the overlap regions of the mineralized fibrils leading to the banded periodic appearance, with the repeat motif corresponding to the D-period of the fibrils [21]. Bone apatite nanocrystals are calcium- (and hydroxide-) deficient, with a ratio of Ca/P < 1.67, which is the theoretical value for the stoichiometric hydroxyapatite mineral $(Ca_{10}(PO_4)_6(OH)_2)$. Other interesting features of bone apatite are the low crystallinity degree, the presence of ionic substituents in its crystal structure (4–6 wt.% carbonate, 0.9 wt.% Na, 0.5 wt.% Mg and others) and the typical plate-like morphology [4].

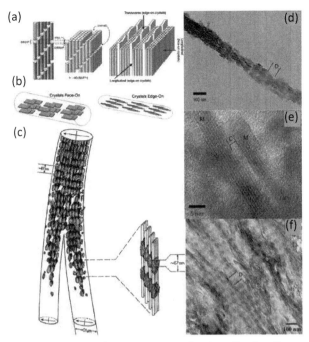

**Figure 3.4** The structural organization of mineralized collagen fibrils. (a) Model of mineralized collagen fibrils showing the arrays of the plate-like apatite crystals in the channels formed in staggered arranged collagen fibrils. (b) Face-on and edge-on projections of the crystals in the mineralized fibril. (c) Drawing of two mineralized collagen fibrils in avian tendon. (d) TEM micrograph of an isolated mineralized collagen fibril from human dentin. (e) HR-TEM micrograph of two edge-on crystals in the mineralized collagen fibril. (f) TEM micrograph of an array of the mineralized fibrils from human dentin.

The crystals are extremely small; in fact, they are probably the smallest biologically formed crystals. In addition, the crystals may change in size and composition with age [22]. Therefore, it is very difficult to determine the exact crystal dimensions in native occurring mineralized collagen fibrils. Although many methods, including TEM, XRD, AFM, and small-angle X-ray scattering (SAXS) measurements, have been used to analyze the apatite crystal size in mineralized collagen fibrils [20, 23–28], it is clear that the values of crystal size from different measurements are not consistent; however, the most accepted dimensions can vary in the resulting ranges: 20–50 nm in length, 15–30 nm in width, and thickness of 1.5–4 nm.

The third level is composed of arrays of mineralized collagen fibrils. These fibrils are almost always associated as bundles or other arrangements, often aligned along their long axis. However, the organization of these fibrils in different bone types varies significantly, reflecting the differences in their functional properties [8].

The fourth level is composed of the different patterns of fibril arrays. At this level the conspicuous diversity in structure occurs, with fibril arrays organized in a variety of patterns. These patterns can be parallel arrays, woven arrangements, plywood like structures, and radial arrays [8].

Cylindrical structures called osteons make up the fifth level. Bones themselves, as opposed to dentin, cementum, scales, and most mineralized tendons, often undergo internal remodeling [29]. This process involves the excavating out of large tunnels by teams of specialized cells called osteoclasts. These tunnels are then refilled by osteoblasts, starting with the deposition of a thin layer of cement on the existing excavated surface, followed by layers of lamellar bone. The process stops when the tunnel is almost completely filled, leaving a narrow channel at the center that function as a blood vessel [30]. In fact, other even smaller capillary-like features (canaliculi) are also built into the structure. These canaliculi are numerous and house the cells (osteocytes) that remain within the bone material itself. The canaliculi tend to radiate out from the central blood vessel. Thus the structure of an osteon is basically onion-like in cross section with layers of lamellae surrounding a central hole; in longitudinal section they are cylindrical [31].

The sixth level is formed by the spongy (trabecular or cancellous) and the compact (cortical) bone tissues. Cancellous bone is extremely porous (75–95 wt.% porosity) and provides space for marrow and blood vessels, but has much lower compressive strength [32]. Cortical bone is otherwise the dense outer layer (5–10 wt.% porosity) that allows many functions of bone [11].

The seventh level is simply the whole bone.

As previously described, the mammalian body contains numerous mineralized tissues, but dental enamel is the tissue with the most robust mechanical properties. In fact, enamel is the hardest material formed by vertebrates and is the most mineralized tissue present in the body [33]. Mature enamel is composed of highly crystalline carbonated-hydroxyapatite crystals for the 95–97% by weight and less than 1% of organic material. The high degree of mineralization makes enamel a fascinating model to understand the fundamental mineralization processes that occur within an extracellular matrix. Enamel is different from bone and dentin in terms of architecture, pathology, and biological mechanisms mediating its formation. Additionally mature enamel is a-cellular and it cannot be resorbed or remodeled. As a result, enamel regeneration cannot occur in vivo and is therefore an attractive biological target for tissue regeneration therapies.

The mammalian tooth is composed of four distinct structures: enamel, dentin, pulp, and cementum [34]. Enamel makes up the uppermost 1–2 mm of the tooth crown and contains a high mineral amount, giving it a high modulus but also making it susceptible to cracking. Dentin lies below the enamel and is tougher, forming the bulk of the tooth and absorbing stresses from enamel, preventing its fracture [35]. The mineral composition and structure of dentin is similar to that of bone. The cementum is the mineralized layer that surrounds the root of the tooth covering the dentin layer and some of the enamel layer. The cementum allows for the anchoring of the tooth to the alveolar bone (jawbone) through the periodontal ligament. The enamel and dentin tissues give rise to a tough, crack-tolerant and abrasion-resistant tissue through their unique architectures and mineral compositions. Enamel is highly patterned and consists of organized interweaving bundles of crystallites (called rods or prisms). It has a reported toughness higher than that of crystalline stoichiometric hydroxyapatite, indicating that the organization of the crystallites is essential for enamel function [36]. Due to the high mineral content and minimal presence of organic matter, enamel is brittle. Interestingly, the architecture of the enamel crystallites can deflect a propagating crack preventing it from reaching the dentin-enamel junction (DEJ), which also has been shown to resist delamination of the tissues despite their differences in composition [37]. The mechanical properties of enamel, dentin, and the DEJ are not completely understood and they comprise at present a significant area of research. The comprehension of the properties of these tissues could serve to stimulate further studies to develop more robust materials for dental applications as well as to inspire fabrication of materials not only for biological applications.

Similar to bone, enamel possesses a complex architecture, which can be divided into several hierarchical levels from the nano- to the macroscale [38]. On the nanoscale, the protein-protein and protein-mineral interactions in the presence of supersaturated ions create a highly organized array of crystallites of hydroxyapatite that grow preferentially along their $c$-axis [39]. The sizes of these crystallites depend on the stage of the mineralization. The crystallites grow primarily in length during the secretory stage and continue to grow in width and thickness during the maturation stage. The assembly of amelogenin proteins has been shown to be crucial for the proper development of enamel crystallites [40]. Disruption of the assembly alters formation at the nanoscale, subsequently affecting larger length scales and giving rise to a diseased or malformed enamel phenotype. On the mesoscale level, there are three main structural components: the rod, the interrod and the aprismatic enamel. The main component of enamel on the mesoscale includes rods, which are bundles of aligned crystallites that are "woven" into intricate architectures that are approximately 3–5 μm in diameter (Fig. 3.5) [41, 42].

The second structural component of the enamel matrix is the interrod (or interprismatic) enamel, which surrounds and packs between the rods. The difference between the rod and the interrod is the orientation of hydroxyapatite crystals; the rod contains aligned crystallites, whereas the mineral in the interrod is less ordered. These structures coalesce to form the tissue of enamel, which can resist high forces and damage by crack deflection. The third structure, aprismatic enamel, refers to the structures containing hydroxyapatite crystals that show no mesoscale or macroscale alignment. The macroscale architecture includes specific zones of enamel that have unique characteristics, which contribute to the whole tissue. The enamel adjacent to the DEJ exhibits a gradual transition from dentin to enamel. Aprismatic regions of enamel have been proposed to be primitive areas of the tooth serving as a toughening mechanism due to their flexible nature. Several authors have identified these aprismatic areas to be located adjacent to the DEJ and at the incisal surface of both deciduous and permanent human enamel. The Tomes' process, a unique structure present at the secretory pole of an enamel-forming cell, is responsible for aligned mineral formation in the prismatic enamel [43]. The absence of this process may give rise to the aprismatic zone in the tooth.

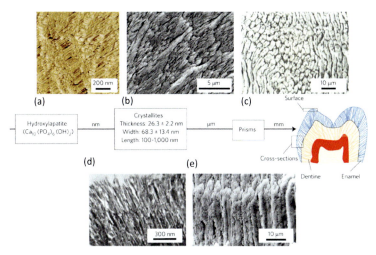

**Figure 3.5** The enamel is composed of three-dimensionally organized nanosized hydroxyapatite crystallites (a, b, d) that are arranged into micrometer-sized prisms (c, e). (a) Atomic force microscope and (b and c) scanning electron microscope images of the enamel surface. (d) Transmission electron microscope and (e) scanning electron microscope images of a cross section of the enamel.

In the body of mammals, osteoblasts and odontoblasts cells fix calcium and phosphate ions and then precipitate biological apatite onto organic matrices. This is the process of physiological biomineralization that is restricted to the specific sites in the skeletal tissues, including growth plate cartilage, bones, and teeth. Unfortunately, owing to ageing, to various diseases and under certain pathological conditions, blood vessels and some internal organs are calcified as well [44]. This process is called pathological calcification or ectopic mineralization and leads to morbidity and mortality. In general, any type of abnormal accumulation of CaPs in wrong places is accounted for a disruption of systemic defense mechanism against calcification [45].

Unwanted depositions always lead to various diseases, e.g., soft tissue calcification (in damaged joints, blood vessels, dysfunctional areas in the brain, diseased organs, scleroderma, prostate stones), kidney and urinary stones [46], dental pulp stones and dental calculus [47], salivary stones, gall stones, pineal gland calcification, atherosclerotic arteries and veins [48], coronary calcification, cardiac skeleton, damaged cardiac valves, calcification on artificial heart valves [49], carpal tunnel, cataracts, malacoplakia, calcified menisci, dermatomyositis, and others. All these cases are examples of a calcinosis, which might be described as a formation of CaP deposits in any soft tissue [50]. Contrary to the mineral phases of the normal calcifications, which consist of only one type of CaP, the mineral phases of abnormal and/or pathological calcifications are found to occur as single or mixed phases of other types of CaPs and/or other phosphatic and non-phosphatic compounds, in addition to or in place of biological apatite [51]. This occurs because the pH of the solution is often relatively low in the places of pathological calcifications. However, in some cases, the chemical composition of an unwanted inorganic phase might depend on the age of the pathological calcification and its location. It is interesting to note that the mineral phases of animal calculus (e.g., from dog) was found to consist of calcium carbonate andbiological apatite, while human calculi do not contain calcium carbonate. Some findings suggested that the mechanisms and factors regulating the physiological biomineralization might be similar to those influencing the ectopic mineralization: both were initiated by various organics (i.e., membrane-enclosed particles released from the plasma membrane of mineralization competent cells), which were present [52].

## 3.3 Nanocrystalline Apatite

In contrast to stoichiometric hydroxyapatite (HA) [$Ca_{10}(PO_4)_6(OH)_2$], which is a stoichiometric apatitic phase that is the most thermodynamically stable and least soluble CaP at physiological conditions, nanocrystalline apatites are nonstoichiometric (Ca/P ratio less than 1.67) and calcium (and OH)-deficient, and may incorporate substituted ions in the crystal lattice (i.e., Na, Mg, K, Sr, Zn, etc.) [4, 5]. The calcium and hydroxide deficiencies are mainly responsible for the higher solubility exhibited by these nanocrystalline apatites compared with HA. They are also able to mature when submitted to humid environments; as a result, "mature" bone crystals in vertebrates are less soluble and reactive than embryonic (young) bone mineral crystals [53].

From a chemical point of view, the composition of nano-crystalline apatites differs significantly from that of HA. The global chemical composition of biological apatites (or their synthetic analogues) has been a somewhat controversial topic in recent decades but can generally be described as follows:

$$Ca_{10-x} (PO_4)_{6-x} (HPO_4 \text{ or } CO_3)_x (OH \text{ or } \frac{1}{2}CO_3)_{2-x} \text{ with } 0 \leq x \leq 2$$

Very immature nanocrystals, however, may depart from this generic formula. This formula underlines the presence of vacancies in both Ca and OH sites. For example, Legeros et al. [54] analyzed various cortical bone samples, suggesting the following relatively homogeneous composition, which reveals a high vacancy content:

$$Ca_{8.3} (PO_4)_{4.3} (HPO_4 \text{ or } CO_3)_{1.7}(OH \text{ or } \frac{1}{2}CO_3)_{0.3}$$

Minor substitutions are also found in biological apatites that involve monovalent cations (especially Na and K), for example. In this case, charge compensation mechanisms must be taken into account. Recent advances in the characterization of apatite nanocrystals have been achieved through the use of spectroscopic techniques and, in particular, through Fourier transform infrared (FT-IR) spectroscopy. The FT-IR method is useful in characterizing the local chemical environment of phosphate, carbonate, and hydroxide ions as well as water molecules. Detailed analyses of the phosphate groups by FT-IR have allowed identifying additional bands in nanocrystalline apatites, which cannot be attributed to phosphate groups of the regular apatitic environment [55, 56]. Rey has referred to these chemical environments as "non-apatitic" environments [5].

Several complementary characterization techniques (i.e., solid-state NMR and Raman [57, 58]) have been recently applied to study apatites nanocrystals (whether biological or their synthetic analogs prepared under physiologically inspired conditions) and they may be described by an apatitic core (often non-stoichiometric) and a structured "non-apatitic" surface hydrated layer containing water molecules and rather labile ions (e.g., $Ca^{2+}$, $HPO_4^{2-}$, $CO_3^{2-}$), as illustrated in Fig. 3.6.

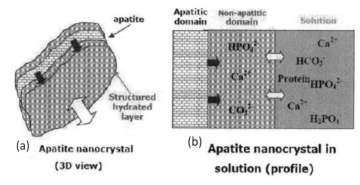

**Figure 3.6** (a) Schematic model of a biomimetic apatite nanocrystals and (b) interaction with surrounding biological fluids.

The presence of this hydrated surface layer is thought to be responsible for most of the properties of biomimetic apatites, and in particular their high surface reactivity in relation with biological surrounding fluids (which is probably directly linked to a high mobility of ionic species contained within this layer, as witnessed by fast surface ion exchange reactions).

As previously mentioned, nanocrystalline apatites represent the main inorganic constituent of hard tissues in vertebrates. Therefore, much attention has been lately focused on the study of their peculiar physical-chemical characteristics and, thereafter, on the possibility to imitate bone mineral for the development of new "advanced" synthetic biomaterials with improved biological properties. Moreover, the possibility to synthesize in laboratory synthetic biomimetic compounds makes it possible to consider these systems as a good bone mineral "model," enabling then to investigate, on the one hand, the interaction between bone-like apatite nanocrystals and the components of surrounding fluids (ions, proteins...) and, on the other hand, to follow surface interactions with drugs aimed at being delivered in vivo.

In the last years, many different strategies have been employed and developed for the preparation of synthetic nanosized apatite crystals. The most common preparation method is the stoichiometric titration of an aqueous calcium solution with a solution of phosphoric acid up to neutrality [59–61]. Several additional methods have been successfully employed, including wet-chemical precipitation [62–64], sol–gel synthesis [65], co-precipitation [66], hydrothermal synthesis [67–69], rapid or continuous precipitation from solution [70], mechanochemical synthesis [71], microwave processing [72, 73], vapor diffusion [74–76], emulsion-based syntheses [77], and other methodologies producing nanocrystals of various shapes and sizes [78, 79] (Fig. 3.7). However, the preparation of biomimetic nanocrystalline apatites is still considered a scientific and technological challenge [80]. As explained previously, biological apatites are known for their high content of defects affecting the lattice parameters, crystal morphology, crystallinity, solubility and thermal stability [81]. Moreover, the surface of biological apatite crystals is rarely smooth, a characteristic that is strictly connected to its biological significance. It is hypothesized that the exceptional roughness of these crystals, comprising surface irregularities in the order of size of single unit cells, may correspond to the tendency to increase protein binding in the biomineralization process [82, 83]. Recent studies have also demonstrated that a rough surface improves the biocompatibility of the material and has a positive effect on inflammatory reactions [84].

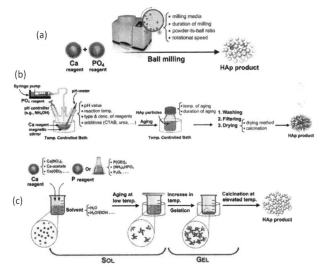

**Figure 3.7** Preparation of apatite (HAp) nanoparticles via (a) mechanochemical method, (b) conventional chemical precipitation and (c) sol–gel process.

Using as main criteria the structural and morphological control, the apatite crystallization methods can be rationally divided into the use of high and low temperature. The synthesis at high temperature usually involves the homogenization of precursor compounds, such as $Ca_3(PO_4)_2$ and $Ca(OH)_2$, and their annealing at about 1000°C. The advantage is the possibility to set the final stoichiometry of the product, whereas the main downsides are the long processing times and high annealing temperatures. In general, when using this method the Ca/P ratio is a fundamental parameter; in fact, if the initial molar ratio of Ca/P is not well configured to 1.67, other CaP phases could appear such as $\alpha$- or $\beta$-tricalcium phosphate (TCP) when the Ca/P value is lower than the stoichiometric one ratio and CaO when the Ca/P value is higher. The $\alpha$-TCP phase is normally formed at temperatures around 1200°C, whereas the $\beta$-TCP phase is formed at lower temperatures, up to 900°C. In addition to the high levels of energy consumption, another major downside of high temperature methods is the difficulty to prepare uniform and nanosized crystals [85].

On the other hand, the synthetic methods at low temperature offer the advantage to produce nanosized crystals, but the disadvantage may be in some cases the presence of transient and metastable phases in the final product. To investigate the effect of temperature on the chemical-physical features of nanosized apatite, Sakhno et al. have characterized two apatites synthesized with the same approach but at two different temperatures (40 and 95°C) [86]. The apatite synthesized at lower temperature displayed platelet-like morphology and constituted by a crystalline core coated with an amorphous surface layer of 1–2 nm. Increasing the temperature of synthesis, the platelet morphology was retained but the apatite nanoparticles exhibited a higher degree of crystallinity (evaluated by XRD). HR-TEM observations revealed that, in this case, the crystalline order was extended up to the particles surfaces, exhibiting clearly the planes (010), (100), and (001). Infrared spectroscopy was used to investigate the surface hydration of both materials, in terms of adsorbed $H_2O$ molecules and surface hydroxyl groups, as well as the Lewis acidity of surface cations, by removing the adsorbed water and adsorbing the molecular probe CO. For both features, strong similarities between amorphous and crystalline surfaces were found. However, interestingly the apatite synthesized at 95°C having a more crystalline surface appeared more able to physisorb multilayers of water in a larger extent than the less crystallized samples.

The main disadvantage of synthetic methods involving low temperature is the possible crystallization of transient phases.

The use of organic compounds acting as templates during crystallization is another interesting strategy that has received increasing attention over the last decade for the generation of inorganic structures with nano dimensions. In this domain, an interesting approach to achieve a well structural control of apatite is the one-step modification using calcium-chelating agents during the synthesis, and for this purpose carboxylate anions (oxalate, acetate, citrate) appear as the most promising additives due to their affinity for calcium ions [87–89]. Recently, Nancollas et al. suggested that the use of citrate in the crystallization of nanocrystalline apatite can be considered an interesting strategy inspired from nature to control the synthesis of this material [90]. In fact, solid-state NMR studies have reconsidered the role of citrate in stabilizing the size and morphology of biological apatites of bone, where it accounts for about the 5.5 wt.% of the total organic component. In this regard, Delgado-Lopez and co-workers recently proposed a very interesting novel protocol to obtain bio-inspired citrate-covered nanocrystalline apatite [88]. Fully biocompatible nanocrystalline apatites (ranging from 20 to 200 nm) were prepared by thermal decomplexing batch crystallization method. This method consisted in the thermal decomplexation of metastable calcium/citrate/phosphate solutions at 80°C. The increase of the temperature caused the destabilization the calcium-citrate complex providing a gradual release of $Ca^{2+}$ ions into the solution, which in the presence of phosphate groups allowed the formation of $[CaPO_4]^-$ and $[CaHPO_4]^0$, that are the growth units of apatite. Size, crystallinity degree, and composition of the nanoparticles can be tailored varying the maturation time as well as pH and concentration of reagents in the mother solution.

## 3.4 Nanocrystalline Apatite for Bone Regeneration and Nanomedical Applications

In the last years, clinical approaches for the treatment of critical connective tissues defects (bone, cartilage, etc.) by using inert prostheses is being replaced by new methods of regenerative medicine based on the use of biomimetic and bioactive scaffolds with the ability to transfer specific information to cells [91–93]. Modern bone grafts not only should replace the missing bones but also be intrinsically osteoinductive acting as scaffolds for guided bone growth [94].

The major motivation behind the use of apatites as material for health care is their chemical similarity to the mineral component of mammalian bones and teeth, as widely described above. As a result, in addition to being non-toxic, they are biocompatible, not recognized as foreign materials in the body and, most importantly, exhibit bioactive behavior and integration into living tissue according to the same biological processes active in remodeling healthy bone [95]. In this way, nanocrystalline apatites can play an important role in the bioactivity of implants (biomaterials). Formation of a bone-like apatite layer on the surface of implants can determine whether these materials can adequately integrate into the host living tissue [96]. In fact, this process leads to an intimate chemical bond between the implants and bone, termed osteointegration. Furthermore, CaPs are also known to well support osteoblast adhesion and proliferation [97]. Thus, apatite-based biomaterials are now used in a number of different bone applications throughout the body, covering all areas of the skeleton [98]. Applications include dental implants, percutaneous devices and use in periodontal treatment, treatment of bone defects, fracture treatment, total joint replacement (bone augmentation), orthopedics, cranio-maxillofacial reconstruction, otolaryngology, and spinal surgery. Depending on the desired characteristics of the material (resorbable or not, highly bioactive or not, etc.), apatites with different chemical-physical properties might be synthesized and used [99]. However, the major limitations in the use of apatites as load-bearing biomaterials are mainly related to their poor mechanical properties; specifically, they are too brittle with a poor fatigue resistance. The poor mechanical behavior is more evident for highly porous ceramics scaffolds because porosity greater than 100 μm is considered a fundamental requirement for proper vascularization and bone cell colonization [100]. That is why in bone repair applications, apatites are generally used as fillers and coatings and in combination with polymers in the hybrid scaffolds.

In general, nanostructured biomaterials offer more improved performances in comparison to their larger particle-sized counterparts due to their higher surface-to-volume ratios and unusual chemical synergistic effects at the nanoscale. Such nanostructured systems can constitute a chemical "bridge" between single molecules and bulk material systems. Nanosized apatites have also demonstrated higher bioactivity than coarser crystals. For example, Kim et al. found that osteoblasts attached with a significantly higher degree to nanosized apatite/gelatin biocomposites than to their micrometer-sized analogues [101]. Increased osteoblast adhesion on nanocrystalline apatite coatings on titanium, compared to traditionally used plasma-sprayed apatite coatings, was also discovered by other researchers [102]. The proliferation and osteogenic differentiation of periodontal ligament cells were found to be promoted when an apatitic nanophase was used, compared to dense hydroxyapatite ceramics [103]. In particular, increased osteoblast adhesion was revealed on nanosized CaPs with higher Ca/P ratios [104]. Moreover, a histological analysis revealed advanced biocompatibility and osteointegration of bone graft substitutes when nanosized apatite was employed in bio-hybrid composites [105]. Other results showed that nanosized apatite could improve cell attachment and mineralization in vivo, which suggests that it may be a better candidate for clinical use in terms of bioactivity and cell response. The size effects of apatite on bone-related cells as well as the influence of crystallinity have been studied [106]. Different apatite nanocrystals, typically of $20 \pm 5$, $40 \pm 10$, and $80 \pm 12$ nm diameter, were prepared and their effects on the proliferation of two types of bone-related cells, marrow mesenchymal stem cells (MSCs), and osteosarcoma cells (U2OS and MG63), were studied. The results showed improved cytophilicity of the nanophase compared to the conventional HA. Greater cell viability and proliferation of MSCs were measured for the apatite nanocrystals, remarkably so for 20 nm sized particles. However, the opposite phenomenon occurred for bone tumor cells when apatite nanoparticles were co-cultured with cells. Apatite nanoparticles can inhibit proliferation of U2OS and MG63 cells, the strength of the inhibition being inversely proportional to the particle size, i.e., smaller nanoparticles possess greater ability to prevent cell proliferation.

Apatite is also known for its ability to bind a wide variety of biomolecules (proteins, amino-acids, peptides) and most therapeutic agents for bone diseases (antibiotics, growth factors, anticancer, and antiosteoporosis drugs) [59, 60, 82, 83, 107–112]. Furthermore, nanocrystalline apatite holds larger load amounts of drugs because of its larger specific surface areas and low degree of crystallinity than coarse particles. A main challenge for innovative bone substitute biomaterials is their functionalization with bioactive molecules that can transfer information and act specifically on the biological environment. In other words, the implanted biomaterial can act as a local scaffold for cell invasion and formation of functional tissue and, in the meantime, deliver previously loaded biomolecules. In this way apatite nanocrystals can enhance their osteointegration or osteoinduction properties and also stimulate specific cellular responses at a molecular level.

One of the most efficient strategies to improve the bone forming ability of biomaterials is their association with bone morphogenetic proteins [113]. Different techniques to conjugate drugs with CaP biomaterials have been reported: Adsorption and impregnation allow the therapeutic agent to be grafted on the surface of the biomaterial, whereas centrifugation and vacuum based-techniques enable it to enter pores [114]. Generally bioactive molecules, such as growth factors, are incorporated in biomaterials by simple impregnation followed by drying, and the type of bonding with the substrate and the release rate are often undetermined [115]. Such associations do not allow the chemical bonding of the growth factor to the biomaterial and thus the release rate is difficult to control. For example, precipitation and clustering of the growth factor molecules may occur and the release is only determined by local dissolution and diffusion rules. The uncontrolled release of growth factors has been related to an accelerated resorption of bone tissue as well as of the implant. Since growth factors agents can stimulate the degradation as well as the formation of bone (depending on their local concentrations), they could damage the osteoconductivity of the coated-implant surface [116].

Similarly, bisphosphonates, well-established molecules as successful antiresorptive agents for the prevention and treatment of post-menopausal osteoporosis [117, 118], affecting bone remodeling, could also block the bone repair process. In fact, high concentration of BPs could have detrimental effects on the fixation of the implant over longer periods of time. Zoledronate, one of the most used bisphosphonates, grafted to apatite coating on titanium implants showed a dose-dependent effect on the inhibition of resorption activity according to the amount of zoledronate loaded [119]. Local and slow administration of the antineoplastic drug methotraxate (MTX) is also useful to avoid systemic side effects, and because its time effect (the sensitivity of cells to this drug increases with time) is greater than dose effect [120]. Adsorption, on the contrary, leads to stable association and control of the amount of bioactive molecules contained in the solid implant, and thus of the dose released. Generally, the release is rather low because most of the bioactive molecules adsorbed are irreversibly bound and they are not spontaneously released in a cell culture media [121]. They can only be displaced by mineral ions and/or soluble proteins with a stronger affinity for apatite surfaces but in a predictable manner, or by cell activity [121]. This characteristic has been observed for various growth factors like bone morphogenetic protein (BMP-2) or vascular endothelial growth factor (VEGF) [113, 120], antiosteoporisis agents [122, 123], and anticancer drugs as methotraxate and cisplatin [115, 124]. It has been reported that slow release of MTX from CaP is not only due to the porosity of the inorganic matrix (as in most of the cases) but also mainly due to the adsorption of MTX [115].

A local release system of antibiotics could be used to prevent post-surgical infections favoring early osteointegration of prosthesis. The release of different antibiotics incorporated in apatitic CaP coatings on titanium implant using biomimetic method was studied [125]. Since the antibiotics containing carboxylic groups (i.e., cephalothin) were better adsorbed than others into CaP biomaterials, these molecules are slowly released from the carrier [125].

Palazzo et al. [126] showed that adsorption and release kinetics of three drugs (cisplatin, alendronate and di(ethylendiam ineplatinum) medronate) are controlled by the surface properties of the nanocrystalline apatitic support such as surface area and surface charge, as well as the charge on the adsorbed molecules and their mode of interaction with the apatitic surface. These properties of biomimetic nanocrystalline apatites suggest the possibility to functionalize the surface of such nanocrystals with different linking agents, such as bisphosphonates for example, to anchor biologically active molecules for specific therapeutic application, or to improve the biocompatibility of bone-implantable biomaterials for hard-tissue engineering and regeneration technologies.

Nanoparticles are promising tools to target cells, e.g., for tumor treatment. Due to their size, they can penetrate the cell wall. This has constituted the scientific discipline "nanomedicine" where cell-specific addressing by functionalized nanoparticles is of high interest, e.g., for cancer treatment and imaging [127]. In fact, the functionalities of nanoparticulate delivery systems provide the opportunity (i) to prolong the circulation in the bloodstream and hence to increase the likelihood of accumulation at tumor sites via EPR effect (Fig. 3.8), (ii) to specifically target cells or tissues of interest via functionalization with ligands specific for cell surface receptors, (iii) to respond to local stimuli in vivo (such as responses to changes in temperature and pH), and (iv) to overcome the cell membrane barrier and avoid the enzyme filled lysosomes where degradation occurs [128, 129].

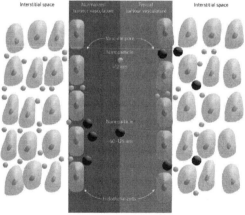

**Figure 3.8** The blood vessels in a typical tumor contain pores of various sizes, which allow nanoparticles of different sizes (black and grey) to enter the tumor (right). However, these pores also cause the interstitial fluid pressure to increase, which limits convective transport of nanoparticles into the tumor. Decreasing the size of these pores (a process called vascular normalization) increases convection and the interstitial penetration of small (~12 nm) nanoparticles (left). However, for larger nanoparticles (~60–125 nm) this increase in convection is overridden by an increase in steric and hydrodynamic hindrances.

Consequently, desired features of the ideal delivery system include (i) non-toxic starting materials and degradation products, (ii) small size (in the range of 10–100 nm) and large surface area for improved uptake, (iii) encapsulation of the active agent within the delivery system (as opposed to surface decoration or adsorption where the active agent is not protected from the environment), (iv) colloidal stability of the delivery system (to prevent agglomeration in vivo during transport), (v) suitable clearance mechanism (to avoid side effects due to drug loaded particles), (vi) long clearance times (to allow adequate time for the delivery system to reach target cells and undergo endocytosis), (vii) controlled release of an active agent (such as a pH trigger), and (viii) targetability of the delivery system (to enable delivery of particles to cells of choice) [130].

Moreover, active targeting moieties can also be incorporated into the nanocarriers to specifically enhance their internalization by the target cells. Most of the ligands used to achieve this aim act by binding to specific structures overexpressed by neoplastic cells. Subsequent receptor-mediated endocytosis leads to the uptake of the targeting moiety, along with the nanoparticle and its attached drug payload. Various types of targeting moieties have been studied to promote the receptor-mediated endocytosis of drug loaded nanoparticles: (i) folic acid (a small molecular weight compound that binds to the membrane receptor overexpressed in a variety of tumors) [131]; (ii) peptides ligands (because of the overexpression of receptors of hypothalamic peptides, such as somatostatin, in a variety of neoplastic tissues); (iii) antibodies (after binding to their cancer-cell-specific membrane antigen most antibodies are internalized by endocytosis) [132].

As drug carriers, apatite nanoparticles have some advantageous properties: (i) favorable biodegradability and biocompatibility; (ii) solubility and less toxicity with respect to silica, quantum dots, carbon nanotubes, or magnetic particles; (iii) more stability/ robustness than liposomes. Taken together, these properties predispose apatite nanoparticles for a more controlled and reliable drug delivery. Contrary to liposomes and other micelle-based carriers, which are subject to dissipation below specific critical concentrations (a clear obstacle to their intravenous administration), CaP-based systems and, particularly, those with Ca/P molar ratio close to that of stoichiometric hydroxyapatite, are negligibly soluble in blood, which is by itself supersaturated with respect to hydroxyapatite. Another property of apatite nanoparticles is their higher biocompatibility and pH-dependent dissolution as compared to polymers [133].

It is important to highlight that here we do not consider nanocrystalline CaP ceramics (bulk systems) but only dispersed systems (colloids). The dissolution of CaPs is accelerated at low pH media, such as those typically found in endo-lysosomes and in the vicinity of tumors, providing an advantage in the delivery of drugs into malign zones or cell organelles. They are also able to permeate the cell membrane and dissolve into the cell, which makes them an attractive candidate for non-viral intracellular gene delivery or transfection [134, 135]. CaPs dissolve into their ionic constituents ($Ca^{2+}$ and $PO_4^{3-}$), which are already present in relatively high concentration (1–5 mM) in cells and in the bloodstream [136]. Their dissolution actively allows preventing undesirable nanoparticle accumulation in cells and tissues; a setback often encountered with inorganic and metallic nanoparticle systems. The rapid increase of intracellular $Ca^{2+}$ above physiological concentrations can lead to apoptosis; however, this concentration never reaches a critical value [137]. Another important advantage of CaPs is the low production costs and excellent storage abilities (not easily subjected to microbial degradation). Unlike most other ceramics, nanosized CaPs can be prepared in situ, under ambient conditions, in a wide array of morphologies, from spheres to platelets to rods to fibers. CaPs can also be prepared with a variety of phase compositions thereby enabling fine tuning of the dissolution properties at the structural level as well [6].

CaP nanoparticles have been recently also used in the imaging by organic dyes and lanthanides, and at the same time to deliver a variety of drugs [138–140]. Apatite nanoparticles have been shown to exhibit better fluorescence properties than their amorphous counterparts when doped with lanthanides because of rigid confinement of the lanthanide ions in the crystalline structure of these nanoparticles [141, 142]. Composite nanoparticles assembling lipids and polymers in combination with CaP cores or shells have shown promise in the delivery of hydrophobic dyes and oligonucleotides [143]. The use of all of these compositions and architectures in biomedical applications takes advantage of the many properties of CaPs that make these materials successful as imaging and drug delivery agents.

Very recent interesting studies have also utilized CaP nanoparticles to deliver oligonucleotides [144, 145]. The major reasons that make direct gene delivery an inefficient process are the rapid clearance from the body and the extracellular enzymatic degradation by plasma nucleases [146, 147]. Naked DNA and siRNA are negatively charged, and the electrostatic repulsion with the anionic cell membrane further reduces their transfection efficiency [137]. Therefore, a suitable carrier is necessary for effective transfection [148, 149]. Although viral gene delivery is very widely used, non-viral gene delivery is getting special attention due to safety concerns associated with viral gene delivery, such as immunotoxicity, intercellular trafficking, and possibility of mutation [150]. CaP nanoparticles have proven to be effective for non-viral intracellular gene delivery or transfection [151–153], and gene silencing through small interfering RNAs (siRNAs). DNA or RNA binding to CaP nanoparticles occurs through electrostatic interaction between $Ca^{2+}$ in the nanocarrier and phosphate groups in DNA or RNA structure [154]. In intracellular gene delivery method, the genes are delivered to tumor/cancer-specific cells. These genes can then kill the cells by replacing the existing genes, or may promote certain enzyme activity that is capable of inducing cytotoxicity to the cells.

## Acknowledgments

The authors acknowledge the PNR-CNR aging program 2012–2014 and the Flagship project Nanomax (PNR-CNR 2011–2013).

## References

1. Dorozhkin SV, Epple M. Biological and medical significance of calcium phosphates. *Angew Chem Int Ed,* 2002; **41**: 3130–3146.

2. Dorozhkin SV. A detailed history of calcium orthophosphates from 1770s till 1950. *Mater Sci Eng C,* 2013; **33**: 3085–3110.

3. Dorozhkin SV. Nanosized and nanocrystalline calcium orthophosphates. *Acta Biomater,* 2010; **6**: 715–734.

4. Gómez-Morales J, Iafisco M, Delgado-López JM, Sarda S, Drouet C. Progress on the preparation of nanocrystalline apatites and surface

characterization: Overview of fundamental and applied aspects. *Prog Cryst Growth Characterization Mater,* 2013; **59**: 1–46.

5. Rey C, Combes C, Drouet C, Cazalbou S, Grossin D, Brouillet F, et al. Surface properties of biomimetic nanocrystalline apatites; applications in biomaterials. *Prog Cryst Growth Characterization Mater,* 2014; **60**: 63–73.

6. Bose S, Tarafder S. Calcium phosphate ceramic systems in growth factor and drug delivery for bone tissue engineering: A review. *Acta Biomater,* 2012; **8**: 1401–1421.

7. Loveridge N. Bone: More than a stick. *J Animal Sci,* 1999; **77**: 190–196.

8. Boskey AL. Mineralization of bones and teeth. *Elements,* 2007; **3**: 385–391.

9. Mellon SJ, Tanner KE. Bone and its adaptation to mechanical loading: A review. *Int Mater Rev,* 2012; **57**: 235–255.

10. Palmer LC, Newcomb CJ, Kaltz SR, Spoerke ED, Stupp SI. Biomimetic systems for hydroxyapatite mineralization inspired by bone and enamel. *Chem Rev,* 2008; **108**: 4754–4783.

11. Fratzl P, Gupta HS, Paschalis EP, Roschger P. Structure and mechanical quality of the collagen-mineral nano-composite in bone. *J Mater Chem,* 2004; **14**: 2115–2123.

12. Weiner S, Wagner HD. The material bone: Structure-mechanical function relations. *Ann Rev Mater Sci,* 1998; **28**: 271–298.

13. Prockop DJ, Fertala A. The collagen fibril: The almost crystalline structure. *J Struct Biol,* 1998; **122**: 111–118.

14. Shoulders MD, Raines RT. Collagen structure and stability. *Ann Rev Biochem,* 2009; **78**: 929–958.

15. Brodsky B, Ramshaw J. The collagen triple-helix structure. *Matrix Biol* 1997; **15**: 545–54.

16. Kadler KE, Holmes DF, Trotter JA, Chapman JA. Collagen fibril formation. *Biochem J,* 1996; **316**: 1–11.

17. Wang X, Liu Z, Cui F. *Biomimetic Synthesis of Self-Assembled Mineralized Collagen-Based Composites for Bone Tissue Engineering. Biomimetics*: John Wiley & Sons, Inc., 2013. pp. 23–50.

18. Ramírez-Rodríguez G, Iafisco M, Tampieri A, Gómez-Morales J, Delgado-López J. pH-responsive collagen fibrillogenesis in confined droplets induced by vapour diffusion. *J Mater Sci Mater Med,* 2014; **25**: 2305–2312.

19. Sanders HM, Iafisco M, Pouget EM, Bomans PH, Nudelman F, Falini G, et al. The binding of CNA35 contrast agents to collagen fibrils. *Chem Commun (Camb)*, 2011; **47**: 1503–1505.

20. Watson ML, Robinson RA. Collagen-crystal relationships in bone. II. Electron microscope study of basic calcium phosphate crystals. *Am. J. Anat*, 1953; **93**: 25–59.

21. Beniash E. Biominerals—hierarchical nanocomposites: The example of bone. *Wiley Interdisciplinary Rev Nanomed Nanobiotechnol*, 2011; **3**: 47–69.

22. Rey C, Combes C, Drouet C, Lebugle A, Sfihi H, Barroug A. Nanocrystalline apatites in biological systems: Characterisation, structure and properties. *Materialwissenschaft und Werkstofftechnik* 2007; **38**: 7.

23. Robinson RA. An electron-microscopic study of the crystalline inorganic component of bone and its relationship to the organic matrix. *J Bone Joint Surg Am*, 1952; **34-A**(2): 389–435.

24. Fernandez-Morán H, Engström A. Electron microscopy and X-ray diffraction of bone. *Biochim Biophys Acta*, 1957; **23**: 260–264.

25. Jackson SA, Cartwright AG, Lewis D. The morphology of bone mineral crystals. *Calcif Tissue Res,* 1978; **25**: 217–222.

26. Norio M, Morio A, Yoshio T. Quantitative analysis of small-angle x-ray scattering of bone: Determination of sizes of its collagen and apatite components. *Jap J Appl Phys,* 1981; **20**: 699.

27. Fratzl P, Fratzl-Zelman N, Klaushofer K, Vogl G, Koller K. Nucleation and growth of mineral crystals in bone studied by small-angle x-ray scattering. *Calcif Tissue Int*, 1991; **48**: 407–413.

28. Ziv V, Weiner S. Bone crystal sizes: A comparison of transmission electron microscopic and x-ray diffraction line width broadening techniques. *Connect Tissue Res,* 1994; **30**: 165–175.

29. Hadjidakis DJ, Androulakis II. Bone Remodeling. *Ann N Y Acad Sci,* 2006; **1092**: 385–396.

30. Manolagas SC. Birth and death of bone cells: Basic regulatory mechanisms and implications for the pathogenesis and treatment of osteoporosis. *Endocr Rev*, 2000; **21**: 115–137.

31. McNamara LM, Majeska RJ, Weinbaum S, Friedrich V, Schaffler MB. Attachment of osteocyte cell processes to the bone matrix. *Anat Rec Adv Integr Anat Evol Biol*, 2009; **292**: 355–363.

32. Rho JY, Kuhn-Spearing L, Zioupos P. Mechanical properties and the hierarchical structure of bone. *Med Eng Phys,* 1998; **20**: 92–102.

33. Whittaker DK. Structural variations in the surface zone of human tooth enamel observed by scanning electron microscopy. *Arch Oral Biol,* 1982; **27**: 383–392.

34. Tamerler C, Sarikaya M. Molecular biomimetics: Genetic synthesis, assembly, and formation of materials using peptides. *MRS Bull,* 2008; **33**: 504–512.

35. Arsenault AL, Robinson BW. The dentino-enamel junction: A structural and microanalytical study of early mineralization. *Calcif Tissue Int,* 1989; **45**: 111–121.

36. White SN, Luo W, Paine ML, Fong H, Sarikaya M, Snead ML. Biological organization of hydroxyapatite crystallites into a fibrous continuum toughens and controls anisotropy in human enamel. *J Dent Res,* 2001; **80**: 321–326.

37. Imbeni V, Kruzic JJ, Marshall GW, Marshall SJ, Ritchie RO. The dentin-enamel junction and the fracture of human teeth. *Nat Mater,* 2005; **4**: 229–232.

38. Paine ML, White SN, Luo W, Fong H, Sarikaya M, Snead ML. Regulated gene expression dictates enamel structure and tooth function. *Matrix Biol,* 2001; **20**: 273–292.

39. Wen HB, Moradian-Oldak J, Fincham AG. Dose-dependent modulation of octacalcium phosphate crystal habit by amelogenins. *J Den. Res.,* 2000; **79**: 1902–1906.

40. Fang P-A, Conway JF, Margolis HC, Simmer JP, Beniash E. Hierarchical self-assembly of amelogenin and the regulation of biomineralization at the nanoscale. *Proc Natll Acad Sci,* 2011; **108**: 14097–14102.

41. Cui FZ, Ge J. New observations of the hierarchical structure of human enamel, from nanoscale to microscale. *J Tissue Eng Regen Med,* 2007; **1**: 185–191.

42. Hannig M, Hannig C. Nanomaterials in preventive dentistry. *Nat Nanotechnol,* 2010; **5**: 565–569.

43. Kodaka T, Nakajima F, Higashi S. Structure of the so-called "prismless" enamel in human deciduous teeth. *Caries Res,* 1989; **23**: 290–296.

44. Daculsi G, Bouler JM, Legeros RZ. Adaptive crystal formation in normal and pathological calcifications in synthetic calcium phosphate and related biomaterials. *Int Rev Cytol,* 1997; **172**: 129–191.

45. Kazama JJ, Amizuka N, Fukagawa M. Ectopic calcification as abnormal biomineralization. *Ther Apher Dial,* 2006; **10**: S34–S38.

46. Achilles W, Jockel U, Schaper A, Burk M, Riedmiller H, Khan SR, et al. In vitro formation of "urinary stones": Generation of spherulites

of calcium phosphate in gel and overgrowth with calcium oxalate using a new flow model of crystallization. *Scanning Microsc,* 1995; **9**: 577–586.

47. Hayashizaki J, Ban S, Nakagaki H, Okumura A, Yoshii S, Robinson C. Site specific mineral composition and microstructure of human supra-gingival dental calculus. *Arch Oral Biol,* 2008; **53**: 168–174.

48. Marra SP, Daghlian CP, Fillinger MF, Kennedy FE. Elemental composition, morphology and mechanical properties of calcified deposits obtained from abdominal aortic aneurysms. *Acta Biomater,* 2006; **2**: 515–520.

49. Gigi A, Compostella L, Fichera AM, Foresti E, Gazzano M, Ripamonti A, et al. Structural and chemical characterization of inorganic deposits in calcified human mitral valve. *J Inorg Biochem,* 1988; **34**: 75–82.

50. Laird DF, Mucalo MR, Yokogawa Y. Growth of calcium hydroxyapatite (Ca-HAp) on cholesterol and cholestanol crystals from a simulated body fluid: A possible insight into the pathological calcifications associated with atherosclerosis. *J Colloid Interface Sci,* 2006; **295**: 348–363.

51. Wesson JA, Ward MD. Pathological biomineralization of kidney stones. *Elements,* 2007; **3**: 415–421.

52. Kirsch T. Determinants of pathological mineralization. *Curr Opin Rheumatol,* 2006; **18**: 174–180.

53. Rey C, Combes C, Drouet C, Sfihi H, Barroug A. Physico-chemical properties of nanocrystalline apatites: Implications for biominerals and biomaterials. *Mater Sci Eng C Biomimetic Supramol Syst,* 2007; **27**: 198–205.

54. Legros R, Balmain N, Bonel G. Age-related changes in mineral of rat and bovine cortical bone. *Calcif Tissue Int,* 1987; **41**: 137–144.

55. Rey C, Collins B, Goehl T, Dickson IR, Glimcher MJ. The carbonate environment in bone mineral: A resolution-enhanced Fourier transform infrared spectroscopy study. *Calcif Tissue Int,* 1989; **45**: 157–164.

56. Rey C, Shimizu M, Collins B, Glimcher MJ. Resolution-enhanced fourier transform infrared spectroscopy study of the environment of phosphate ion in the early deposits of a solid phase of calcium phosphate in bone and enamel and their evolution with age: 2. Investigations in the $V_4$ $PO_4$ domain. *Calcif Tissue Int,* 1991; **49**: 383–388.

57. Jäger C, Welzel T, Meyer-Zaika W, Epple M. A solid-state NMR investigation of the structure of nanocrystalline hydroxyapatite. *Magn Reson Chem,* 2006; **44**: 573–580.

58. Pasteris JD, Wopenka B, Freeman JJ, Rogers K, Valsami-Jones E, van der Houwen JAM, et al. Lack of OH in nanocrystalline apatite as a function of degree of atomic order: Implications for bone and biomaterials. *Biomaterials,* 2004; **25**: 229–238.

59. Iafisco M, Varoni E, Di Foggia M, Pietronave S, Fini M, Roveri N, et al. Conjugation of hydroxyapatite nanocrystals with human immunoglobulin G for nanomedical applications. *Colloid Surf B,* 2012; **90**: 1–7.

60. Iafisco M, Palazzo B, Martra G, Margiotta N, Piccinonna S, Natile G, et al. Nanocrystalline carbonate-apatites: Role of Ca/P ratio on the upload and release of anticancer platinum bisphosphonates. *Nanoscale,* 2012; **4**: 206–217.

61. Iafisco M, Bosco R, Leeuwenburgh SCG, van den Beucken JJJP, Jansen JA, Prat M, et al. Electrostatic spray deposition of biomimetic nanocrystalline apatite coatings onto titanium. *Adv Eng Mater,* 2012; **14**: B13–B20.

62. Wang J, Shaw LL. Morphology-enhanced low-temperature sintering of nanocrystalline hydroxyapatite. *Adv Mater,* 2007; **19**: 2364–2369.

63. Ganesan K, Epple M. Calcium phosphate nanoparticles as nuclei for the preparation of colloidal calcium phytate. *N J Chem,* 2008; **32**: 1326–1330.

64. Zhang Y, Lu J. A simple method to tailor spherical nanocrystal hydroxyapatite at low temperature. *J Nanoparticle Res,* 2007; **9**: 589–594.

65. Ben-Nissan B, Choi AH. Sol-gel production of bioactive nanocoatings for medical applications. Part 1: An introduction. *Nanomedicine,* 2006; **1**: 311–319.

66. Tas AC. Synthesis of biomimetic Ca-hydroxyapatite powders at 37°C in synthetic body fluids. *Biomaterials,* 2000; **21**: 1429–1438.

67. Ashok M, Kalkura SN, Sundaram NM, Arivuoli D. Growth and characterization of hydroxyapatite crystals by hydrothermal method. *J Mater Sci Mater M,* 2007; **18**: 895–898.

68. Guo XY, Gough JE, Xiao P, Liu J, Shen ZJ. Fabrication of nanostructured hydroxyapatite and analysis of human osteoblastic cellular response. *J Biomed Mater Res A,* 2007; **82A**: 1022–1032.

69. Chaudhry AA, Haque S, Kellici S, Boldrin P, Rehman I, Fazal AK, et al. Instant nano-hydroxyapatite: A continuous and rapid hydrothermal synthesis. *Chem Commun* 2006; **21**: 2286–2288.

70. Gómez-Morales J, Torrent-Burgues J, Boix T, Fraile J, Rodríguez-Clemente R. Precipitation of stoichiometric hydroxyapatite by a continuous method. *Cryst Res Technol* 2001; **36**: 15–26.

71. Yeong KCB, Wang J, Ng SC. Mechanochemical synthesis of nanocrystalline hydroxyapatite from CaO and $CaHPO_4$. *Biomaterials*, 2001; **22**: 2705–2712.

72. Krishna DSR, Siddharthan A, Seshadri SK, Kumar TSS. A novel route for synthesis of nanocrystalline hydroxyapatite from eggshell waste. *J Mater Sci Mater M*, 2007; **18**: 1735–1743.

73. Lak A, Mazloumi M, Mohajerani MS, Zanganeh S, Shayegh MR, Kajbafvala A, et al. Rapid formation of mono-dispersed hydroxyapatite nanorods with narrow-size distribution via microwave irradiation. *J Am Ceram Soc*, 2008; **91**: 3580–3584.

74. Iafisco M, Delgado-Lopez JM, Gomez-Morales J, Hernandez-Hernandez MA, Rodriguez-Ruiz I, Roveri N. Formation of calcium phosphates by vapour diffusion in highly concentrated ionic micro-droplets. *Cryst Res Technol*, 2011; **46**: 841–846.

75. Gómez-Morales J, Delgado-López JM, Iafisco M, Hernández-Hernández A, Prat M. Amino acidic control of calcium phosphate precipitation by using the vapor diffusion method in microdroplets. *Cryst Growth Des*, 2011; **11**: 4802–4809.

76. Iafisco M, Gómez Morales J, Hernandez-Hernandez, MA, Garcia-Ruiz, JM, Roveri, N. Biomimetic carbonate-hydroxyapatite nanocrystals prepared by vapor diffusion. *Adv Eng Mater*, 2010; **12**: B218–B223.

77. Phillips MJ, Darr JA, Luklinska ZB, Rehman I. Synthesis and characterization of nano-biomaterials with potential osteological applications. *J Mater Sci Mater M*, 2003; **14**: 875–882.

78. Layrolle P, Lebugle A. Characterization and reactivity of nanosized calcium phosphates prepared in anhydrous ethanol. *Chem Mater*, 1994; **6**: 1996–2004.

79. Ye F, Guo HF, Zhang HJ. Biomimetic synthesis of oriented hydroxyapatite mediated by nonionic surfactants. *Nanotechnology*, 2008; **19**: 245605.

80. Sadat-Shojai M, Khorasani M-T, Dinpanah-Khoshdargi E, Jamshidi A. Synthesis methods for nanosized hydroxyapatite with diverse structures. *Acta Biomater*, 2013; **9**: 7591–7621.

81. Iafisco M, Varoni E, Battistella E, Pietronave S, Prat M, Roveri N, et al. The cooperative effect of size and crystallinity degree on

the resorption of biomimetic hydroxyapatite for soft tissue augmentation. *Int J Artif Organs*, 2010; **33**: 765–774.

82. Iafisco M, Sabatino P, Lesci IG, Prat M, Rimondini L, Roveri N. Conformational modifications of serum albumins adsorbed on different kinds of biomimetic hydroxyapatite nanocrystals. *Colloids Surf B Biointerfaces*, 2010; **81**: 274–284.

83. Iafisco M, Foggia MD, Bonora S, Prat M, Roveri N. Adsorption and spectroscopic characterization of lactoferrin on hydroxyapatite nanocrystals. *Dalton Trans*, 2011; **40**: 820–827.

84. Müller B. Tailoring biocompatibility: Benefitting patients. *Mater Today* 2010; **13**: 58.

85. Uskoković V, Uskoković DP. Nanosized hydroxyapatite and other calcium phosphates: Chemistry of formation and application as drug and gene delivery agents. *J Biomed Mater Res Part B Appl Biomater,* 2011; **96B**: 152–191.

86. Sakhno Y, Bertinetti L, Iafisco M, Tampieri A, Roveri N, Martra G. Surface hydration and cationic sites of nanohydroxyapatites with amorphous or crystalline surfaces: A comparative study. *J Phys Chem C*, 2010; **114**: 16640–16648.

87. Achelhi K, Masse S, Laurent G, Saoiabi A, Laghzizil A, Coradin T. Role of carboxylate chelating agents on the chemical, structural and textural properties of hydroxyapatite. *Dalton T*, 2010; **39**: 10644–10651.

88. Delgado-Lopez JM, Iafisco M, Rodriguez I, Tampieri A, Prat M, Gomez-Morales J. Crystallization of bioinspired citrate-functionalized nanoapatite with tailored carbonate content. *Acta Biomater,* 2012; **8**: 3491–3499.

89. Li CF. Crystalline behaviors of hydroxyapatite in the neutralized reaction with different citrate additions. *Powder Technol* 2009; **192**: 1–5.

90. Xie B, Nancollas GH. How to control the size and morphology of apatite nanocrystals in bone. *Proc Natl. Acad Sci U S A*, 2010; **107**: 22369–22370.

91. Iafisco M, Sandri M, Panseri S, Delgado-López JM, Gómez-Morales J, Tampieri A. Magnetic bioactive and biodegradable hollow Fe-doped hydroxyapatite coated poly(L-lactic) acid micro-nanospheres. *Chem Mater,* 2013; **25**: 2610–2617.

92. Iafisco M, Palazzo B, Ito T, Otsuka M, Senna M, Delgado-Lopez J, et al. Preparation of core–shell poly(L-lactic) acid-nanocrystalline apatite hollow microspheres for bone repairing applications. *J Mater Sci Mater Med*, 2012; **23**: 2659–2669.

93. Tampieri A, Sprio S, Sandri M, Valentini F. Mimicking natural bio-mineralization processes: A new tool for osteochondral scaffold development. *Trends Biotechnol*, 2011; **29**: 526–535.

94. Tampieri A, Sprio S, Sandri M, Valentini F. Mimicking natural bio-mineralization processes: A new tool for osteochondral scaffold development. *Trends Biotechnol*, 2011; **29**: 526–535.

95. Iafisco M, Delgado-Lopez JM, Varoni EM, Tampieri A, Rimondini L, Gomez-Morales J, et al. Cell surface receptor targeted biomimetic apatite nanocrystals for cancer therapy. *Small*, 2013; **9**: 3834–3844.

96. Kokubo T, Takadama H. How useful is SBF in predicting in vivo bone bioactivity? *Biomaterials*, 2006; **27**: 2907–2915.

97. Vallet-Regí M, Ruiz-Hernández E. Bioceramics: From bone regeneration to cancer nanomedicine. *Adv Mater*, 2011; **23**: 5177–5218.

98. Dorozhkin SV. Bioceramics of calcium orthophosphates. *Biomaterials*, 2010; **31**: 1465–1485.

99. Zhou H, Lee J. Nanoscale hydroxyapatite particles for bone tissue engineering. *Acta Biomater*, 2011; **7**: 2769–2781.

100. Navarro M, Michiardi A, Castaño O, Planell JA. Biomaterials in orthopaedics. *J R Soc Interface*, 2008; **5**: 1137–1158.

101. Kim H-W, Kim H-E, Salih V. Stimulation of osteoblast responses to biomimetic nanocomposites of gelatin–hydroxyapatite for tissue engineering scaffolds. *Biomaterials*, 2005; **26**: 5221–5230.

102. Zhang L, Chen Y, Rodriguez J, Fenniri H, Webster TJ. Biomimetic helical rosette nanotubes and nanocrystalline hydroxyapatite coatings on titanium for improving orthopedic implants. *Int J Nanomed*, 2008; **3**: 323–333.

103. Sun WB, Chu CL, Wang J, Zhao HT. Comparison of periodontal ligament cells responses to dense and nanophase hydroxyapatite. *J Mater Sci Mater Med*, 2007; **18**: 677–683.

104. Ergun C, Liu H, Webster TJ, Olcay E, Yilmaz Ş, Sahin FC. Increased osteoblast adhesion on nanoparticulate calcium phosphates with higher Ca/P ratios. *J Biomed Mater Res Part A*, 2008; **85**: 236–241.

105. Zhou DS, Zhao KB, Li Y, Cui FZ, Lee IS. Repair of segmental defects with nano-hydroxyapatite/collagen/PLA composite combined with mesenchymal stem cells. *J Bioactive Compatible Polym*, 2006; **21**: 373–384.

106. Cai Y, Liu Y, Yan W, Hu Q, Tao J, Zhang M, et al. Role of hydroxyapatite nanoparticle size in bone cell proliferation. *J Mater Chem*, 2007; **17**: 3780–3787.

107. Palazzo B, Walsh D, Iafisco M, Foresti E, Bertinetti L, Martra G, et al. Amino acid synergetic effect on structure, morphology and surface properties of biomimetic apatite nanocrystals. *Acta Biomater*, 2009; **5**: 1241–252.

108. Iafisco M, Palazzo B, Falini G, Foggia MD, Bonora S, Nicolis S, et al. Adsorption and conformational change of myoglobin on biomimetic hydroxyapatite nanocrystals functionalized with alendronate. *Langmuir*, 2008; **24**: 4924–4930.

109. Varoni EM, Iafisco M, Rimondini L, Prat M. Development of a targeted drug delivery system: Monoclonal antibodies adsorption onto bonelike hydroxyapatite nanocrystal surface. *Adv Mat Res*, 2012; **409**: 175–180.

110. Iafisco M, Margiotta N. Silica xerogels and hydroxyapatite nanocrystals for the local delivery of platinum–bisphosphonate complexes in the treatment of bone tumors: A mini-review. *J Inorg Biochem*, 2012; **117**: 237–247.

111. Rodríguez-Ruiz I, Delgado-López JM, Durán-Olivencia MA, Iafisco M, Tampieri A, Colangelo D, et al. pH-responsive delivery of doxorubicin from citrate–apatite nanocrystals with tailored carbonate content. *Langmuir*, 2013; **29**: 8213–8221.

112. Iafisco M, Palazzo B, Marchetti M, Margiotta N, Ostuni R, Natile G, et al. Smart delivery of antitumoral platinum complexes from biomimetic hydroxyapatite nanocrystals. *J Mater Chem*, 2009; **19**: 8385–8392.

113. Autefage H, Briand-Mesange F, Cazalbou S, Drouet C, Fourmy D, Goncalves S, et al. Adsorption and release of BMP-2 on nanocrystalline apatite-coated and uncoated hydroxyapatite/beta-tricalcium phosphate porous ceramics. *J Biomed Mater Res Part B Appl Biomater*, 2009; **91B**: 706–715.

114. Gautier H, Daculsi G, Merle C. Association of vancomycin and calcium phosphate by dynamic compaction: in vitro characterization and microbiological activity. *Biomaterials*, 2001; **22**: 2481–2487.

115. Lebugle A, Rodrigues A, Bonnevialle P, Voigt JJ, Canal P, Rodriguez F. Study of implantable calcium phosphate systems for the slow release of methotrexate. *Biomaterials*, 2002; **23**: 3517–3522.

116. Liu YL, Enggist L, Kuffer AF, Buser D, Hunziker EB. The influence of BMP-2 and its mode of delivery on the osteoconductivity of implant surfaces during the early phase of osseointegration (vol. 28, pg 2677, 2007). *Biomaterials*, 2007; **28**: 5399.

117. Nancollas GH, Tang R, Phipps RJ, Henneman Z, Gulde S, Wu W, et al. Novel insights into actions of bisphosphonates on bone:

Differences in interactions with hydroxyapatite. *Bone*, 2006; **38**: 617–627.

118. Alghamdi HS, Bosco R, Both SK, Iafisco M, Leeuwenburgh SCG, Jansen JA, et al. Synergistic effects of bisphosphonate and calcium phosphate nanoparticles on peri-implant bone responses in osteoporotic rats. *Biomaterials*, 2014; **35**: 5482–5490.

119. Peter B, Pioletti DP, Laib S, Bujoli B, Pilet P, Janvier P, et al. Calcium phosphate drug delivery system: Influence of local zoledronate release on bone implant osteointegration. *Bone*, 2005; **36**: 52–60.

120. Midy V, Hollande E, Rey C, Dard M, Plouet J. Adsorption of vascular endothelial growth factor to two different apatitic materials and its release. *J Mater Sci Mater Med*, 2001; **12**: 293–298.

121. Errassif F, Menbaoui A, Autefage H, Benaziz L, Ouizat S, Santran V, et al. Adsorption on apatitic calcium phosphates: Applications to drug delivery. In: Narayan R, Singh M, McKittrick J, eds. *Advances in Bioceramics and Biotechnologies*: Wiley-VCH Verlag GmbH & Co. KGaA 2010.

122. Yoshinari M, Oda Y, Ueki H, Yokose S. Immobilization of bisphosphonates on surface modified titanium. *Biomaterials*, 2001; **22**: 709–715.

123. McLeod K, Kumar S, Smart RSC, Dutta N, Voelcker NH, Anderson GI, et al. XPS and bioactivity study of the bisphosphonate pamidronate adsorbed onto plasma sprayed hydroxyapatite coatings. *Appl Surf Sci*, 2006; **253**: 2644–2651.

124. Barroug A, Kuhn LT, Gerstenfeld LC, Glimcher MJ. Interactions of cisplatin with calcium phosphate nanoparticles: in vitro controlled adsorption and release. *J Orthop Res*, 2004; **22**: 703–708.

125. Stigter M, Bezemer J, de Groot K, Layrolle P. Incorporation of different antibiotics into carbonated hydroxyapatite coatings on titanium implants, release and antibiotic efficacy. *J Control Release*, 2004; **99**: 127–137.

126. Palazzo B, Iafisco M, Laforgia M, Margiotta N, Natile G, Bianchi CL, et al. Biomimetic hydroxyapatite-drug nanocrystals as potential bone substitutes with antitumor drug delivery properties. *Adv Funct Mater*, 2007; **17**: 2180–188.

127. Pietronave S, Iafisco M, Locarno D, Rimondini L, Maria Prat M. Functionalized nanomaterials for diagnosis and therapy of cancer. *J Appl Biomater Biomech*, 2009; **7**: 77–89.

128. Hillaireau H, Couvreur P. Nanocarriers' entry into the cell: Relevance to drug delivery. *Cell Mol Life Sci*, 2009; **66**: 2873–2896.

129. Cheng CJ, Saltzman WM. Nanomedicine: Downsizing tumour therapeutics. *Nat Nano*, 2012; **7**: 346–347.

130. Adair JH, Parette MP, Altýnoğlu EI, Kester M. Nanoparticulate alternatives for drug delivery. *ACS Nano*, 2010; **4**: 4967–4970.

131. Russell-Jones G, McTavish K, McEwan J, Rice J, Nowotnik D. Vitamin-mediated targeting as a potential mechanism to increase drug uptake by tumours. *J Inorg Biochem*, 2004; **98**: 1625–1633.

132. Bildstein L, Dubernet C, Couvreur P. Prodrug-based intracellular delivery of anticancer agents. *Adv Drug Deliver Rev*, 2011; **63**: 3–23.

133. Uskokovic V, Uskokovic DP. Nanosized hydroxyapatite and other calcium phosphates: Chemistry of formation and application as drug and gene delivery agents. *J Biomed Mater Res B Appl Biomater*, 2011; **96**: 152–191.

134. Epple M, Ganesan K, Heumann R, Klesing J, Kovtun A, Neumann S, et al. Application of calcium phosphate nanoparticles in biomedicine. *J Mater Chem*, 2010; **20**: 18–23.

135. Bisht S, Bhakta G, Mitra S, Maitra A. pDNA loaded calcium phosphate nanoparticles: Highly efficient non-viral vector for gene delivery. *Int J Pharm*, 2005; **288**: 157–168.

136. Wang S, McDonnell EH, Sedor FA, Toffaletti JG. pH effects on measurements of ionized calcium and ionized magnesium in blood. *Arch Pathol Lab Med*, 2002; **126**: 947–950.

137. Reischl D, Zimmer A. Drug delivery of siRNA therapeutics: potentials and limits of nanosystems. *Nanomed Nanotechnol Biol Med,* 2009; **5**: 8–20.

138. Kester M, Heakal Y, Fox T, Sharma A, Robertson GP, Morgan TT, et al. Calcium phosphate nanocomposite particles for in vitro imaging and encapsulated chemotherapeutic drug delivery to cancer cells. *Nano Lett*, 2008; **8**: 4116–4121.

139. Altýnoğlu EI, Russin TJ, Kaiser JM, Barth BM, Eklund PC, Kester M, et al. Near-infrared emitting fluorophore-doped calcium phosphate nanoparticles for in vivo imaging of human breast cancer. *ACS Nano*, 2008; **2**: 2075–2084.

140. Tabaković A, Kester M, Adair JH. Calcium phosphate-based composite nanoparticles in bioimaging and therapeutic delivery applications. *Wiley Interdisciplinary Rev Nanomed Nanobiotechnol,* 2012; **4**: 96–112.

141. Mondejar SP, Kovtun A, Epple M. Lanthanide-doped calcium phosphate nanoparticles with high internal crystallinity and with a shell of DNA as fluorescent probes in cell experiments. *J Mater Chem,* 2007; **17**: 4153–159.

142. Al-Kattan A, Dufour P, Dexpert-Ghys J, Drouet C. Preparation and physicochemical characteristics of luminescent apatite-based colloids. *J Phys Chem C*, 2010; **114**: 2918–2924.

143. Li J, Chen Y-C, Tseng Y-C, Mozumdar S, Huang L. Biodegradable calcium phosphate nanoparticle with lipid coating for systemic siRNA delivery. *J Control Release*, 2010; **142**: 416–421.

144. Sokolova V, Epple M. Synthetic pathways to make nanoparticles fluorescent. *Nanoscale*, 2011; **3**: 1957–1962.

145. Leng AM, Yang J, Liu T, Cui JF, Li XH, Zhu YA, et al. Nanoparticle-delivered VEGF-silencing cassette and suicide gene expression cassettes inhibit colon carcinoma growth in vitro and in vivo. *Tumor Biol*, 2011; **32**: 1103–1111.

146. Xu ZP, Zeng QH, Lu GQ, Yu AB. Inorganic nanoparticles as carriers for efficient cellular delivery. *Chem Eng Sci*, 2006; **61**: 1027–1040.

147. Pouton CW, Seymour LW. Key issues in non-viral gene delivery. *Adv Drug Deliv Rev*, 2001; **46**: 187–203.

148. Yazaki Y, Oyane A, Sogo Y, Ito A, Yamazaki A, Tsurushima H. Control of gene transfer on a DNA-fibronectin-apatite composite layer by the incorporation of carbonate and fluoride ions. *Biomaterials,* 2011; **32**: 4896–4902.

149. Tan SJ, Kiatwuthinon P, Roh YH, Kahn JS, Luo D. Engineering nanocarriers for siRNA delivery. *Small*, 2011; **7**: 841–856.

150. Sun B, Yi M, Yacoob CC, Nguyen HT, Shen H. Effect of surface chemistry on gene transfer efficiency mediated by surface-induced DNA-doped nanocomposites. *Acta Biomater*, 2012; **8**: 1109–1116.

151. Olton D, Li J, Wilson ME, Rogers T, Close J, Huang L, et al. Nanostructured calcium phosphates (NanoCaPs) for non-viral gene delivery: Influence of the synthesis parameters on transfection efficiency. *Biomaterials*, 2007; **28**: 1267–1279.

152. Maitra A. Calcium phosphate nanoparticles: Second-generation nonviral vectors in gene therapy. *Expert Rev Mol Diagn*, 2005; **5**: 893–905.

153. Kumta PN, Sfeir C, Lee D-H, Olton D, Choi D. Nanostructured calcium phosphates for biomedical applications: Novel synthesis and characterization. *Acta Biomater*, 2005; **1**: 65–83.

154. Chen W-Y, Lin M-S, Lin P-H, Tasi P-S, Chang Y, Yamamoto S. Studies of the interaction mechanism between single strand and double-strand DNA with hydroxyapatite by microcalorimetry and isotherm measurements. *Colloids Surf A Physicochem Eng Aspects,* 2007; **295**: 274–283.

# Chapter 4

# New Biomimetic Strategies for Regeneration of Load-Bearing Bones

Simone Sprio, Andrea Ruffini, Massimiliano Dapporto, and Anna Tampieri

*Institute of Science and Technology for Ceramics,*
*National Research Council of Italy,*
*Via Granarolo 64, 48018 Faenza, Italy*

simone.sprio@istec.cnr.it

The regeneration of critical-size bone defects requires the application of a scaffold able to instruct cells towards new tissue formation and remodelling. In the case of load-bearing bone parts, the requirement of high mimicry of native tissue is even more crucial since bone-like mechanical competence is required, besides bone-like chemistry and extensive macro-porous architecture. This chapter highlights some of the most recent advances in materials science addressed to this specific issue; in particular, it is illustrated how nature can inspire biomedical engineers to develop new biomorphic devices with hierarchical structure that can pave the way to new-generation smart devices with outstanding functional properties.

---

*Bio-Inspired Regenerative Medicine: Materials, Processes, and Clinical Applications*
Edited by Simone Sprio and Anna Tampieri
Copyright © 2016 Pan Stanford Publishing Pte. Ltd.
ISBN 978-981-4669-14-6 (Hardcover), 978-981-4669-15-3 (eBook)
www.panstanford.com

## 4.1 Bone Tissue: Structure, Biomechanics and Remodelling

Bone is a dynamic living tissue that possesses the ability to change its mass and structure in response to changes in the biomechanical and biochemical environment. This amazing ability is expressed by Wolff's law [1], on the basis of which the bone structure continuously remodels and organizes itself to become stronger under specific loading by stress-induced orientation of trabeculae. In this respect, the internal architecture of the bone trabeculae undergoes adaptive changes, followed by secondary changes to the external cortical portion of the bone that may also become thicker as a result (Fig. 4.1).

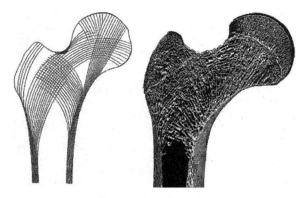

**Figure 4.1** Orientation of bone trabeculae in human femur.

Therefore, during physical stimulations due to the daily human activities bones are subjected to a dynamic process of formation by osteoblast cells and resorption by osteoclasts that, besides maintaining equilibrium in mass and density, also enables the continuous repairing of micro-damages (Fig. 4.2).

The complex behaviour of bones, in response to external stimuli, is made possible by the hierarchical organization of its structure, occurring along several scales from the nano- to the macro-size. Hierarchically organized porous structures enable higher resistance and much more complex mechanical performances in comparison with bodies with similar, but random, porosity extent; besides, multi-scale hierarchy enables increased lightness and elasticity, as well as suitable propagation of the physical stimuli down to the cell level that in turn permits and activates bone remodelling (Fig. 4.3).

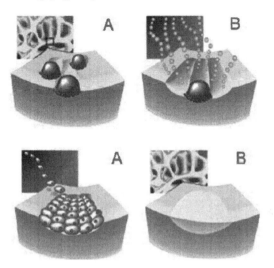

**Figure 4.2** Top: Digestion of the old bone by osteoclasts; bottom: formation of new bone by osteoblasts.

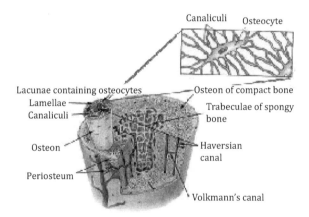

**Figure 4.3** Hierarchical structure of bone.

By a holistic approach, the bones with their complex structure are part of a more extended system: the whole musculo-skeletal system. In fact, bones are compression-resistant elements connected to muscles by tensile-resistant elements (i.e. tendons and ligaments), thus forming a tensegrity structure [2–5], where a complex *ensemble* of compressive and tensile forces, in continuous dynamic equilibrium, is established at the macro-scale and can propagate down to the smallest bone trabeculae, thanks to the hierarchical organization of both bone and ligament tissues.

Tensegrity (i.e. tensional integrity), is a concept introduced by civil engineering and translated to biology by D. Ingber [6], thus helping to elucidate several mechanisms at the basis of cell behaviour under the influence of mechanical stimuli. In this respect the most amazing and fascinating aspect at the basis of the great complexity of human body is that not only the human skeleton is a tensegrity structure, but also our cells have similar internal organization. Indeed, specific investigation clearly highlighted that the cell behaviour is influenced by the elastic response of substrates, thus driving survival/apoptosis or proliferation and/or differentiation [7–9].

In particular, it was found that the elements composing the internal cell structure (cytoskeleton) are closely interconnected so that the mechanical interaction between cells and substrate reflects into modifications in the force fields acting at the cytoplasm level, in turn driving specific changes to cell morphology and behaviour. Therefore, human body is a strongly interacting system organized in a globally integrated three-dimensional architecture, that continuously exchange physical signals propagating from the molecular to the macroscopic scale and vice versa (Fig. 4.4).

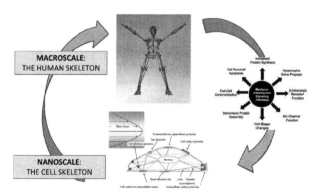

**Figure 4.4** Scheme of interacting tensegrity structures at the macro- and nano level in human body.

The cell sensitivity to mechanical stimuli is expressed particularly in the development of a process known as bone mechano-transduction, which drives bone repair and remodelling [10]. This process involves the osteocytes, which are mature quiescent cells embedded in the bone matrix and mutually connected by protrusions that are sensitive to the shearing forces taking place upon variation of the interstitial fluid flow through the bone canaliculi [11]. These in turn generate electric potentials deforming the cell membranes. Such deformations act as stimuli activating feedback processes that involve the exchange of a cascade of biochemical stimuli yielding remodelling of the bone structure. It is hypothesized that the mechano-sensitivity of bone cells can be triggered by the peculiar organization of pores and the elastic properties of bone [12], in turn related to its multi-scale hierarchical structure.

For most human tissues, and particularly in the case of bone, an effective regeneration is facilitated by the presence of a suitable environment playing the role of a guide triggering cell behaviour. In the case of bones, such a guide has a specific chemical and morphological nature, i.e. bone regeneration should be assisted by a scaffold made of bioactive and bio-resorbable hydroxyapatite (HA) and presenting an open and interconnected porosity favouring angiogenesis and extensive bone ingrowth. However, as already mentioned in this chapter, the regeneration of load-bearing bones requires physical stimulation to develop adequate remodelling into an organized 3-D structure able to withstand complex biomechanical stimuli. This requires new approaches enabling early physical stimulation of implanted scaffolds. In this respect the complete regeneration of load-bearing bones, including limbs and vertebrae, is still an open challenge for surgeons, just because scaffolds presenting a suitable compromise between chemical mimesis, complex pore organization and adequate mechanical strength, are still to be developed.

## 4.2 Main Limitations in Current Approaches for Regeneration of Load-Bearing Bones

In the last decades, in consideration of the ever-increasing life expectancy and more active lifestyles, the number of bone diseases determined by ageing, degenerative diseases or traumas is steadily growing, with a huge and alarming socio-economic impact [13]. Due to this, the effort of materials scientist is increasingly addressed towards the development of new biomaterials and devices enabling bone regeneration and recovery of the functional properties of bone. However, in spite of the good results achieved so far, several critical clinical cases with very significant impact still exist; in this respect, two major categories can be identified: (i) complex fractures in long segmental bones, and (ii) bone diseases related to traumas or metabolic disorders such as osteoporosis (Fig. 4.5).

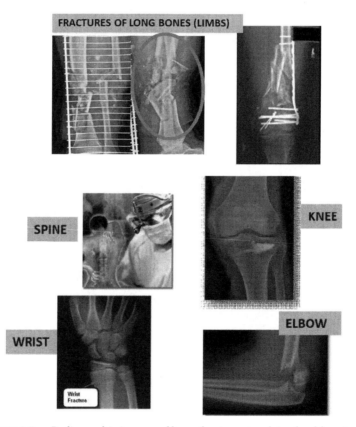

**Figure 4.5** Radiographic images of bone fractures involving load-bearing bones.

These two categories, being related to regeneration of extended, critical-size, bone parts, require smart approaches associated to synthetic scaffolds with features of good mimicry to the host tissues. To this, the most recent approaches pinning on nanotechnology and bio-inspired concepts are particularly promising to develop new smart solutions for regeneration of complex bone districts that conventional therapies are still not able to achieve.

In the case of defects affecting long segmental bones, currently used surgical techniques can be divided in two groups: with or without bone graft. The treatment strategy without graft transplant is the Ilizarov technique, an osteotomy followed by bone distraction that avoids problems related to graft integration relying on the bone regeneration potential, but is highly inconvenient for the patients [14–16]. Therefore, alternative strategies have been developed aiming at accelerating and simplifying the healing process with the use of grafts, with different alternatives including autologous vascularized bone grafts, homologous bone graft, heterologous bone graft (xenograft), or prostheses, each one of them dealing with both specific advantages and drawbacks. The main concerns respectively are donor site morbidity and limited available amount; possible immune response and viral transmission; possible animal-derived pathogen transmission and risk of immunogenic rejection; high invasiveness and surgery-related systemic risks, long recovery time and need of prostheses revision [17–21]. Moreover, due to the damage affecting foreign bone tissue upon pre-implant treatment and purification, heterologous bone parts often retain low regenerative potential and, consequently, the recovery of the bone functionality is difficult, particularly in the case of repair of long bone segments. Particularly in the case of very serious or comminuted fractures affecting long bones, which often involve blood vessels and soft tissues, the patient is often called to withstand numerous and painful reconstructive interventions; in such cases the healing is often impaired by several serious complications. Among these, non-union may affect up to ~50% of cases [22, 23], strongly depending on a number of factors such as the mechanism of injury and type of fracture, associated injuries, comorbidities, age, sex, lifestyles and pharmacological agents. Different types of pseudoarthrosis exist and reflect different pathways of developing this complication [24]. In case of infections, non-union becomes one of the most challenging orthopaedic complications to manage and it may be even a limb-threatening complication [25].

Therefore, the healing of long bones subjected to non-union is still an unsolved problem greatly involving millions of people subjected to serious diseases that jeopardize the ability of deambulation and manipulation. The socio-economic impact of such diseases is so huge that require the establishment of regenerative solutions.

In this respect, several approaches have been described to promote and enhance the bone tissue regeneration, including extracorporeal shock wave therapy (ESWT), ultrasound, electromagnetic, bone morphogenetic proteins (BMPs) and platelet-rich-plasma (PRP) [26]. However, due to the extensive clinical heterogeneity, it is not possible to provide clear recommendations regarding the application of these approaches. The problems remain the need to better understand the most effective treatment options, subject to surgical stabilization as a first step.

Due to these very serious drawbacks, the use of osteoconductive synthetic bone substitutes may offer clear benefits compared to autografts, including less time in the operating room and significantly less pain and recovery time for the patient, and to allografts, avoiding the risk of viral or bacterial infection and possible immune response of the host tissue.

In order to achieve an early osseointegration that enable good stability of the bone/implant construct and the possibility for the patient to stimulate bone regeneration by progressively increasing loading and deambulation, procedures of guided tissue regeneration should be focused on fast and adequate osteogenesis and osteoconductivity. Osteogenesis can be stimulated by scaffolds exhibiting highly exposed active surfaces, favouring cell adhesion and proliferation. In this respect, the mineral part of bone is a nano-sized apatite (general formula: $Ca_{10}(PO_4)_6(OH)_2$) characterized by low crystal order and containing foreign ions (e.g. $CO_3^{2-}$, $Mg^{2+}$, $SiO_4^{4-}$, $Sr^{2+}$, $HPO_4^{2-}$, $Na^+$, $K^+$) which have specific functions in the formation, stabilization and maturation of bone [27, 28]. These features provide the potential for protein linking as well as cell adhesion and proliferation [29–34].

In particular, carbonate ions in the phosphate site of the apatite lattice (i.e. known as the B site) greatly increase the apatite solubility, without changing the surface polar property and the affinity of the osteoblast cells, thus allowing dissolution and re-precipitation of new bone matrix; a very relevant ion present in the structure of newly formed bone is magnesium that greatly enhances the nucleation of the mineral phase, thus accelerating the formation of new tissue. Since decades, synthetic HA phases presenting multiple ion substitutions were synthesized [35, 36]. In particular, co-substitution with carbonate in B position favoured higher bio-availability of osteogenic chemical agents, thus increasing solubility in physiological conditions [36]. The ability of synthetic multi-substituted apatites able to exchange ions with the physiological environment and to be progressively resorbed may enhance cell adhesion and differentiation towards osteogenic phenotype.

Adequate osteoconductivity is provided by the presence of open and interconnected porosity in the bone scaffold, in association with suitable chemical features; therefore a wide open porosity permitting cell colonization and penetration enables early osseointegration and consequent physical stabilization of the bone/implant construct [37, 38]. However, most of the bio-devices today developed exhibits tortuous porosity that hampers the development of extensive angiogenesis and penetration of blood vessels in the inner parts of the scaffold; in consequence, even though a good surface integration occurred, bone penetration is limited to few millimetres from the interface thus penalizing the stability of the bone/implant construct [39]. In such cases, the lack of suitable pore interconnection or scarce driving force for bone and epithelial cells to propagate in inner parts of a scaffold may create spatially discontinuous ingrowth with formation of bone islands throughout the whole scaffold and also necrotic areas. Lack of angiogenesis is among the most serious reasons for non-complete osseointegration of the scaffold; these concerns are particularly serious in the case of scaffolds for long segmental bones [40, 41].

The convergence of the properties of bioactivity, osteoconductivity and mechanical strength in a single implantable bio-device is hampered by two factors:

(1) the sintering process necessary to consolidate 3-D porous ceramic bodies, particularly hydroxyapatite bodies, yields grain growth and strong reduction of the specific surface area that strongly reduce the hydrophilic character and surface reactivity in turn impacting on the bioactivity and resorbability of the scaffold;

(2) hydroxyapatite is intrinsically weak, compared to other ceramic materials; therefore, even in the case of well consolidated bodies, the mechanical stimulation of the HA scaffold in vivo can be problematic, particularly when the scaffold exhibits an extensive open porosity.

Indeed, the concerns related to the poor mechanical strength of hydroxyapatite could be overcome, in the case of fast and extensive bone penetration in the scaffold. Therefore, new regenerative therapies could be designed, based on early integration and progressive recovery of mechanical bio-competence of the new bone. This approach would require a certain hospitalization time but at the advantage of a progressive recovery and healing of the diseased bone.

## 4.3  Regeneration of Long Segmental Bones: New Biomorphic Porous Devices

To date, no suitable solutions have been found for regenerating long and load-bearing bone segments. In this respect, macroporous hydroxyapatite constructs in addition to cultured bone marrow stem cells (BMSCs) were previously tested to treat a series of patients affected by traumatic bone defects, with good osseointegration and satisfactory recovery of deambulation ability [42]. However, the insufficient strength of these scaffolds represented an important limiting factor thus forcing the involved surgeons to apply invasive fixation to prevent ruptures. Indeed, the mechanical strength of a highly porous but "disorganized" scaffold is often insufficient, to manage the in vivo stresses and physiological loadings in a reliable way. Moreover, the costs and legal issues related to the cell culture of autologous patient's cells in clinical procedures still limit the cost-effectiveness of this approach.

Since the unique biomechanical properties of bone mainly depend on its hierarchically organized structure ranging from the molecular to the nano-, micro-, and macro-scales, only scaffolds endowed with a 3D structure capable of exhibiting complex biomechanical performances may activate mechano-transduction processes and yield regeneration of well-organized bone. In consideration of the limits imposed by the ceramic technology, new manufacturing approaches are required for the synthesis of scaffolds with adequate requisites for regeneration of long segmental bones. Indeed, even the most advanced forming techniques are not able to produce hydroxyapatite bodies with the required degree of structural complexity and mechanical features to withstand early loading in vivo. In this respect, since a decade the attention of materials scientists is increasingly directed to the astonishing properties of natural structures and their complex structural organization, with the attempt to find inspiration for new-generation smart devices with strongly improved performances. The complex structure exhibited by living beings such as insects, molluscs, plants is an astonishing example of nanotechnology where the nucleation of inorganic phases onto organic, macromolecular templates gives rise to hybrid structures that cannot be reproduced by any available manufacturing techniques. Indeed, these structures possess a hierarchic organization on multiple size scales that provide high strength and lightness. Among these, ligneous structures exhibit a morphology and organization similar to that of bone, which confer impressive biomechanical properties: for example, some tree branches can withstand very heavy loads and others can be stretched and bent into any shape [43, 44]. Wood can be regarded as a cellular material at the scale of hundred micrometers to centimetres that enable coexistence of elasticity, lightness and strength associated with high porosity extent (Fig. 4.6) [45, 46].

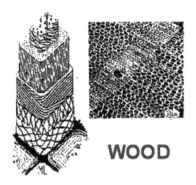
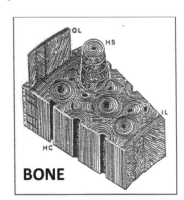

Figure 4.6    Cellular structures of wood and bone.

Therefore, woods may be taken as templates to develop new inorganic devices with bone-like structural features. Indeed, woods are characterized by a very big variety in density and strength as well as in pore organization (Fig. 4.7), so that a main task is to select woods endowed with open porosity and suitable interconnection thus enabling extensive permeability to cells and fluids, and exhibiting at the same time adequate anisotropic mechanical behaviour.

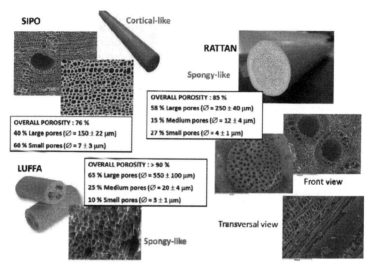

**Figure 4.7** Structure and porosity of various woods.

On this basis, selected wood structures could reproduce different bone portions characterized by different porosity and pore distribution, such as cortical and spongy bone.

Processes for transformation of natural structures into inorganic bodies were already investigated in past studies, thus obtaining 3D bodies in a variety of compositions, through a sequence of chemical and thermal reactions. Particularly, transformation into silicon carbide was obtained by pyrolysis and subsequent infiltration of molten silicon [47–49]. However, the requirement of both bioactivity and bioresorbability imposes that these new approaches are addressed to development of materials able to exhibit positive interface reactions with the physiological environment.

Porous woods like pine and rattan were recently transformed into biomorphic hydroxyapatite by a multi-step process [50] (Fig. 4.8). The multi-step process (Fig. 4.8 top) allowed a precise control of phase composition and degree of crystal order of the final crystallinity as well as of the microstructure, since the different reactions occurred between a gas and the solid template at a molecular level, where calcium, oxygen, carbonate and phosphate ions were progressively added, while building the HA molecules.

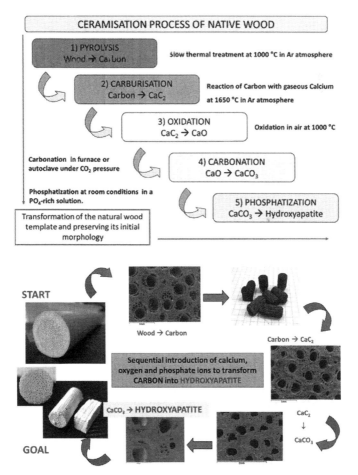

**Figure 4.8**  Multi-step transformation process and intermediate products from wood to HA.

Wood-derived biomorphic HA exhibits a biomimetic phase composition (carbonated HA); the formation of acicular nanometric grains of HA took place by the progressive dissolution of $CaCO_3$ particles in the liquid media containing phosphate ions [50]. This slow process enabled incorporation of carbonate ions in the HA lattice, the maintenance of the original wood microstructure, and the close control of the chemical features of the scaffold, i.e. the Ca/P ratio and the extent of crystal ordering of the HA phase. In particular, the last stage of reaction, transforming biomorphic calcium carbonate into a HA scaffold, was carried out by soaking biomorphic $CaCO_3$ into a phosphate-rich solution, in order to activate phenomena of dissolution and recrystallization of calcium phosphate. The characteristics of the phosphate solution, i.e. temperature and ionic strength, as well as the ratio between $CO_3$ (belonging to the solid biomorphic body) and $PO_4$ ions determine the kinetics of transformation and the characteristics of the final HA body, in terms of foreign ion content, crystal order and Ca/P ratio. As known, hydroxyapatite phase can exhibit a wide range of compositions, in terms of ionic substitutions in the sites of calcium and/or phosphate, and of the Ca/P ratio, also due to the possible existence of calcium vacancies in the HA lattice. The off-stoichiometry of HA phase due to reduced calcium content lower the solubility of HA, thus increasing its potential bioactivity; moreover the partial substitution with foreign ions that can be introduced in the last stage of the phosphatization reaction can make the final HA much closer to the natural bone tissue, thus potentially increasing its therapeutic efficiency. In particular, carbonate ions are introduced in the HA lattice, during reaction of the $CaCO_3$ template, that strongly increases its solubility and favour bio-resorption and osseointegration. Among the existing ligneous sources, rattan possesses a structure particularly suitable for bone scaffolding, i.e. a channel-like porosity very close to the Haversian structure with wide pores having diameter adequate for enhanced cell hosting and 3D colonization (Fig. 4.9), that may help to promote extensive vascularization also throughout large volumes. Moreover, the channel-like structure of rattan resulted in anisotropic mechanical properties with values in the range of the trabecular bone, which reflect the complex bone response to directional loading.

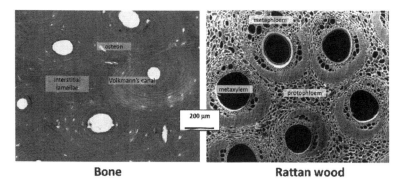

**Figure 4.9** Similarity between channel-like porosity in rattan wood and bone.

The new biomorphic HA scaffolds possess unique characteristics among ceramic biomaterials, and provide significant proof of concept of the potential fallout coming from transformation of natural sources into inorganic devices. In particular, biomorphic transformation enables to obtain consolidated 3D ceramics with complex structures not achievable by any other existing manufacturing processes. This paves the way to new-generation devices with potential of applications in several technological fields. Moreover, contrary to most of the conventional approaches for ceramic development, biomorphic transformation enable direct conversion of existing 3-D bodies into consolidated devices without any need of thermal sintering treatments; therefore, the microstructure of the final device can be designed and maintained at the nano-size, as the grain growth related to high temperature conventional sintering procedures can be prevented.

With respect to these issues, biologic properties shown by wood-derived HA were very promising: Preliminary in vitro investigation of cell adhesion and morphology, carried out by seeding MG63 osteoblast-like cells on rattan-derived HA (1 × $10^5$/ml), reported a nearly complete covering of the scaffold surface after only 7 days (Fig. 4.10) and a good morphology of the attached cells, well spread on the scaffold trabeculae. This confirms the close interaction of cells and healthy state of cells in contact with the surface of wood-derived HA, thus demonstrating the enhanced hydrophilicity of the scaffold.

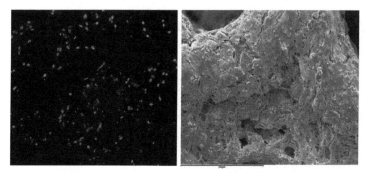

**Figure 4.10**  Covering of the surface of rattan-derived HA scaffold by osteoblast-like cells.

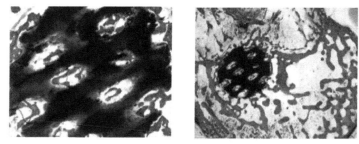

**Figure 4.11**  Bone formation and penetration at one month from implant in rabbit femur.

The high osteogenic and osteoconductive character of the biomorphic HA scaffolds was demonstrated by preliminary in vivo tests, carried out on skeletally mature adult New Zealand White disease-free rabbits. The scaffolds were implanted in critical defects created in the femoral distal epiphysis and evaluated after one-month follow-up. Extensive bone formation and penetration inside the scaffold channels was detected (Fig. 4.11). The newly formed bone tissue around and inside scaffolds had a regular architectural pattern surrounding the implants without connective capsules or gaps. To evaluate features such as bio-resorption ability, as well as the potential of new bone and vascular formation in the case of extended bone defects, longer follow up times are required. In this respect, as the biomorphic HA scaffolds were not consolidated by thermal treatments but upon direct transformation of a solid biomorphic $CaCO_3$, a nano-sized structure was obtained and maintained (Fig. 4.12) thus providing improved hydrophilicity and surface activity as well as enhanced solubility in vivo. Therefore, new-generation biomorphic scaffolds with enhanced surface activity are promising biomaterials for regeneration of extended long segmental bones.

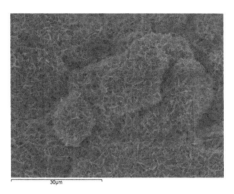

**Figure 4.12** Nano-sized structure of biomorphic HA scaffold.

## 4.4 Treatment of Osteoporosis-Related Fractures: New Biomimetic Injectable Devices

Several bone disorders, such as osteonecrosis or osteopenia related to metabolic diseases such as osteoporosis, require mini-invasive surgery due to the difficulty of intervention and scaffold placement in anatomical regions such as vertebral bodies and femur heads. To this, injectable scaffolds are considered as among the most promising approaches.

*Osteoporosis* is a term whose popularity has rapidly increased during the last decades referring to one of the most common metabolic bone disease. Osteoporosis has been defined as a *skeletal disorder characterized by compromised bone strength predisposing to an increased risk of fracture* [51]: A bone loss over time occurs and generally no symptoms anticipate the fractures. Epidemiological studies show that especially adults are affected by osteoporosis, the post-menopausal women in particular [52], but several interacting factors contribute to the risk of fractures, including clinical, behavioural, nutritional and genetic variables.

The normal bone turnover involves a balance between the processes of bone resorption and bone formation, in which osteoclasts resorb bone by acidification and proteolytic digestion and osteoblasts secrete osteoid, the organic matrix of bone, into the resorption cavity. Normally, except in growing bones, the rates of bone deposition and absorption are equal to each other, so that the total mass of bone remains constant.

The continual deposition and absorption of bone have important physiological functions: bone daily adjusts its strength and shape in accordance with stress patterns; furthermore, the production of new organic matrix is needed as the old organic matrix degenerates, because old bone becomes relatively brittle and weak.

Even if the detailed biochemical pathways underlying osteoporosis are not completely known, it has been widely observed that an imbalance in the activity of the osteoblasts and osteoclasts is involved.

The bones mainly weakened by osteoporosis are the wrist, the hip and the spine [53].

Osteoporotic vertebral bodies are characterized by a highly weakened trabecular bone structure, so that the force needed to cause a vertebral compression fracture is often surprisingly low (Fig. 4.13).

Vertebral fractures are typically localized in the thoraco-lumbar spine segment, between the dorsal kyphosis and the lumbar lordosis.

The fracture risk increases with age and generally an immediate stabilization is needed to avoid pain, disability and detrimental compressions of the spinal cord [54].

The treatment of vertebral compression fractures has, for many years until the advent of minimally invasive surgery, consisted of bed rest and analgesics.

Plaster jackets have sometimes been used for early mobilization of the patients, but proof of their effectiveness has not been demonstrated with much evidence in the literature.

Surgical treatment is normally not indicated, unless a neurological deficit is present or imminent.

Also several drugs have been commercially proposed, such as bisphosphonates, alendronates and strontium-containing molecules (e.g. strontium ranelate) because of evidence of strontium's ability to re-establish the correct balance between osteoblast and osteoclast activity [55, 56].

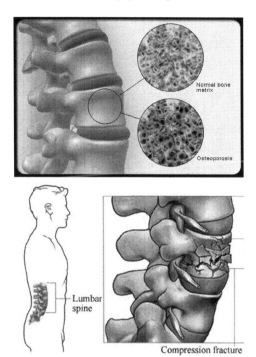

**Figure 4.13** Bone weakening and fracture upon metabolic diseases such as osteoporosis (http://www.medicinenet.com/osteoporosis_pictures_slideshow/article.htm; https://uvahealth.com/services/orthopedics/conditions/vertebral-compression-fracture).

However, the pharmacological approaches often result in deleterious systemic effects [57], even on bone mineralization, due to reduction in calcium absorption and possible alterations of the properties of the mineral bone [58].

For that reason in the past years, the interest of research in designing new clinical approaches for the stabilization of the damaged vertebral body has grown, especially due to the economic burden of the osteoporosis-related fractures.

Minimally invasive surgery techniques offer many benefits for the patient over traditional surgery, such us fewer associated injuries, quicker recovery time and less pain. Moreover, shorter hospital stays are needed, often allowing outpatient treatments that result in the reduction of health costs [59].

In the 1990s, a surgical procedure different from the previous, termed *vertebroplasty*, was introduced to medically treat vertebral compression fractures: This is a percutaneous technique during which a bone cement is injected in the vertebral body to provide immediate pain relief by stabilization.

Inflatable bone tamps can be used, prior to the injection of cement, to create a void in the vertebral body: In this case, the technique is known as *balloon vertebroplasty* or *kyphoplasty*.

The cement will follow the path of least resistance and the procedure is monitored directly under fluoroscopic control (Fig. 4.14).

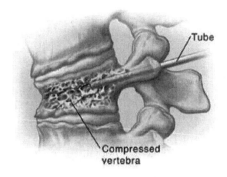
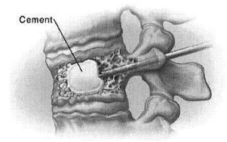

**Figure 4.14** Injection of bone cement into a compressed vertebra (http://www.fairview.org/healthlibrary/Article/40123).

Bone cements are pastes obtained by mixing a powder and a liquid, with ability to self-harden in a few minutes, to fill voids generated by fractures, to augment and stabilize the weakened vertebra, restoring it to its anatomical shape and biomechanical functionality.

The properties of an ideal bone cement are easy injectability, high radiopacity, a setting dough viscosity that does not change much between mixing and delivery into the vertebral body, an adequate resorption rate according to the bone metabolism, and mechanical properties comparable to those of an healthy vertebral body.

For that purpose, a wide range of bone cements have been designed and tested.

To date, vertebroplasty has been carried out almost exclusively with polymethylmethacrylate (PMMA)-based cement.

The use of acrylic bone cements leads to pain relief and a rapid strengthening of the damaged vertebral bodies, because of fast setting of the paste upon injection, and high mechanical performance after a few hours.

In spite of their widespread use, acrylic cements exhibit, however, several drawbacks, such as exothermic polymerization reaction, excessive stiffness, toxic monomer (MMA) release and lack of suitable porosity.

The increased number of indications for vertebroplasty, also in the treatment of traumatic fractures, has caused the mean patient age to decrease [60]: For a young and active population, the PMMA biocompatibility problems are unacceptable.

An ideal regenerative bone cement should exhibit a bone-like composition associated with an open and interconnected porosity permitting cell colonization and proliferation of new mature bone inside the injected cement mass.

In the 1980s, Brown and Chow [60, 61] and LeGeros [62] discovered calcium phosphate cements (CPCs), promising candidates for injectable materials for bone.

The first commercial CPC products were introduced in the 1990s for the treatment of maxillo-facial defects [63, 64] as well as for the treatment of fractures [65]. Since then, new cement formulations have been developed that fulfil specific requirements for other applications, such as bone augmentation [66, 67], reinforcement of osteoporotic bones [68], fixation of metallic implants in weakened bone [69] and spinal fractures and vertebroplasty [70].

The CPCs do not show the typical drawbacks related to the use of acrylic cements; their main advantages arise from the excellent biocompatibility and in vivo osteoconductivity, the ability to harden in vivo through a low-temperature setting reaction, as well as the possibility of loading them with drugs, proteins or growth factors.

However, major critical issues of CPCs still limiting their use are the long setting times at physiological conditions and the low mechanical strength [71].

CPCs are hydraulic cements. In general, all CPCs are formed by a combination of one or more calcium orthophosphate powders, which upon mixing with a liquid phase, usually water or an aqueous solution, form a paste that is able to set and harden after being injected as a result of a dissolution-precipitation process (Fig. 4.15).

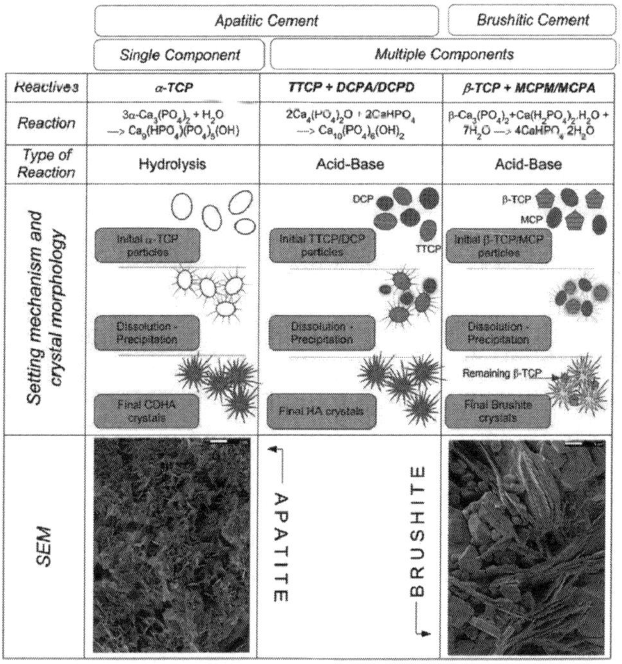

**Figure 4.15** Reactions yielding formation and setting of CPCs [72].

The entanglement of the precipitated crystals is responsible for cement hardening. Despite the large number of possible formulations, the CPCs developed up to now have only two different end products, precipitated hydroxyapatite (HA) or brushite (DCPD).

This, in fact, is a predictable situation since hydroxyapatite is the most stable calcium phosphate at pH > 4.2 and brushite the most stable one at pH < 4.2.

Different approaches can be used for the synthesis of CPCs:

- Monocomponent CPCs, in which a single calcium phosphate compound, alpha tricalcium phosphate ($\alpha$-TCP) hydrolyses to CDHA without varying the Ca/P ratio, according to the equation:

$$3\alpha\text{-Ca}_3(PO_4)_2 + H_2O \rightarrow Ca_9(HPO_4)(PO_4)_5OH$$

- Multicomponent CPCs, in which two or more calcium phosphates, some more acidic and the other basic, set following an acid–base reaction.

When set, CPCs consist of a network of calcium phosphate crystals, with a chemical composition and crystal size that can be tailored to closely resemble the biological hydroxyapatite occurring in living bone.

The setting reaction that gives rise to the solid consists in three stages: dissolution of the reactants, nucleation of the new phase (either apatite or brushite) and crystal growth.

During dissolution, the raw powders release calcium and phosphate ions, generating a supersaturation in the solution. Once the ionic concentration reaches a critical value, the nucleation of the new phase occurs, generally surrounding the powder particles.

A similar setting reaction in CPCs is not exothermic, and therefore allows the incorporation of different drugs and biological molecules, making them good candidates for drug delivery applications [73].

Not only the total interconnected porosity is relevant for the loading and delivery of drugs, but also the pore dimensions and pore size distribution within the cement, as well as its specific surface area (SSA). These parameters vary with the processing conditions of the cements, such as the liquid-to-powder (L/P) ratio and the particle size of the starting powder, as shown in Fig. 4.16.

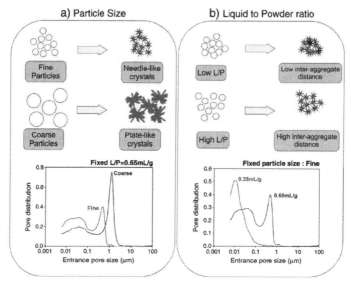

**Figure 4.16** Formation of CPCs nanoparticles under different conditions [72].

Among the various approaches reported so far for the synthesis of CPCs, the one based on the hydrolysis and transformation of $\alpha$-Ca$_3$(PO$_4$)$_2$ ($\alpha$TCP) into elongated calcium-deficient hydroxyapatite (CD-HA) particles is particularly interesting and promising [74].

The main source of interest in this approach is that the process is isothermal and not subjected to pH variations that can penalize cell survival. Moreover CD-HA, the end-product of the hardened cement, is characterized by increased bioactivity and bio-resorbability compared with stoichiometric HA [75] and can be endowed with specific biological functions related to new bone formation and organization by tailored ion substitution (e.g. with Mg$^{2+}$, CO$_3^{2-}$, SiO$_4^{4-}$, Sr$^{2+}$) [76].

In particular, strontium is attracting a big interest due to its claimed ability, as previously cited, of re-establishing the correct balance between osteoblast and osteoclast activity, altered by metabolic diseases such as osteoporosis.

With respect to injectable bone cements, recent papers described the development of Sr-containing CPCs based on commercial $\alpha$-TCP and soluble salts containing strontium (e.g.

$SrCO_3$, $SrHPO_4$) [77–79], one of which [78] has been also tested in ovariectomized rats [80].

The use of multiple inorganic components in CPCs can make difficult the optimization of rheological properties related to flowability, injectability, cohesion that in turn influence setting time, porosity and mechanical performances. This is one of the main concerns penalizing the development of CPCs for clinical use.

One of the most important properties of CPCs is bioactivity. Bioactivity, together with the perfect adaptability of the cement paste during implantation, leads to a stable connection between defect and implant, speeding up bone healing process. Once implanted, CPCs can be resorbed by two different mechanisms: active resorption regulated by living cells like macrophages or osteoclasts, and/or passive resorption via chemical dissolution or hydrolysis in the body fluids.

A local administration of strontium in osteoporotic bone can be achieved by the resorption of an apatitic Sr-substituted bone cement: In this case, the strontium ions are introduced in the crystal lattice of $\alpha$TCP during synthesis, carried out by solid-state reaction between monetite, calcium carbonate and strontium carbonate [81].

The introduction of strontium ions in the crystal lattice can be demonstrated by crossing mainly two analysis: the chemical analysis of the synthesized powder (ICP-OES), to compare the molar amount of strontium before and after the synthesis, and the x-ray diffraction analysis (XRD). The latter, because of different ionic dimensions of strontium and calcium (ionic radii: $Sr^{2+}$ = 1.13 Å, $Ca^{2+}$ = 1.00 Å), can give information about the volumetric increase of the $\alpha$TCP lattice, reflecting in shifted diffraction patterns to lower diffraction angles and broadening of the peaks with increased Sr contents, and about the absence of other Sr-containing secondary phases [81].

The composition of the setting solution should be designed with the purpose of improving the cement osteoconductivity, e.g. by the addition of a small amount of bio-soluble polymers, such as sodium alginate. The presence of sodium alginate enhance the injectability and cohesion of the paste, providing at the same time a soluble structure that can in vivo dissolve and promote cell adhesion and proliferation.

Ideally, when CPC is resorbed, it is progressively replaced by new bone in vivo. The replacement arises with the resorption of the cement surface in compliance with the kinetic of bone growth, thus avoiding gaps between implant and tissue, and guiding bone formation.

Due the unique features of such novel bioactive ion-doped CPC, new regenerative therapies based on regenerative injectable bone cements may be established in the near future, with improved recovery of the quality of life of patients and with reduced risks related to systemic administration of strontium-based drugs.

## 4.5 Conclusions and Future Perspectives

Today, the development of regenerative biomaterials strongly targets on the attainment of a close mimicry of natural tissues, to activate an active cross-talk with cells and stimulate the regenerative process. A bone-like chemical composition and complex, hierarchically organized microstructure that provide cell-conducive porosity and enhanced mechanical performances are key features that can enable the regeneration of extensive, load-bearing bone parts. However, the intrinsic features of the bioactive materials employed for bone scaffolding often make difficult the simultaneous fulfilment of all these requirements and this is one of the main reasons why clinical needs related to long and load-bearing bone healing are still unmet.

In this respect, the establishment of roadmaps for the development of new materials and processes enabling the convergence of all the features required for long bone regeneration will be a primary activity for materials scientists in the incoming years. In particular, the inspiration from nature is now increasingly considered as one of the most promising criteria to follow. In fact, new emerging concepts of fabrication, based on transformation of native structures into biomorphic devices, can overcome the limitations of conventional manufacturing that, particularly in the case of ceramic, bone-like materials, is not able to provide highly organized structures with details defined at the micron size. In this respect, due to the innumerable examples of natural structures exhibiting smart properties that are not achievable by conventional fabrication approaches, there are virtually no limits to the potential applications of biomorphic materials in various high-impact fields other than the biomedical one.

## Acknowledgments

The authors would like to acknowledge the PNR-CNR Aging Program 2012–2014 for the funding of the research presented in this work.

## References

1. Wolff J., Maquet P., Furlong R. (1986), *The Law of Bone Remodelling* (Springer-Verlag).

2. Ingber D. E. (1993), Cellular tensegrity: Defining new rules of biological design that govern the cytoskeleton. *J. Cell. Sci.,* **104**, pp. 613–627.

3. Ingber D. E. (2008), Tensegrity and mechanotransduction, *J. Bodywork Mov. Ther.*, **12**(3), pp. 198–200.

4. Wang N., Butler J. P., Ingber D. E. (1993), Mechanotransduction across the cell surface and through the cytoskeleton. *Science*, **260**(5111), pp. 1124–1127.

5. Chen C. S., Ingber D. E. (1999), Tensegrity and mechanoregulation: From skeleton to cytoskeleton. *Osteoarthr. Cartilage,* **7**, pp. 81–94.

6. Ingber D. E. (1998), The architecture of life. *Sci. Am.,* **278**(1), pp. 48–57.

7. Li J., Han D., Zhao Y.-P. (2014), Kinetic behaviour of the cells touching substrate: The interfacial stiffness guides cell spreading. *Sci. Rep.,* **4**, 3910.

8. Cameron A. R., Frith J. E., Cooper-White J. J. (2011), The influence of substrate creep on mesenchymal stem cell behaviour and phenotype. *Biomaterials*, **32**(26), pp. 5979–5993.

9. Wells R. G. (2008), The role of matrix stiffness in regulating cell behavior. *Hepatology,* **47**, pp. 1394–1400.

10. Pavalko F. M., Norvell S. M., Burr D. B., Turner C. H., Duncan R. L., Bidwell J. P. (2003), A model for mechanotransduction in bone cells: the load-bearing mechanosomes. *J. Cell. Biochem.,* **88**, pp. 104–112.

11. Sikavitsas V. I. (2001), Biomaterials and bone mechanotransduction. *Biomaterials,* **22**, pp. 2581–2593.

12. Bilezikian J. P., Raisz L. G., Rodan G. A. (2002), *Principles of Bone Biology*, 3rd ed., vol. 1 (Academic Press, San Diego) 1.

13. Sprio S., Sandri M., Iafisco M., Panseri S., Filardo G., Kon E., Marcacci M., Tampieri A. (2014), Composite biomedical foams for engineering bone tissue, *Biomedical Foams for Tissue Engineering Applications*, Woodhead Publishing Limited, Cambridge (UK), pp. 249–280.

14. Filardo G., Kon E., Tampieri A., Cabezas-Rodríguez R., Di Martino A., Fini M., Giavaresi G., Lelli M., Martínez-Fernández J., Martini L., Ramírez-Rico J., Salamanna F., Sandri M., Sprio S., Marcacci M. (2014), New bio-ceramization process applied to vegetable hierarchical structures for bone regeneration: An experimental model in sheep. *Tissue Eng. Part A,* **20**(3–4), pp. 763–773.

15. Goldstrohm G. L., Mears D. C., Swartz W. M. (1984), The results of 39 fractures complicated by major segmental bone loss and/or leg length discrepancy. *J. Trauma,* **24**(1), pp. 50–58.

16. Paderni S., Terzi S., Amendola L. (2009), Major bone defect treatment with an osteoconductive bone substitute. *Chir Organi Mov.,* **93**(2), pp. 89–96.

17. Stevenson S. (1987), The immune response to osteochondral allografts in dogs. *J. Bone Joint Surg. Am.,* **69**(4), pp. 573–582.

18. Lord C. F., Gebhardt M. C., Tomford W. W., Mankin H. J. (1988), Infection in bone allografts. Incidence, nature, and treatment. *J. Bone Joint Surg. Am.,* **70**(3), pp. 369–376.

19. Mankin H. J., Gebhardt M. C., Tomford W. W. (1987), The use of frozen cadaveric allografts in the management of patients with bone tumors of the extremities. *Orthop. Clin. North Am.,* **18**(2), pp. 275–289.

20. Alman B. A., De Bari A., Krajbich J. I. (1995), Massive allografts in the treatment of osteosarcoma and Ewing sarcoma in children and adolescents. *J. Bone Joint Surg. Am.,* **77**(1), pp. 54–64.

21. Berrey B. H. Jr, Lord C. F., Gebhardt M. C., Mankin H. J. (1990), Fractures of allografts. Frequency, treatment, and end-results. *J. Bone Joint Surg. Am.,* **72**(6), pp. 825–833.

22. Giannoudis P. V., Atkins R. (2007), Management of long-bone non-unions. *Injury,* **38**(Suppl 2), pp. S1–S2.

23. Kanakaris N. K., Giannoudis P. V. (2007), The health economics of the treatment of long-bone non-unions. *Injury,* **38**(Suppl 2), p. S77.

24. Calori G. M., Albisetti W., Agus A., Iori S., Tagliabue L. 2007. Risk factors contributing to fracture nonunions. *Injury Int J Care Injured,* **38S**: pp. S11–S18.

25. Motsitsi N. S. (2008), Management of infected nonunion of long bones: The last decade (1996–2006), *Injury,* **39**, pp. 155–160.

26. Longo U. G., Trovato U., Loppini M., Rizzello G., Khan W. S., Maffulli N., Denaro V. (2012), Tissue engineered strategies for pseudoarthrosis. *Open Orthop. J.*, **6**, pp. 564–570.

27. LeGeros R. Z., LeGeros J. P. (1984), Phosphate minerals in human tissues, eds. Nriagu J. O., Moore P. B. (*Phosphate Minerals.* Springer-Verlag, New York).

28. LeGeros R. Z. (1991), Calcium phosphates in oral biology and medicine. *Monogr. Oral Sci.*, **15**, pp. 1–201.

29. Kandori K., Fudo A., Ishikawa T. (2002), Study on the particle texture dependence of proteinadsorption by using synthetic micrometer-sized calcium hydroxyapatite particles. *Colloids Surf.*, **24**, pp. 145–153,

30. Capriotti L. A., Beebe T. P. Jr., Schneider J. P. (2007), Hydroxyapatite surface-induced peptide folding. *J. Am. Chem. Soc.*, **129**, pp. 5281–5287.

31. Corno M., Rimola A., Bolis V., Ugliengo P. (2010), Hydroxyapatite as a key biomaterial: Quantum-mechanical simulation of its surfaces in interaction with biomolecules. *Phys. Chem. Chem. Phys.*, **12**, pp. 6309–6329.

32. Webster T., Siegel R., Bizios R. (1999), Osteoblast adhesion on nanophase ceramics. *Biomaterials*, **20**, pp. 1221–1227.

33. Webster T., Ergun C., Doremus R., Siegel R., Bizios R. (2000), Enhanced functions of osteoblasts on nanophase ceramics. *Biomaterials*, **21**, pp. 1803–1810.

34. Webster T., Ergun C., Doremus R., Siegel R., Bizios R. (2001), Enhanced osteoclast-like cell functions on nanophase ceramics. *Biomaterials*, **22**, pp. 1327–1333.

35. Landi E., Tampieri A., Celotti G., Langenati R., Sandri M., Sprio S. (2005), Nucleation of biomimetic apatite in synthetic body fluids: Dense and porous scaffold development. *Biomaterials*, **26**(16), pp. 2835–2845.

36. Sprio S., Tampieri A., Landi E., Sandri M., Martorana S., Celotti G., Logroscino G. (2008), Physico-chemical properties and solubility behaviour of multi-substituted hydroxyapatite powders containing silicon. *Mater. Sci. Eng. C*, **28**, pp. 179–187.

37. Daculsi G. (1998), Biphasic calcium phosphate concept applied to artificial bone, implant coating and injectable bone substitute. *Biomaterials*, **19**, pp. 1473–1478.

38. Kessler S., Mayr-Wohlfart U., Ignatius A., Puhl W., Claes L., Günther K. P. (2003), Der Einfluss von bone morphogenetic protein-2

(BMP-2), vascular endothelial growth factor (VEGF) und basischem fibroblastenwachstumsfaktor (b-FGF) auf osteointegration, degradation und biomechanische eigenschaften eines synthetischen knochenersatzstoffes. *Z. Orthop.*, **141**, pp. 472–480.

39. Conor T. B., O'Kelly K. U. (2010), Fabrication and characterization of a porous multidomain hydroxyapatite scaffold for bone tissue engineering investigations, *J. Biomed. Mater. Res. Part B: Appl. Biomater.*, **93B**, pp. 459–467.

40. Babis G. C., Soucacos P. N. (2005), Bone scaffolds: The role of mechanical stability and instrumentation. *Int. J. Care Injured*, **36S**, pp. S38–S44.

41. Sprio S., Ruffini A., Valentini F., D'Alessandro T., Sandri M., Panseri S., Tampieri A. (2011), Biomimesis and biomorphic transformations: New concepts applied to bone regeneration. *J. Biotechnol.*, **156**(4), pp. 347–355.

42. Quarto R., Mastrogiacomo M., Cancedda R., Kutepov S. M., Mukhachev V., Lavroukov A., Kon E., Marcacci M. (2001), Repair of large bone defects with the use of autologous bone marrow stromal cells. *N. Engl. J. Med.*, **344**(5), pp. 385–386.

43. Fratzl P., Weinkamer R. (2007), Nature's hierarchical materials. *Prog. Mater. Sci.*, **52**, pp. 1263–1334.

44. Wegst U. G. K., Ashby M. F. (2004), The mechanical efficiency of natural materials. *Philos. Mag.*, **84**, pp. 2167–2181.

45. Gibson E. J. (1992), Wood: A natural fibre reinforced composite. *Met. Mater.*, **6**, pp. 333–336.

46. Lucas P. W., Darvell B. W., Lee P. K. D., Yuen T. D. B., Choong M. F. (1995), The toughness of plant cell walls. *Philos. Trans. Roy. Soc.*, **B 348**, pp. 363–372.

47. Greil P., Lifka T., Kaindl A. (1998), Biomorphic cellular silicon carbide ceramics from wood: I. processing and microstructure. *J. Eur. Ceram. Soc.*, **18**, pp. 1961–1973.

48. Greil P., Lifka T., Kaindl A. (1998), Biomorphic cellular silicon carbide ceramics from wood: II. Mechanical properties. *J. Eur. Ceram. Soc.*, **18**, pp. 1975–1983.

49. Parfen'eva L. S., Orlova T. S., Kartenko N. F., Sharenkova N. V., Smirnov B. I., Smirnov I. A., Misiorek H., Jezowski A., Varela-Feria F. M., Martinez-Fernandez J. De Arellano-Lopez A. R. (2005), *Phys. Solid State*, **47**(7), pp. 1216–1220.

50. Tampieri A., Sprio S., Ruffini A., Celotti G., Lesci I. G., Roveri N. (2009), From Wood to Bone: Multi-step process to convert wood hierarchical structures into biomimetic hydroxyapatite scaffolds for bone tissue engineering. *J. Mater. Chem.*, **19**(28), pp. 4973–4980.

51. Osteoporosis Prevention, Diagnosis, and Therapy (2000), NIH Consens Statement Online March 27–29, **17**(1), 1–36.

52. Stetzer E. (2011), Identifying risk factors for osteoporosis in young women. *Internet J. Allied Health Sci. Pract.*, **9**(4).

53. Siris et al. (2014), The clinical diagnosis of osteoporosis: A position statement from the National Bone Health Alliance Working Group. *Osteoporos. Int.*, **25**, pp. 1439–1443.

54. Wilcox R. K., Boerger T. O., Allen D. J., Barton D. C., Limb D., Dickson R. A., Hall R. M. (2003), A dynamic study of thoracolumbar burst fractures. *J. Bone Joint Surg. Am.*, **85-A**(11), pp. 2184–2189.

55. Dahl S. G., Allain P., Marie P. J., Mauras Y., Boivin G., Ammann P., Tsouderos Y., Delmas P. D., Christiansen C. (2001), Incorporation and distribution of strontium in bone. *Bone,* **28**, 446–453.

56. Marie P. J., Ammann P., Boivin G., Rey C. (2001), Mechanisms of action and therapeutic potential of strontium in bone. *Calcif. Tissue Int.*, **69**, pp. 121–129.

57. Kennel K. A., Drake M. T. (2009), Adverse effects of bisphosphonates: Implications for osteoporosis management, *Mayo Clin. Proc.*, **84**(7), pp. 632–638.

58. Grynpas M. D., Hamilton E., Cheung R., Tsouderos Y., Deloffre P., Hott M., Marie P. J. (1996), Strontium increases vertebral bone volume in rats at a low dose that does not induce detectable mineralization defect. *Bone,* **18**, pp. 253–259.

59. Park et al. (2007), Minimally invasive surgery: The evolution of fellowship. *Surgery*, **142**, pp. 505–511, discussion 511–513.

60. Verlaan J. J., Diekerhof C. H., Buskens E., van der Tweel I., Verbout A. J., Dhert W. J., Oner F. C. (2004), Surgical treatment of traumatic fractures of the thoracic and lumbar spine: A systematic review of the literature on techniques, complications, and outcome. *Spine (Phila Pa 1976)*, **29**(7), pp. 803–814.

61. Brown W. E., Chow L. C. (1983), A new calcium phosphate setting cement. *J. Dent. Res.*, **62,** p. 672.

62. LeGeros R. Z., Chohayeb A., Shulman A. (1982), Apatitic calcium phosphates: Possible dental restorative materials. *J. Dent. Res.*, **61,** p. 343.

63. Friedman C. D., Costantino P. D., Takagi S., Chow L. C. (1998), Bone Source hydroxyapatite cement: A novel biomaterial for craniofacial skeletal tissue engineering and reconstruction. *J. Biomed. Mater. Res.*, **43**, pp. 428–432.

64. Kamerer D. B., Hirsch B. E., Snyderman C. H., Costantino P., Friedman C. D. (1994), Hydroxyapatite cement: A new method for achieving watertight closure in transtemporal surgery. *Am. J. Otol.*, **15**, pp. 47–49.

65. Constantz B. R., Ison I. C., Fulmer M. T., Poser R. D., Smith S. T., VanWagoner M. (1995), Skeletal repair by in situ formation of the mineral phase of bone, *Science*, **267**, pp. 1796–1799.

66. Horstmann W. G., Verheyen C. C. P. M., Leemans R. (2003), An injectable calciumphosphate cement as a bone-graft substitute in the treatment of displaced lateral tibial plateau fractures. *Injury*, **34**, pp. 141–144.

67. Welch R. D., Zhang H., Bronson D. G. (2003), Experimental tibial plateau fractures augmented with calcium phosphate cement or autologous bone graft. *J. Bone Joint Surg.*, **85**, p. 222.

68. Maestretti G., Cremer C., Otten P., Jakob R. P. (2007), Prospective study of standalone balloon kyphoplasty with calcium phosphate cement augmentation in traumatic fractures. *Eur. Spine J.*, **16**, pp. 601–610.

69. Mermelstein L. E., Chow L. C., Friedman C. D., Crisco J. J. (1996), The reinforcement of cancellous bone screws with calcium phosphate cement. *J. Orthop. Trauma*, **10**, pp. 15–20.

70. Takemasa R., Kiyasu K., Tani T., Inoue S. (2007), Validity of calcium phosphate cement vertebroplasty for vertebral non-union after osteoporotic fracture with middle column involvement, *Spine J.*, **7**, p. 148S.

71. Khairoun I., Boltong M., Driessens F. C. M., Planell J. (1998), Some factors controlling the injectability of calcium phosphate bone cements. *J. Mater. Sci. Mater. Med.*, **9**, pp. 425–428.

72. Ginebra M. P., Canal C., Espanol M., Pastorino D., Montufar E. B. (2012), Calcium phosphate cements as drug delivery materials. *Adv. Drug Deliv. Rev.*, **64**, pp. 1090–1110.

73. Ginebra M. P., Traykova T., Planell J. A. (2006), Calcium phosphate cements: Competitive drug carriers for the musculoskeletal system? *Biomaterials*, **27**, pp. 2171–2177.

74. Bohner M. (2000), Calcium orthophosphates in medicine: From ceramics to calcium phosphate cements. *Injury-Int. J. Care Injured*, **31** Suppl 4, pp. 37–47.

75. Mavropoulos E., Rossi A. M., da Rocha N. C. C., Soares G. A., Moreira J. C., Moure G. T. (2003), Dissolution of calcium-deficient hydroxyapatite synthesized at different conditions. *Mater. Characterization,* **50**, pp. 203–207.

76. Landi E., Logroscino G., Proietti L., Tampieri A., Sandri M., Sprio S. (2008), Biomimetic Mg-substituted hydroxyapatite: From synthesis to in vivo behaviour. *J. Mater. Sci. Mater. Med.,* **19**, pp. 239–247.

77. Alkhraisat M. H., Moseke C., Blanco L., Barralet J. E., Lopez-Carbacos E., Gbureck U. (2008), Strontium modified biocements with zero order release kinetics. *Biomaterials,* **29**, pp. 4691–4697.

78. Baier M., Staudt P., Klein R., Sommer U., Wenz R., Grafe I., Meeder P. J., Nawroth P. P., Kasperk C. (2013), Strontium enhances osseointegration of calcium phosphate cement: A histomorphometric pilot study in ovariectomized rats. *J. Orthopaedic Surg. Res.,* **8**, p. 16.

79. Schumacher M., Henss A., Rohnke M., Gelinsky M. (2013), A novel and easy-to-prepare strontium(II) modified calcium phosphate bone cement with enhanced mechanical properties. *Acta Biomater.,* **9**, pp. 7536–7544.

80. Thormann U., Ray S., Sommer U., ElKhassawna T., Rehling T., Hundgeburth M., Henss A., Rohnke M., Janek J., Lips K. S., Heiss C., Schlewitz G., Szalay G., Schumacher M., Gelinsky M., Schnettler R., Alt V. (2013), Bone formation induced by strontium modified calcium phosphate cement in critical-size metaphyseal fracture defects in ovariectomized rats. *Biomaterials,* **34**, pp. 8589–8598.

81. Saint-Jean S. J., Camire C. L., Nevsten P., Hansen S., Ginebra M. P. (2005), Study of the reactivity and in vitro bioactivity of Sr-substituted alpha-TCP cements. *J. Mater. Sci. Mater. Med.,* **16**, 993–1001.

## Chapter 5

# New Bio-Inspired Processes for Synthesis and Surface Treatments of Biomaterials

**Frank A. Müller**

*Otto-Schott-Institute of Materials Research (OSIM),*
*Friedrich-Schiller-University of Jena,*
*Löbdergraben 32, 07743 Jena, Germany*

frank.mueller@uni-jena.de

## 5.1  Introduction

After implantation, biomaterials interact through their surfaces with the living organism. Therefore, the outer surface of a biomaterial plays a key role in controlling interactions between the biological system and an artificial material [1]. The physical and chemical states of a material for instance influence the fixation of an implant in the surrounding bone tissue [2, 3]. Properties like the composition of the surface and its topography or roughness are of particular relevance for the amount and kind of proteins that adsorb to the materials surface. They also affect the wetting behavior of physiologic fluids that in turn influence cell controlled mechanisms like adhesion, proliferation and differentiation as well as the formation of extracellular matrix [4–8].

---

*Bio-Inspired Regenerative Medicine: Materials, Processes, and Clinical Applications*
Edited by Simone Sprio and Anna Tampieri
Copyright © 2016 Pan Stanford Publishing Pte. Ltd.
ISBN 978-981-4669-14-6 (Hardcover), 978-981-4669-15-3 (eBook)
www.panstanford.com

Load-bearing implants (e.g., endoprosthesis, dental implants, orthopedic fixation devices), which are in direct contact to bone, should ideally bond to their bony surrounding without the formation of a fibrous tissue interface. However, this is often observed for various bioinert materials (e.g., titanium alloys). Calcium phosphates, in particular hydroxyl apatite (HA, $Ca_{10}(PO_4)_6(OH)_2$), could fulfill this requirement due to its close resemblance to the inorganic part of bone tissue. However, due to its weak mechanical properties HA cannot be considered for load-bearing applications. For this reason, several physico-chemical [9], morphological [10], and bioorganic [11] modifications of metallic implant surfaces have been investigated to provide materials with osteoconductive and osteoinductive behavior, respectively. The commercially most widespread method to realize this is plasma spraying of HA. However, these coatings show some disadvantages compromising their long-term stability [12–14]. The problems are mainly related to delamination, an insufficient adhesion of the coating and in controlling the composition of calcium phosphates at process temperatures exceeding 10,000°C. Moreover, the method cannot be used to coat porous materials due to its line-of-sight characteristic.

It is generally accepted that the in vitro apatite formation from simulated body fluid (SBF), which resembles the inorganic part of human blood plasma, represents an indicator for the in vivo bioactivity of a material [15]. Beyond that, the utilization of SBF allows to coat materials surfaces with a biomimetic apatite whose structure and composition is close to biological apatite.

## 5.2 Biomimetic Apatite

**Definition:** *Biomimetic apatite, precipitated under physiological conditions from a simulated body fluid (SBF), mimics the chemical, physical and structural properties of biological bone apatite. After an implantation into a bony defect it adopts the metabolic function of bone and allows the substantial integration of the implant.*

The bone tissue of vertebrates represents a composite material grown by a biomineralization process. It consists of 65 mass-% carbonated hydroxy apatite (CHA), 25 mass-% proteins (mainly collagen I) and water [16]. The main function of bone is related to the structural and mechanical support of the skeletal apparatus.

Beyond that, bone constitutes a storage and hauling mechanism for the two essential elements phosphorus and calcium. Due to the solubility of bone apatite under physiological conditions, bone is able to regenerate in case of fracture and to respond to mechanical load by bone formation and resorption, respectively. Bone apatite contains carbonate ions (3–9 mass-%) substituting the phosphate ions (B-type CHA) as well as the hydroxy ions (A-type CHA) of the HA crystal [17]. Figure 5.1 illustrates ionic substitutions of biological or biomimetic apatite with a composition of $Ca_{10-x-y}Mg_y(HPO_4)_{x-z}(CO_3)_z(PO_4)_{6-x}(OH)_{2-x-w}(CO_3)_{w/2}$ ($0 \leq x, y \leq 1$; $z, w \leq x$) compared to stoichiometric HA. CHA crystals are plate-shaped with dimensions in the range of 25 to 50 nm and a thickness of 2 to 5 nm [16]. The dimensions on the nanoscale, the low crystallinity, and the non-stoichiometric composition are important features for the solubility and resorption capacity of biological apatite, which significantly exceed that of stoichiometric synthetic apatite and consequently facilitates the dynamic remodeling of bone tissue [18, 19]. The [001]-direction (c-axis) represents the preferred growth orientation of CHA crystals. This direction is oriented parallel to the longitudinal axis of the collagen fibrils [20–22]. This hierarchical feature is an important characteristic for the biomineralization of calcium phosphates [23].

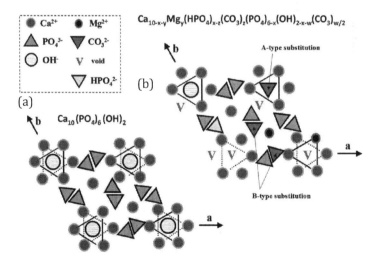

**Figure 5.1** Projection of the (001) plane of (a) stoichiometric hydroxyapatite and (b) ionic substitutions in bone apatite or biomimetic apatite.

Stoichiometric HA, which can be synthesized by wet-chemical precipitation or by solid-state reactions at elevated temperatures [23], represents the most stable calcium orthophosphate with the lowest solubility at pH > 4.2 [24]. Therefore, HA only inadequately supports the dynamic remodeling processes of bone after an implantation. On the other hand, biomimetic apatite, which precipitated under physiological conditions and which mimics the structural and chemical properties of bone apatite represents an interesting alternative due to its capacity to be actively integrated into the physiological bone remodeling processes.

## 5.3 Literature Survey

In the year 1971, Hench et al. developed a glass in the system $SiO_2$-$CaO$-$P_2O_5$-$Na_2O$ that was the first synthetic material allowing a direct bond to living tissue [25]. Over the years, further glass and ceramic compositions capable of firmly bonding to bone in vivo were developed [26–29]. These materials are classified as bioactive ceramics [30]. One common characteristic of these materials is related to the time-dependent surface modification after implantation [31]. A biologically active carbonated hydroxyl apatite layer (CHA) forms on the surface. Due to its close chemical and structural relationship to the inorganic part of bone this layer is able to bond directly to the surrounding tissue [32]. The following definition of bioactive materials was given by Hench [32]:

*"A layer of biologically active CHA must form for a bond with tissues to occur. This is the common characteristic of all the known bioactive implant materials."*

In the year 1991, Kokubo extended this definition [15]. A further requirement for a bioactive material is, that the in vivo apatite formation can be reproduced in a SBF with a composition similar to the inorganic part of human blood plasma. Hence, an indicator for the bioactivity of a material is the capacity to form apatite on its surface in SBF.

The development of recent SBF solutions goes back to the composition of *Earle's Balanced Salt Solution* (EBSS) [33] and *Hank's Balanced Salt Solution* (HBSS) [34], which origin in a physiological salt solution that Ringer developed in the year 1883 [35]. Table 5.1 summarizes the ionic composition of blood plasma and synthetic physiological solutions. SBF, that was first mentioned by Kokubo in the year 1990 [36] can be considered as a TRIS (tris-hydroxymethyl-aminomethane)-HCl buffered variation of HBSS with a molar Ca/P ratio of 2.5 instead of 1.62. Both show a very low $HCO_3^-$ concentration of 4.2 mmol/l, which significantly deviates from the $HCO_3^-$ content in human blood plasma (27 mmol/l). The reason for this deviation results from an increasing instability of SBF with increasing $HCO_3^-$ content [37], which on the other hand depends on the recipe of preparation and the utilized salts [38]. In 1999, Bayraktar and Tas were the first to obtain a physiological $HCO_3^-$ concentration of 27 mmol/l in TRIS-HCl buffered SBF [39]. Bigi et al. were the first to prepare physiological SBF by using a HEPES (2-(4-(2-hydroxyethyl)-1-piperazinyl)ethane sulfonic acid)-NaOH buffer [40]. However, it was shown that HEPES buffered systems become unstable during storage. They release $CO_2$, which decreases the carbonate concentration and increases the value of pH [41].

**Table 5.1** Ionic concentration of human blood plasma and of synthetic physiological solutions (mmol/l)

|  | Blood plasma | Ringer | EBSS | HBSS | Kokubo c-SBF | Tas SBF | Bigi SBF | Kokubo r-SBF |
|---|---|---|---|---|---|---|---|---|
| $Na^+$ | 142.0 | 130.0 | 143.5 | 142.1 | 142.0 | 142.0 | 141.5 | 142.0 |
| $K^+$ | 3.6–5.5 | 4.0 | 5.37 | 5.33 | 5.0 | 5.0 | 5.0 | 5.0 |
| $Ca^{2+}$ | 2.1–2.6 | 1.4 | 1.8 | 1.26 | 2.5 | 2.5 | 2.5 | 2.5 |
| $Mg^{2+}$ | 1.5 |  | 0.8 | 0.9 | 1.5 | 1.5 | 1.5 | 1.5 |
| $Cl^-$ | 95–107 | 109.0 | 123.5 | 146.8 | 147.8 | 125.0 | 124.5 | 103.0 |
| $HCO_3^-$ | 27.0 |  | 26.2 | 4.2 | 4.2 | 27.0 | 27.0 | 27.0 |
| $HPO_4^{2-}$ | 0.6–1.5 |  | 1.0 | 0.78 | 1.0 | 1.0 | 1.0 | 1.0 |
| $SO_4^{2-}$ | 0.5 |  | 0.8 | 0.41 | 0.5 | 0.5 | 0.5 | 0.5 |
| Ca/P | 2.5 |  | 1.8 | 1.62 | 2.5 | 2.5 | 2.5 | 2.5 |
| Buffer |  |  |  |  | TRIS | TRIS | HEPES | HEPES |
| pH | 7.4 | 6.5 | 7.2–7.6 | 6.7–6.9 | 7.2–7.4 | 7.4 | 7.4 | 7.4 |

The biomimetic coating of bioinert material surfaces by exposure to SBF was first described by Tanahashi et al. in the year 1994 [42]. To initiate the nucleation of apatite, various organic substrates in direct contact to bioactive glass particles of the system $CaO\text{-}SiO_2\text{-}MgO\text{-}P_2O_5\text{-}CaF_2$ were exposed to SBF. In a second step, the thus treated substrates were exposed to 1.5 SBF with ionic concentrations 50% above the physiological ones to accelerate crystal growth. After 24 h a homogeneous apatite layer precipitated on the substrates. It was shown that thus coated polyether sulfone (PESF) substrates substantially bonded to the surrounding bone tissue after implantation into the tibia of rats [43]. In 1999, this system was refined by Miyaji et al. [44]. They utilized a sodium silicate solution instead of bioactive glass particles to activate polyethylene terephthalate (PET) substrates [44]. This method was also suitable to coat complex geometries and porous structures with biomimetic apatite. Rhee and Tanaka activated collagen membranes [45] and cellulose fibers [46] with citric acid to initiate the formation of biomimetic apatite from 1.5 SBF. Varma et al. used a phosphorylation and subsequent activation in $Ca(OH)_2$ to coat chitosan with biomimetic apatite from 1.5*SBF [47]. Zhu et al. investigated the influence of surface charges of functional groups on the apatite formation from 1.5 SBF and found that the heterogeneous nucleation of calcium phosphates favors negatively charged surfaces [48]. Habibovic et al. were the first to utilize $CO_2$ treated 5 SBF to further accelerate the precipitation of biomimetic apatite [49]. Barrere et al. investigated the influence of the crystal growth inhibitors $Mg^{2+}$ [50] and $HCO_3^-$ [51], and Tas and Bhaduri utilized a combination of 10 SBF and $NaHCO_3$ to coat $Ti_6Al_4V$ substrates within 2 h with a 20 µm thick calcium phosphate layer [52]. Dorozhkin et al. used a diffusion chamber to keep the concentration of 4 SBF constant [53].

The motivation to coat bioinert materials biomimetically is to functionalize them with a bone-like, carbonate containing (max. 9 mass-%) apatite with a molar Ca/P ratio between 1.33 and 1.8. However, the utilization of highly supersaturated SBF leads to the precipitation of calcium phosphates with a significantly increased carbonate contend of up to 40 mass-% and molar Ca/P ratios as high as 2.7 [53–55]. These materials do not fulfill the requirements of a bone-like structure and composition.

## 5.4   In vitro Apatite Formation

After implantation into a bony defect bioactive materials form a CHA layer on their surface. This layer bonds directly to bone. The formation of a CHA layer can be reproduced in vitro by using SBF with a composition similar to the inorganic part of human blood plasma.

## 5.4.1 Simulated Body Fluid

Simulated body fluid for in vitro bioactivity tests were prepared by pipetting calculated amounts of concentrated solutions of KCl, NaCl, $NaHCO_3$, $MgSO_4 \cdot 7H_2O$, $CaCl_2$, TRIS (tris-hydroxymethyl aminomethane), $NaN_3$, and $KH_2PO_4$ into double distilled water [56]. This procedure allows to prepare SBF with an equal $HCO_3^-$ content like in human blood plasma (27 mmol/l). However, to evaluate the influence of the $HCO_3^-$ concentration on the formation and composition of biomimetic apatite various SBF solutions with $HCO_3^-$ concentrations ranging from 5 to 27 mmol/l were prepared. Table 5.2 summarizes the ionic concentrations of the SBF solutions. The pH value of the SBF solutions was adjusted to 7.3–7.4 at 37°C. The test samples were freely suspended in SBF for up to 21 days. The surface to volume ratio S/V was 0.05 $cm^{-1}$.

**Table 5.2** Ionic concentrations of different SBF solutions (mmol/l)

|  | SBF5 | SBF10 | SBF15 | SBF20 | SBF27 |
|---|---|---|---|---|---|
| $Na^+$ | 142.0 | 142.0 | 142.0 | 142.0 | 142.0 |
| $K^+$ | 5.0 | 5.0 | 5.0 | 5.0 | 5.0 |
| $Ca^{2+}$ | 2.5 | 2.5 | 2.5 | 2.5 | 2.5 |
| $Mg^{2+}$ | 1.0 | 1.0 | 1.0 | 1.0 | 1.0 |
| $Cl^-$ | 131.0 | 126.0 | 121.0 | 116.0 | 109.0 |
| $HCO_3^-$ | 5.0 | 10.0 | 15.0 | 20.0 | 27.0 |
| $HPO_4^{2-}$ | 1.0 | 1.0 | 1.0 | 1.0 | 1.0 |
| $SO_4^{2-}$ | 1.0 | 1.0 | 1.0 | 1.0 | 1.0 |

**Supersaturation**: It is known that solutions mimicking human blood plasma are supersaturated with respect to HA [57]. The degree of supersaturation $S$ with respect to different calcium phosphates can be calculated according to Eq. 5.1 [58].

$$S = (IA/K_{sp})^{1/n}, \tag{5.1}$$

where IA is the ionic activity, $K_{sp}$ is the solubility product and $n$ is the number of ions in a formula unit. The solubility products of different calcium phosphates at 37°C are listed in Table 5.3 [59–61].

**Table 5.3** Solubility product of various apatites

| | | $-\log K_{sp}$ |
|---|---|---|
| $Ca_{10}(PO_4)_6(OH)_2$ | HA | 117.2 |
| $Ca_{10}(PO_4)_6(CO_3)_{0.5}OH$ | CHA (A-type) | 115.6 |
| $Ca_9(HPO_4)_{0.5}(CO_3)_{0.5}(PO_4)_5OH$ | CHA (B-type) | 111.54 |

The IA values for compounds described in Table 5.3 are given by the Eqs. 5.2–5.4:

$$HA: IA = [Ca^{2+}]^{10} [PO_4^{3-}]^6 [OH^-]^2 \, a_1^2 a_2^{10} a_3^6 \tag{5.2}$$

$$CHA \text{ (A-type): } IA = [Ca^{2+}]^{10} [PO_4^{3-}]^6 [CO_3^{2-}]^{0.5} [OH^-] \, a_1 a_2^{10.5} a_3^6 \tag{5.3}$$

$$CHA \text{ (B-type): } IA = [Ca^{2+}]^9 [HPO_4^{2-}]^{0.5}[CO_3^{2-}]^{0.5}[PO_4^{3-}]^6[OH^-] \, a_1 a_2^{10} a_3^5$$
$$\tag{5.4}$$

The activity coefficient $a_z$ of a $z$-valent ion (e.g., $z = 1$ for $OH^-$, $z = 2$ for $Ca^{2+}$, etc.) was calculated using the modified Debye–Huckel equation proposed by Davis [62]:

$$-\log a_z = A \, z^2 \, [I^{1/2}/(1 + I^{1/2}) - 0.3I] \tag{5.5}$$

It was proven that Eq. 5.5 is valid for ionic strengths up to 0.2 mol/l [63]. In that case the constant $A$ is equal to 0.515 [63]. The total ionic strength $I$ of the solution is given by

$$I = 0.5\Sigma z_i^2 c_i, \tag{5.6}$$

where $z_i$ is the charge of the $i$ ion and $c_i$ is the concentration in mol/l listed in Table 5.2. The concentration of $CO_3^{2-}$, $HPO_4^{2-}$, and $PO_4^{3-}$ was calculated using the equilibrium constants for reaction 5.7, 5.8, and 5.9, respectively [64].

$$H_2PO_4^- \leftrightarrow HPO_4^{2-} + H^+ \quad pK_1 = 7.18 \tag{5.7}$$

$$HPO_4^{2-} \leftrightarrow PO_4^{3-} + H^+ \quad pK_2 = 12.19 \tag{5.8}$$

$$HCO_3^- + OH^- \leftrightarrow CO_3^{2-} + H_2O \quad pK_3 = 10.25 \tag{5.9}$$

The values for the degree of supersaturation in SBF solutions and human blood plasma assuming a physiological pH of 7.4 with respect to the compounds listed in Table 5.3 are depicted in Fig. 5.2. The solutions are supersaturated with respect to all phases discussed. While the changes in the degree of supersaturation with respect to HA are negligible, the degree of supersaturation with respect to A- and B-type CHA varied depending on the content of $HCO_3^-$ ions in the SBF solution. All SBF solutions are most saturated with respect to B-type carbonated apatite $Ca_9(HPO_4)_{0.5}(CO_3)_{0.5}(PO_4)_5OH$ [24]. The calculations described above generally indicate that the formation of carbonate-containing apatite from SBF is more likely than the formation of stoichiometric hydroxy apatite.

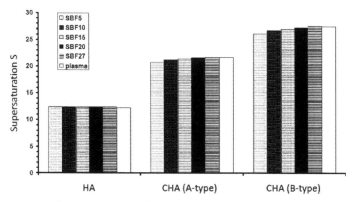

**Figure 5.2**  Supersaturation of SBF with respect to various apatites.

## 5.4.2 Bioactive Surfaces

The preparation of bioactive titanium surfaces, capable to form apatite during exposure to SBF, was first described by Kim et al. in 1996 [65]. The bioinert material was treated in NaOH and subsequently annealed at 600°C to create a crystalline sodium titanate layer on its surface able to induce the nucleation of calcium phosphate by ionic exchange.

Alternatively, the surface of bioinert titanium can be activated using a two-step wet-chemical treatment in HCl and NaOH [66, 67]. These surfaces served as a model substrate for all further investigations. Figure 5.3 shows SEM micrographs of a titanium surface after acid etching (Fig. 5.3a) and after a subsequent

NaOH activation (Fig. 5.3b). The surface topography resulting from acid etching remains intact and is overlaid by an additional substructure on the nanoscale. EDX analyses reveal that titanium, oxygen, and sodium are present in the surface [68]. The mean macro roughness increased from 1.4 ± 0.3 µm for titanium to 6.6 ± 1.9 µm for chemically modified titanium. At the same time, the contact angle decreased from 97° to 5° [69].

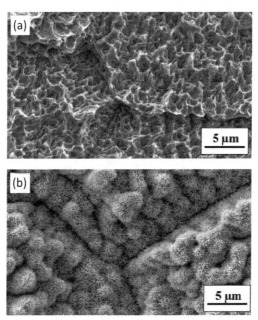

**Figure 5.3** Surface of chemically modified titanium (a) after HCl etching and (b) after a subsequent NaOH activation.

Using TEM-SAED analysis it was shown that according to Eqs. 5.10–5.12

$$3TiO_2 + 2NaOH \rightarrow Na_2Ti_3O_7 + H_2O \qquad (5.10)$$

$$6TiO_2 + 2NaOH \rightarrow Na_2Ti_6O_{13} + H_2O \qquad (5.11)$$

$$2TiH_2 + 2NaOH + 10H_2O \rightarrow Na_2Ti(OH)_4 + TiO_2 \cdot 9H_2O + H_2, \qquad (5.12)$$

modified titanium surfaces consist of nanocrystalline $Na_2Ti_3O_7$ and $Na_2Ti_6O_{13}$ as well as an additional amorphous phase [70].

In vivo investigations revealed that these surfaces led to a significantly increased bone-implant contact [69]. Materials of the same composition have also been prepared by sol-gel synthesis [71]. They also demonstrated in vitro bioactivity in SBF. This behavior can be explained by ionic exchange processes leading to the incorporation of calcium into the materials surface and to an increase of the ionic activity near the surface [66].

### 5.4.3 Structure and Properties of Biomimetic Apatite

#### 5.4.3.1 Nucleation and crystal growth

The before mentioned model substrates were exposed to SBF. After 2 days in SBF isolated spheroids with a diameter of approximately 5 µm formed on the surface of bioactive titanium (Fig. 5.4). The spheroids consist of calcium, magnesium, phosphorus, and oxygen.

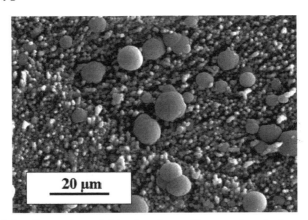

**Figure 5.4** Formation of biomimetic apatite on chemically modified titanium after 2 days in SBF.

The change in the Gibbs free energy $\Delta G$ represents the driving force for the nucleation and growth of a solid phase from a supersaturated solution [72]

$$\Delta G = -RT \ln S, \tag{5.13}$$

where $R$ is the gas constant, $T$ is the absolute temperature and $S$ is the degree of supersaturation. Normally, the heterogeneous nucleation on a substrate is favored, because the required change in the Gibbs free energy is smaller than for a homogeneous nucleation from solution (Eqs. 5.14–5.16) [72].

$$\Delta G_{het} = \phi \Delta G_{hom} \tag{5.14}$$

with

$$\phi = (2 + \cos\theta)(1 - \cos\theta)^2/4 \tag{5.15}$$

and

$$\cos\theta = (\gamma_{SL} - \gamma_{SN})/\gamma_{NL}, \tag{5.16}$$

where $\theta$ is the contact angle between the nucleus and the substrate and $\gamma_{NL}$, $\gamma_{SN}$, $\gamma_{SL}$ are the interface free energies between nucleus and solution, substrate and nucleus, and substrate and solution, respectively.

The nucleation rate $J_{KB}$ can be calculated according to Eq. 5.17 [72, 73]

$$J_{KB} = K \exp(-\Delta G_N^*/kT), \tag{5.17}$$

where $k$ is the Boltzmann constant, $K$ is a kinetic factor and $\Delta G_N^*$ is the activation energy. $\Delta G_N^*$ can be calculated according to Eq. 5.18:

$$\Delta G_N^* = \beta v^2 \sigma^3 / (kT \ln(S))^2 \tag{5.18}$$

where $\beta$ is a geometry factor, $v$ is the molar volume and $\sigma$ is the free energy for the formation of a critical nucleus [73]. With increasing supersaturation $S$ and decreasing interfacial free energy $\sigma$, the decrease of the activation energy $\Delta G_N^*$ leads to a significantly increased nucleation rate. This means that $J_{KB}$ can be controlled by adjusting the composition and supersaturation of the SBF solution.

During the subsequent crystal growth, the increase of the layer thickness depends on material transport processes in the SBF solution. The flow density $J_F$ depends on the gradient of concentration (grad $c$) in the instant vicinity of the crystal surface. It can be calculated according to Eq. 5.19 [74]:

$$J_F = D \operatorname{grad} c = D \, dc/dz, \tag{5.19}$$

where $D$ is the coefficient of diffusion and $z$ is the distance from the crystal surface.

The molar Ca/P ratio of SBF (2.5) exceeds that one of HA (1.67). Therefore, the growth rate of the apatite crystals depends on the time-depending change of the concentration $c_{p,t}$ of $PO_4^{3-}$ ions in the SBF solution [75]:

$$-dc_{p,t}/dt \infty (c_{p,t})^3 \qquad (5.20).$$

Consequently, the surface to volume ratio S/V has to be small enough (<0.05 cm$^{-1}$) to assure that sufficient $PO_4^{3-}$ ions are available in the SBF solution. In the case of an unknown surface area, the exposure to SBF should be performed under dynamic conditions.

Figure 5.5 shows the SEM micrograph and the corresponding EDX spectrum of the surface of bioactive titanium that was exposed to SBF for 2 weeks [68]. Independent of the $HCO_3^-$ content of the SBF solution, the precipitated layers consist of nanoscale calcium phosphate platelets, which form aggregates with a diameter of up to 20 µm. Traces of $Mg^{2+}$ and $Na^+$ ions indicate the substitution of $Ca^{2+}$. This is in good agreement with the composition of non-stoichiometric biological apatite in bone, which also contains minor amounts of $Mg^{2+}$, $Na^+$, $CO_3^{2-}$, $HPO_4^{2-}$, $F^-$, or $Cl^-$ [76].

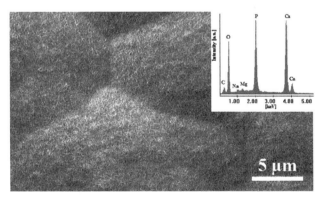

**Figure 5.5** Formation of biomimetic apatite on chemically modified titanium after 14 days in SBF [68].

The coatings were characterized by XRD analysis. They consist of hydroxy apatite of low crystallinity (Fig. 5.6a). The crystallite size in the c-direction of the apatite crystals was calculated from the (002) peak broadening at 26° using the Scherrer equation

[56, 77]. With increasing $HCO_3^-$ concentration of the SBF solution the crystallite size decreased from 26 nm for SBF5 to 19 nm for SBF27 (Fig. 5.6b). $HCO_3^-$ is known to support the heterogeneous nucleation of CHA by increasing the supersaturation of the SBF solution. This leads to a higher density of nuclei and consequently to decreased crystal growth rates. Therefore, $HCO_3^-$ is described to be a grain growth inhibitor [51].

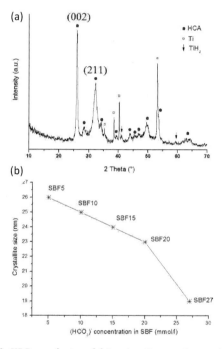

**Figure 5.6** (a) XRD analysis of biomimetic apatite and (b) crystallite sizes of biomimetic apatite in dependence of the $HCO_3^-$ concentration in SBF [56].

The TEM micrograph in Fig. 5.7a illustrates the surface transformation during chemical pretreatment and exposure to SBF [68]. The rough titanium hydride surface formed during acid etching. The subsequent NaOH treatment resulted in a nanoscaled sodium titanate surface (see also Fig. 5.3). During exposure to SBF $Ca^{2+}$ replaced the $Na^+$ ions in the surface and induced the formation of biomimetic apatite. The crystals have a size between 5 × 5 × 20 and 5 × 25 × 200 nm³ [68] and are in the same range as those found in mammalian bone (5 × 25 × 100 nm³) [16].

Figure 5.7b shows the corresponding SAED spectra [68]. All distances of the nanocrystalline structure correspond exactly to hexagonal HA with $a_0$ = 0.944 nm and $c_0$ = 0.688 nm (JCPDS 9-432).

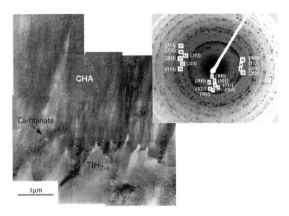

**Figure 5.7** (a) Cross-sectional TEM view of precipitated biomimetic apatite on a bioactive titanium substrate and (b) corresponding SAED analysis [68].

### 5.4.3.2 Carbonate substitution

Figure 5.8a shows FTIR spectra of apatite coatings precipitated from different SBF solutions [56]. The bands can be assigned to the characteristic bending and stretching modes of the $PO_4^{3-}$ group, the $HPO_4^{2-}$ group, and the $CO_3^{2-}$ group in B-type CHA [78]. The Raman spectra in Fig. 5.8b also show the characteristic $PO_4^{2-}$ peaks at 950 cm$^{-1}$ and 1050 cm$^{-1}$ [79, 80]. Additionally, the band at 3567 cm$^{-1}$ can be assigned to the OH$^-$ group in hydroxyl apatite. In SBF27 this band disappeared which indicates an additional A-type substitution where the OH$^-$ group is replaced by $CO_3^{2-}$.

The ratio of the FTIR absorption bands at 1420 cm$^{-1}$ and 604 cm$^{-1}$ can be used to quantify the $CO_3^{2-}$ substitution. The $CO_3^{2-}$ concentration $y$ in the biomimetic apatite can be calculated according to LeGeros [81] by using Eq. 5.21

$$y = 10.134x + 0.2134, \qquad (5.21)$$

where $x$ is the ratio of the absorption bands $A(CO_3^{2-})/A(PO_4^{3-})$ [56]. Table 5.4 summarizes the $CO_3^{2-}$ content of apatite precipitated from different SBF solutions. The highest $CO_3^{2-}$ content amounts to 9.1 mass-% in the layer precipitated from SBF27.

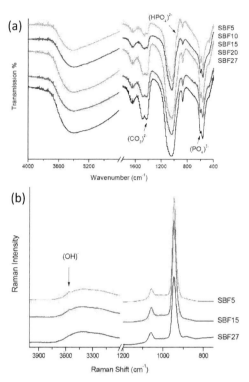

**Figure 5.8** (a) FTIR and (b) Raman spectra of biomimetic apatite precipitated from SBF solutions with different $HCO_3^-$ concentration [56].

**Table 5.4** Carbonate content of apatite precipitated from SBF (mass-%)

|  | SBF5 | SBF10 | SBF15 | SBF20 | SBF27 |
|---|---|---|---|---|---|
| $CO_3^-$ | 2.5 | 3.2 | 5.7 | 6.2 | 9.1 |

The general formula for Ca-deficient HA can be written as

$$Ca_{10-x}(HPO_4)_x(PO_4)_{6-x}(OH)_{2-x} \qquad (5.22)$$

with $0 \leq x \leq 1$. For stoichiometric HA ($x = 0$) the molar Ca/P ratio is 1.67. If $HPO_4^{2-}$ is incorporated into the structure, the Ca/P ratio decreases to a minimum of 1.5 at $x = 1$. $CO_3^{2-}$ can easily substitute $HPO_4^{2-}$ due to the same charge. This results in a Ca/P ratio of 1.8 for a complete substitution. Beyond that, $Mg^{2+}$ can substitute up to 10 Mol-% of $Ca^{2+}$ [82]. Thus, the formula can be written as

$$Ca_{10-x-y}Mg_y(HPO_4)_{x-z}(CO_3)_z(PO_4)_{6-x}(OH)_{2-x}, \quad (5.23)$$

with $0 \leq x, y, z \leq 1$. The molar Ca/P ratio ranges from 1.33 ($x, y = 1$ and $z = 0$) to 1.6 ($x, y, z = 1$). For a maximum $CO_3^{2-}$ substitution ($z = 1$) the carbonate content is equal to 6.4 mass-%. The carbonate content of apatite precipitated from SBF5, SBF10, SBF15, and SBF20 was below this level. Using Raman analysis, it was shown that with an increasing content of $HCO_3^-$ in the SBF solution the substitution of $CO_3^{2-}$ for $OH^-$ occurred. Considering an additional A-type substitution, the formula can be written as

$$Ca_{10-x-y}Mg_y(HPO_4)_{x-z}(CO_3)_z(PO_4)_{6-x}(OH)_{2-x-w}(CO_3)_{w/2}. \quad (5.24)$$

The theoretical maximum amount of carbonate substitution in this AB-type CHA for $w = 1$ is equal to 10 mass-%. In the case of SBF27, which is the solution with the composition most similar to human blood plasma, the carbonate content of the precipitated apatite amounts to 9.1 mass-%. Hence, it can be assumed that the A-sites are occupied after the B-sites are completely substitution [56]. Moreover, this means that only by using SBF27 it is possible to achieve an AB-type substitution, which is also present in human bone tissue.

### 5.4.3.3 Growth orientation

In vertebrates bone the apatite crystals are orientated with their c-axis [001] along the direction of collagen fibers. This means they are aligned parallel to the lines of principal stress [16, 18]. Thus, they optimally contribute to the high compression strength of bone. XRD analysis of biomimetically precipitated CHA crystals reveal that they preferentially grow in the direction of their crystallographic c-axis (Fig. 5.6a) [68]. A significant increase in the intensity of the (002) peaks can be detected when compared to the intensities of the (211), (112), and (300) peaks (rings 8–10 in Fig. 5.7b). The calculated peak intensity ratio $I(002)/I(211)$ amounts to 2.5 for biomimetic apatite precipitated from SBF. This significantly exceeds that one of untextured HA powder samples with a ratio of 0.4. Thus, the $I(002)/I(211)$ ratio of biomimetic apatite is in the range that was found in the longitudinal direction of a rabbit ulna (3.4) (long bone) and in the direction along the bone surface in rabbit skull (2.0) (flat bone) [83].

The same preferred growth orientation can be deduced from TEM observations [68]. From the SAED pattern shown in Fig. 5.7b, it is evident that diffraction rings are incomplete (e.g., #5 of the basal (002) plane and #12 of the prismatic {310} planes). These incomplete rings form arcs rotated with respect to each other by an angle of 90°. The preferred orientation of the CHA crystals along their c-axis [001] is identical with the direction of the maximum intensity of the basal arcs of ring #5. The high-magnification TEM image in Fig. 5.9a was analyzed by an auto-correlation method. For this purpose, the image was superposed with its copy translated by vectors of various orientations and lengths [68]. The intensity of each correlation was then plotted as a function of the corresponding translation vector. This yields a map where the brightest regions correspond to the highest degree of correlation (Abb. 5.9b). The highest auto-correlation intensity is not only obtained for small translation vectors but also for displacement vectors parallel to the average growth direction. Thus, the elongation of the bright zone in the vertical z direction indicates a preferred orientation of the crystals in this direction (Abb. 5.9c).

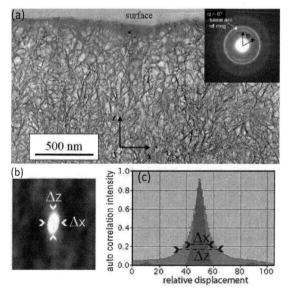

**Figure 5.9** (a) Cross-sectional TEM micrograph of biomimetic apatite and corresponding SAED analysis, (b) and (c) auto correlation intensities [68].

## 5.5 Conclusions

Novel SBF solutions with a high stability and with a composition equal to the inorganic part of human blood plasma have been developed. Utilizing these solutions under physiological conditions in combination with a bioactive surface (e.g., HCl-NaOH-treated Ti) facilitates the precipitation of a biomimetic apatite with a composition, structure, and growth orientation equal to biological bone apatite.

This procedure also represents a novel approach to coat bioinert materials with a bonelike carbonated apatite layer. Therefore, it is a promising alternative to the common plasma spraying technique, which can only deliver stoichiometric hydroxyapatite of low solubility. The targeted control of thermodynamic and kinetic parameters also allows to accelerate the mineralization process and to prepare biomimetic apatite coatings within a few hours [84, 85].

SBF solutions provide an essential contribution for the development of novel in vitro test systems. The utilization of stable SBF solutions significantly increased the reproducibility of bioactivity tests. The combination of in vitro cell tests with SBF solutions represents a promising new approach to evaluate the early stages of bone bonding and to investigate the in vitro response of osteoblasts [86].

Biomimetic apatite is of particular interest for applications in bone regeneration due to its close relationship to bone apatite [69]. Beyond that, however, it has already been demonstrated that porous structures biomimetically coated with apatite represent promising new scaffold materials for osteochondral tissue engineering [87].

## References

1. DF Williams, Tissue-biomaterials interactions, *J Mater Sci*, **22** (1987) 3421–3445.

2. T Albrektson, PI Brenemark, HA Hansson, B Ivarsson, U Johsson, Ultrastructural analysis of the interface zone of titanium and gold implants, in: *Clinical Applications of Biomaterials* (ed. AJC Lee, T Albrektsson, PI Brenemark), Wiley, Chichster (1982), pp. 167–177.

3. S Szmukler-Moncler, T Testori, JP Bernard, Etched implants: A comparative study analysis of four implant systems, *J Biomed Mater Res*, **B69** (2004) 46–57.

4. K Kieswetter, Z Schwarz, DD Dean, BD Boyan, The role of implant surface characteristics in the healing of bone, *Crit Rev Oral Biol Med*, **7** (1996) 329–345.

5. F Rupp, L Schneideler, D Rehbein, D Axmann, J Geis-Gerstofer, Roughness induced dynamic changes of wettability of acid etched titanium implants, *Biomaterials*, **25** (2004) 1429–1438.

6. M Lampin, C Warocquier, C Legris, M Degrange, MF Sigot-Luizard, Correlation between substratum roughness and wettability, cell adhesion, and cell migration, *J Biomed Mater Res*, **36** (1997) 99–108.

7. DD Deligianni, N Katsala, S Ladas, D Sotiropoulou, J Amedee, YF Missirlis, Effect of surface roughness of the titanium alloy Ti–6Al–4V on human bone marrow cell response and on protein adsorption, *Biomaterials*, **22** (2001) 1241–1251.

8. F Rupp, L Schneideler, N Olshanska, M de Wild, M Wieland, J Geis-Gerstorfer, Enhancing surface free energy and hydrophilicity through chemical modification of microstructured titanium implant surface, *J Biomed Mater Res*, **A76** (2006) 323–334.

9. BD Ratner, AS Hoffmann, Physicochemical surface modification of materials used in medicine, in: *Biomaterials Science: An Introduction to Materials in Medicine*, 2nd ed. (ed. BD Ratner, AS Hoffman, FJ Schoen, JE Lemons), Elsevier, Amsterdam (2004), pp. 201–218.

10. JA Jansen, AF von Reum, Textured and porous materials, in: *Biomaterials Science: An Introduction to Materials in Medicine* (ed. BD Ratner, AS Hoffman, FJ Schoen, JE Lemons), 2nd ed., Elsevier, Amsterdam (2004), pp. 218–225.

11. AS Hoffman, JA Hubbell, Surface-immobilized biomolecules, in: *Biomaterials Science: An Introduction To Materials in Medicine* (ed. BD Ratner, AS Hoffman, FJ Schoen, JE Lemons), 2nd ed., Elsevier, Amsterdam (2004), pp. 225–232.

12. S Radin, P Ducheyne, The effect of plasma sprayed induced changes in the characteristics of the in vitro stability of calcium phosphate ceramic, *J Mater Sci Mater Med*, **1** (1990) 119–124.

13. CPAT Klein, P Patka, HBM van der Lubbe, JGC Wolke, K de Groot, Plasma sprayed coating of tetracalcium phosphate, hydroxyapatite, and $\alpha$-TCP on titanium alloys: An interfacial study, *J Biomed Mater Res*, **21** (1991) 53–65.

14. CY Chang, BC Wang, E Chang, BC Wu, The influence of plasma spraying parameters on the characteristics of hydroxyapatite coating, *J Mater Sci Mater Med*, **6** (1996) 249–257.

15. T Kokubo, Bioactive glass ceramics: Properties and applications, *Biomaterials*, **12** (1991) 155–163.

16. S Weiner, HDWagner, The material bone: Structure-mechanical function relations, *Ann Rev Mater Sci*, **28** (1998) 271–298.

17. B Wopenka, JD Pasteris, A mineralogical perspective on the apatite in bone, *Mater Sci Eng*, **C25** (2005) 131–143.

18. M Vallet-Regí, JM González-Calbet, Calcium phosphates as substitution of bone tissues, *Prog Sol State Chem*, **32** (2004) 1–31.

19. E Landi, A Tampieri, G Celotti, R Langenati, M Sandri, S Sprio, Nucleation of biomimetic apatite in synthetic body fluid: Dense and porous scaffold development, *Biomaterials*, **26** (2005) 2835–2845.

20. WJ Schmidt, Über die Kristallorientierung in Zahnschmelz, *Naturwissenschaften*, **24** (1936) 361.

21. JP Nightingale, P Lewis, Pole figures of the orientation of apatite in bones, *Nature*, **232** (1971) 334–335.

22. SW White, DJS Hulmes, A Miller, PA Timmins, Collagen–mineral axial relationship in calcified turkey leg tendon by X-ray and neutron diffraction, *Nature*, **266** (1977) 421–425.

23. SV Dorozhkin, M Epple, Biological and medical significance of calcium phosphates, *Angew Chem Int Ed*, **41** (2002) 3130–3146.

24. JC Elliot, *Structure and Chemistry of the Apatites and Other Calcium Orthophosphates*, Elsevier Press, Amsterdam, Niederlande (1994).

25. LL Hench, RJ Splinter, WC Allen, TK Greenlee Jr, Bonding mechanisms at the interface of ceramic prosthetic materials, *J Biomed Mater Res*, **2** (1971) 117–141.

26. U Gross, V Strunz, The interface of various glasses and glass-ceramics with a bony implantation bed, *J Biomed Mater Res*, **19** (1985) 251–271.

27. W Hohland, W Vogel, K Naurnann, J Gummel, Interface reactions between machinable bioactive glass-ceramics and bone, *J Biomed Mater Res*, **19** (1985) 303–312.

28. M Jarcho, Calcium phosphate ceramics as hard tissue prosthetics, *Clin Orthop Relat Res*, **157** (1981) 259–278.

29. T Nakamura, T Yamamuro, S Higashi, T Kokubo, S Itoo, A new glass-ceramic for bone replacement: Evaluation of its bonding to bone tissue, *J Biomed Mater Res*, **19** (1985) 685–698.

30. T Yamamuro, LL Hench, J Wilson (eds.), *Handbook on Bioactive Ceramics: Bioactive Glasses and Glass-Ceramics*, vol. I. CRC Press, Boca Raton, FL (1990).

31. LL Hench, J Wilson, *An Introduction to Bioceramics*, World Scientific, London, UK (1993).

32. LL Hench, Bioceramics, *J Am Ceram Soc*, **81** (1998) 1705–1728.

33. W Earle, Production of malignancy in vitro. IV. The mouse fibroblast cultures and changes in the living cells, *J Natl Cancer Inst*, **4** (1943) 165–212.

34. JH Hanks, RE Wallace, Relation of oxygen and temperature in the preservation of tissues by refrigeration, *Proc Soc Exp Biol Med*, **71** (1949) 196–200.

35. S Ringer, A further contribution regarding the influence of the different constituents of the blood on the contraction of the heart, *J Physiol*, **4** (1883) 29–42.

36. T Kokubo, Surface chemistry of bioactive glass-ceramics, *J Non-Cryst Solids*, **120** (1990) 138–151.

37. A Oyane, K Onuma, A Ito, HM Kim, T Kokubo, T Nakamura, Formation and growth of clusters in conventional and new kinds of simulated body fluids, *J Biomed Mater Res*, **65A** (2003) 339–348.

38. S Jalota, SB Bhaduri, AC Tas, Effect of carbonate content and buffer type on calcium phosphate formation in SBF solutions, *J Mater Sci Mater Med*, **17** (2006) 697–707.

39. D Bayraktar, AC Tas, Chemical preparation of carbonated calcium hydroxyapatite powders at 37°C in urea-containing synthetic body fluids, *J Eur Ceram Soc*, **19** (1999) 2573–2579.

40. A Bigi, E Boanini, S Panzavolta, N Roveri, Biomimetic growth of hydroxyapatite on gelatin films doped with sodium polyacrylate, *Biomacromolecules*, **1** (2000) 752–756.

41. EI Dorozhkina, SV Dorozhkin, Surface mineralisation of hydroxyapatite in modified simulated body fluid (mSBF) with higher amounts of hydrogencarbonate ions, *Colloids Surf A Physicochem Eng Aspects*, **210** (2002) 41–48.

42. M Tanahashi, T Yao, T Kokubo, M Minoda, T Miyamoto, T Nakamura, T Yamamuro, Apatite coating on organic polymers by a biomimetic process, *J Am Ceram Soc*, **77** (1994) 2805–2808.

43. M Tanahashi, T Kokubo, T Nakamura, Y Katsura, M Nagano, Ultrastructural study of an apatite layer formed by a biomimetic process and its bonding to bone, *Biomaterials*, **17** (1996) 47–51.

44. F Miyaji, HM Kim, S Handa, T Kokubo, T Nakamura, Bonelike apatite coating on organic polymers: Novel nucleation process using sodium silicate solution, *Biomaterials*, **20** (1999) 913–919.

45. SH Rhee, J Tanaka, Hydroxyapatite coating on a collagen membrane by a biomimetic method, *J Am Ceram Soc*, 81 (1994) 3029–3031.

46. SH Rhee, J Tanaka, Hydroxyapatite formation on cellulose cloth induced by citric acid, *J Mater Sci: Mater Med*, **11** (2000) 449–452.

47. HK Varma, Y Yokogawa, FF Espinosa, Y Kawamoto, K Nishizawa, F Nagata, T Kameyama, Porous calcium phosphate coating over phosphorylated chitosan film by a biomimetic method, *Biomaterials*, **20** (1999) 879–884.

48. P Zhu, Y Masuda, K Koumoto, The effect of surface charge on hydroxyapatite nucleation, *Biomaterials*, **25** (2004) 3915–3921.

49. P Habibovic, F Barrere, CA van Blitterswijk, K de Groot, P Layrolle, Biomimetic hydroxyapatite coating on metal implants, *J Am Ceram Soc*, **85** (2002) 517–522.

50. F Barrere, CA van Blitterswijk, K de Groot, P Layrolle, Nucleation of biomimetic Ca–P coatings on $Ti_6Al_4V$ from a SBF × 5 solution: Influence of magnesium, *Biomaterials*, **23** (2002) 2211–2220.

51. F Barrere, CA van Blitterswijk, K de Groot, P Layrolle, Influence of ionic strength and carbonate on the Ca–P coating formation from SBF × 5 solution, *Biomaterials*, **23** (2002) 1921–1930.

52. AC Tas, SB Bhaduri, Rapid coating of $Ti_6Al_4V$ at room temperature with a calcium phosphate solution similar to 10× simulated body fluid, *J Mater Res*, **19** (2004) 2742–2749.

53. SV Dorozhkin, EI Dorozhkina, M Epple, A model system to provide a good in vitro simulation of biological mineralization, *Cryst Growth Des*, **4** (2004) 389–395.

54. Dorozhkina EI, Dorozhkin SV, Structure and properties of the precipitates formed from condensed solutions of the revised simulated body fluid, *J Biomed Mater Res*, **67A** (2003) 578–581.

55. AAP Marques, MCF Magalhaes, RN Correia, Inorganic plasma with physiological $CO_2/HCO_3^-$ buffer, *Biomaterials*, **24** (2003) 1541–1548.

56. L Müller, FA Müller, Preparation of SBF with different $HCO_3^-$ content and its influence on the composition of biomimetic apatites, *Acta Biomater*, **2** (2006) 181–189.

57. PX Zhu, Y Masuda, T Yonezawa, K Koumoto, Investigation of apatite deposition onto charged surface in aqueous solutions using a quarz-crystal microbalance, *J Am Ceram Soc*, **86** (2003) 782–790.

58. GH Nancollas, In vitro studies of calcium phosphate crystallization, in: *Biomineralization* (ed. S Mann, J Webb, RJP Williams), VCH, Weinheim (1989).

59. A Ito, K Maekawa, S Tsutsumi, F Ikazaki, T Tateishi, Solubility product of OH-carbonated hydroxyapatite, *J Biomed Mater Res*, **36** (1997) 522–528.

60. GH Nancollas, In *Biomineralization* (ed. S Mann, J Webb, RJP Williams) VCH Verlagsgesellschaft GmbH, Weinheim (1989), p. 159.

61. R Tang, ZJ Henneman, GH Nancollas, Constant composition kinetics study of carbonated apatite dissolution, *J Cryst Growth*, **249** (2003) 614–624.

62. JW Davies, *Ion Association*, Butterworth Press, London (1962).

63. P Siripphannon, Y Kameshina, A Yasumori, K Okada, S Hayashi, Comparative study of the formation of hydroxyapatite in simulated body fluid under static and flowing system, *J Biomed Mater Res*, **60** (2002) 175–185.

64. LL Hench, GP Latorre, Reaction kinetics of bioactive ceramics—Part IV. Effect of glass and solution composition, In *Biomat 5*. (ed. T Yamamuro, T Kokubo, T Nakamura), Kobonshi Kankokai Inc., Kyoto, Japan (1992), p. 67.

65. H-M Kim, F Miyaji, T Kokubo, T Nakamura, Preparation of bioactive Ti and its alloys via simple chemical surface treatment, *J Biomed Mater Res*, **32** (1996) 409–417.

66. L Jonášová, FA Müller, A Helebrant, J Strnad, P Greil, Biomimetic apatite formation on chemically treated titanium, *Biomaterials*, **25** (2004) 1187–1194.

67. FA Müller, MC Bottino, L Müller, VAR Henriques, U Lohbauer, AHA Bressiani, JC Bressiani, In vitro apatite formation on chemically treated (P/M) Ti-13Nb-13Zr, *Dent Mater*, **24** (2008) 250–256.

68. FA Müller, L Müller, D Caillard, E Conforto, Preferred growth orientation of biomimetic apatite crystals, *J Cryst Growth*, **304** (2007) 464–471.

69. C von Wilmowsky, L Müller, R Lutz, U Lohbauer, F Rupp, FW Neukam, E Nkenke, KA Schlegel, FA Müller, Osseointegration of chemically modified titanium surfaces: An in vivo study, *Adv Eng Mater*, **10** (2008) B61–B66.

70. E Conforto, D Caillard, L Müller, FA Müller, The structure of titanate nanobelts used as seeds for the nucleation of hydroxyapatite at the surface of titanium implants, *Acta Biomater*, **4** (2008) 1934–1943.

71. I Becker, I Hofmann, FA Müller, Preparation of bioactive sodium titanate ceramics, *J Eur Ceram Soc*, **27** (2007) 4547–4553.

72. JW Mullin, *Crystallization*, 3rd ed., Butterworth-Heinemann, Oxford (1993).

73. P Calvert, P Rieke, Biomimetic mineralization in and on polymers, *Chem Mater*, **8** (1996) 1715–1727.

74. AE Nielsen, Electrolyte crystal growth mechanisms, *J Cryst Growth*, **67** (1984) 289–310.

75. KH Prakash, R Kumar, SC Yu, KA Khor, P Cheang, On the kinetics of apatite growth on substrates under physiological conditions, *Langmuir*, **22** (2006) 269–276.

76. D Tadic, F Peters, M Epple, Continuous synthesis of amorphous carbonated apatites, *Biomaterials*, **23** (2002) 2553–2559.

77. SN Danilchenko, OG Kukharenko, C Moseke, IY Protsenko, LF Sukhodub, B Sulkio-Cleff, Determination of the bone mineral crystallite size and lattice strain from diffraction line broadening, *Cryst Res Technol*, **37** (2002) 1234–1240.

78. S Koutsopoulos, Synthesis and characterization of hydroxyapatite crystals: A review study on the analytical methods, *J Biomed Mater Res*, **62** (2002) 600–612.

79. A Krajewski, M Mazzocchi, PL Buldini, A Ravaglioli, A Tinti, P Taddei, C Fagnano, Synthesis of carbonated hydroxyapatites: Efficienty of the substitution and critical evaluation of analytical methods, *J Mol Struct*, **744–747** (2005) 221–228.

80. RM Wilson, JC Elliot, SEP Dowkner, P Rodriguez-Lorenzo, Rietveld refinements and spectroscopic studies of the structure of Ca-deficient apatite, *Biomaterials*, **26** (2005) 1317–1327.

81. RZ LeGeros, *Calcium Phosphates in Oral Biology and Medicine*, Karger, Basel (1991).

82. JK Matthew, J Rakovan, JM Hughes, *Phosphates—Geochemical, Geobiological and Materials Importance*, Reviews in Mineralogy & Geochemistry **48** (2002).

83. T Nakano, K Kaibara, Y Tabata, N Nagata, S Enomoto, E Marukawa, Y Umakoshi, Unique alignment and texture of biological apatite crystallites in typical calcified tissues analyzed by microbeam x-ray diffractometer system, *Bone*, **31** (2002) 479–487.

84. IF Hofmann, L Müller, P Greil, FA Müller, Calcium phosphate nucleation on cellulose fabrics, *Surf Coat Technol*, **201** (2006) 2392–2398.

85. CR Rambo, FA Müller, L Müller, H Sieber, I Hofmann, P Greil, Biomimetic apatite coating on biomorphous alumina scaffolds, *J Mater Sci Eng C*, **26** (2006) 92–99.

86. JB Nebe, L Müller, F Luethen, A Ewald, C Bergemann, E Conforto, FA Müller, Osteoblast response to biomimetically altered titanium surfaces, *Acta Biomater*, **4** (2008) 1985–1995.

87. FA Müller, L Müller, I Hofmann, P Greil, MM Wenzel, R Staudenmaier, Cellulose-based scaffold materials for cartilage tissue engineering, *Biomaterials*, **27** (2006) 3955–3963.

# Chapter 6

# Fibre-Reinforced, Biphasic Composite Scaffolds with Pore Channels and Embedded Stem Cells Based on Alginate for the Treatment of Osteochondral Defects

**F. Despang, C. Halm, K. Schütz, B. Fischer, A. Lode, and M. Gelinsky**

*Centre for Translational Bone, Joint and Soft Tissue Research,*
*University Hospital Carl Gustav Carus*
*and Medical Faculty of Technische Universität Dresden,*
*Fetscherstr. 74, Dresden, Saxony, 01307, Germany*

f.despang@web.de, michael.gelinsky@tu-dresden.de

## 6.1 Osteochondral Defects and the Tissue Engineering Approach

The musculoskeletal system enables humans for an upright position and locomotion by transmitting forces. Bones are likewise beams and levers that are moved by muscles bound by tendons to the hard tissue. Joints, the flexible connections of two or more bones, allow this movement. Here, bones are covered by a thin layer of cartilage, only a few millimetres thick, that is transmitting

---

*Bio-Inspired Regenerative Medicine: Materials, Processes, and Clinical Applications*
Edited by Simone Sprio and Anna Tampieri
Copyright © 2016 Pan Stanford Publishing Pte. Ltd.
ISBN 978-981-4669-14-6 (Hardcover), 978-981-4669-15-3 (eBook)
www.panstanford.com

forces and cushions between the bones and enables motion by reducing the friction in concert with synovia. Cartilage can bear stresses in the range of 2–12 MPa [1] and exhibits a stiffness of 0.3–60 MPa [2–4] depending on the loading frequency. However, cartilage is characterised by a limited regenerative capacity. Hunter concluded already in 1742 that "Cartilage when destroyed, [...] is never recovered" [5]. However, nowadays several surgical techniques are established to support the healing process of an articular cartilage defect depending on the degree of damage such as debridement, microfracturing, autologous chondrocyte transplantation (ACT) or mosaicplasty [6, 7]. What is still valid is that the regenerative capacity of this tissue is low [8] and in many cases total endoprosthesis might be the final solution to improve the quality of life by regaining mobility and recover function of the joint.

Articular cartilage consists of a network of structural proteins, mostly collagen type II but also type IX–XI, and glycosaminoglycans, predominantly aggrecan, which retain water and ions, compensating the charge of the molecules [9]. The proteoglycans can absorb and release a substantial amount of water leading to elasticity. The matrix is synthesised by chondrocytes which originate from mesenchymal stem cells. They are entirely embedded in the matrix and appear in groups of several cells forming chondrons, occupying ca. 1–10 vol.-% of cartilage tissue [6, 10, 11]. The chondrocytes are only supplied by diffusion processes from synovia because this thin tissue lacks vascularisation, and in consequence the transport of nutrients, factors and cells is limited and the exchange rate is low. Therefore, injuries hardly heal without surgical intervention and are still challenging to treat. This is especially true for the heavily loaded knees strained by mechanical, i.e. sportive demands, malposition or trauma as well as metabolic factors or obesity.

In cases where both the cartilage and the underlying bone are destroyed, the patient suffers from an osteochondral defect. Motion and mobility are hindered, and thus the quality of life is reduced. Due to the low metabolic activity and slow matrix production as well as the absence of blood vessels, damage in cartilage progresses over time leading to osteoarthritis where not only articulate cartilage but also subjacent bone is affected. Intrinsic repair based on the direct contact to bone marrow and blood clotting tends to the formation of fibrocartilagenous tissue, which is less capable of bearing forces, breaks down easily as well as being prone to microfractures between healthy and repaired tissue [12, 13]. In order to improve the quality of life of patients with such osteochondral defects, a new promising approach—beyond the classical surgical techniques—has arisen to restore the functionality of the damaged tissue following the idea of tissue engineering [13, 14].

According to this concept, three-dimensional constructs forming substrates for seeded cells are used to foster the tissue regeneration. The carrier first ensures the mechanical stability and serves as scaffold for the cells which have the regenerative potential. Later on, the scaffold is degraded and replaced by new extracellular matrix (ECM) produced by the cells. These cells were first harvested from the patient and expanded in vitro and, if stem cells were applied, differentiated into the desired lineage. The utilisation of mesenchymal stem cells circumvents the limited availability of autologous chondrocytes and enables to keep healthy cartilage undamaged.

In the case of osteochondral defects where two types of tissue are involved, a biphasic scaffold should be applied that is adapted to both tissues. The biphasic scaffolds need to remain complete over the healing process and interfacial rupture should be avoided [7]. Therefore, sometimes a third adaptation layer is introduced to relax the shear stress in the interfacial zone [15]. Biphasic or even multi-layered scaffolds based on collagen with hydroxyapatite (HAP) for the adaptation to the osseous tissue have been previously developed using a freeze-drying method [16, 17]. However, freeze-dried collagen scaffolds exhibit low mechanical strength and stiffness.

Therefore, we have engineered a biphasic but monolithic scaffold based on alginate [16] with two layers adapted to cartilage and bone tissue concerning their composition [18]. Technological parameters were adapted to embed living cells in the chondral layer during the sol-gel process applied for fabrication. Parallel aligned pores that are formed during ionotropic gelation should lead to an improvement of nutrient supply towards the cells and pervade the scaffold through the entire height perpendicularly to the bilayer interface.

The scaffold production technology is based is based on the biopolymer alginate which is suitable for embedding of cells and also can generate a fascinating pore pattern of parallel aligned pores in honeycomb arrangement. Here we report how this biphasic scaffold was further reinforced by fibres.

## 6.2 Scaffolds with Parallel Aligned Pores Generated from the Biopolymer Alginate

### 6.2.1 Biopolymer Alginate and Its Structure Formation Phenomenon of Directed Ionotropic Gelation

The polysaccharide alginate is the structural element of brown algae; however, it is also synthesised by some bacteria [20, 21]. Salts of alginate are obtained by alkaline extraction followed by precipitation with diluted acids [22]. The alginate molecule is a non-branched co-polymer which consists of D-manuronic (M) and L-guluronic (G) acid residues which are intramolecularly bound by $\beta$–1,4-glycosidic linkage. The units are statistically arranged. Each monomer bears a carboxylic and two hydroxy groups which lead to a negative charge at neutral pH and $pK_a$ around 3–4. The functional groups of GG blocks are arranged in a manner that multivalent cations ions can be intermolecularly chelated by alginate chains. Due to its morphological similarity, this structure is named "egg box model". Since the generation of an alginate 3D network is mostly caused by ionic interactions and not by temperature effects, it is called ionotropic gelation. The molecular weight and the M/G ratio, i.e. the quotient of manuronic to guluronic monomer units, and their block-like arrangements affect the properties of the resulting gel. The monomer content and appearance in doublets or triplets in the alginate molecular chain can be quantified by nuclear magnetic resonance spectroscopy (NMR) [23].

Alginate is used as viscosifier and gelling agent in food industry. Wood engineers apply alginate to increase strength as well as to tailor the wetting behaviour and permeability of packing paper [24, 25]. Alginate is also intensively used in the biomedical field [26]. Medical applications comprise those for hard as well as epithelial tissues like dental impression kits like Gilalgin (BK Giulini, Italy) or Tropicalgin (Zhermack, Italy), wound dressings like algiDERM (Bard, USA), Sorbsan (B. Braun Petzold,

Germany), Curasorb (Covidien, USA) or Urgosorb (Urgo, Germany). Furthermore, it is applied in the pharmaceutical area as tablet to treat pyrosis (Gaviscon; Reckitt Benckiser, Germany) or to benefit from retarded release of drugs like Verahexal (Hexal, Germany). Commercially available alginates of food grade might contain residues of heavy metals, bacterial proteins, polyphenols (flavonoids) if they are not specifically cleaned for medical purposes [27]. This might be a source of inflammatory reactions. Systematic investigation on cleaning processes of alginate was carried out by Zimmermann et al. in Würzburg [28, 29].

Most research on alginates in biomedicine is focused on tissue engineering of cartilage [16, 30, 31], wound dressings [32], cell immobilisation within beads or microspheres [33–35] as well as for the controlled release of pharmaceutical agents [36–39]. Furthermore, alginate as biomaterial is intensively investigated concerning e.g. regeneration of nerves [40–42], revascularisation [43] and tissue engineering of bone [44–46]. Especially for the latter, the special feature to generate an anisotropic structure with parallel pore channels is explored which mimics an osteon-like structure and might guide the ingrowth of cells and flow of media. Its well-known application for cell embedding is therefore now translated to 3D scaffolds which allow a more efficient and accurate delivery of cells into a defect.

Parallel-aligned pores are generated when gelling ions diffuse in broad front into the alginate sol. Therefore, an alginate sol is covered with an electrolyte solution containing multivalent cations ions (Fig. 6.1). Immediately at their first contact, a primary membrane of the biopolymer chelated by the cations is formed at the interface. The later sol-gel transition gradually progresses with a lower velocity [47] of approximately 1 mm/h leading to simultaneous separation of phases depending on the concentration of alginate and electrolyte accumulating in the walls or the pore channels, respectively.

The discoverer of this phenomenon, the German colloid chemist Heinrich Thiele, explained the pore formation by the dehydration of the alginate due to charge transfer which appears during complexation [48]. Water as the main reaction product consequently accumulates in droplets that are trapped at the gelation front and pushed into the sol generating the macro structure of channel like pores. Later Kohler et al. presented another model for this phenomenon which is based on observed micro movements ahead of the gel formation front as well as mathematical considerations [49]. In the convection zone, the alginate molecules get pinned to the gel and thereby change their conformation. This leads to a shear force acting on the sol with a molecule transport towards the gel and a solvent-rich phase towards the sol. The hydrodynamic flow is only stable and leads to parallel aligned pores above a critical contraction velocity [50]. This dissipative structure model is based on diffusion and transportation parameters of alginate and the electrolyte ions. Maneval et al. introduced the idea of the spinodal decomposition phenomenon driven by elastic stress fields as key factor for this anisotropic pore formation [51]. A compendium on contributions to this fascinating structuring method is given elsewhere [52].

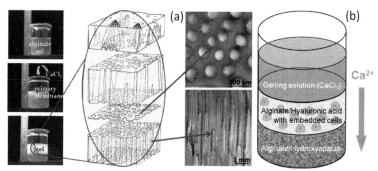

**Figure 6.1** Generation of parallel aligned pores by ionotropic gelation of alginate (drawing adapted from Wenger [19]). (a) Principle of ionotropic gelation and experimental set-up: covering of alginate sol by electrolyte followed by diffusion in broad front into sol leading to gelation, electrolyte filled channels and incorporation of additives into the alginate based walls of scaffolds. (b) Biphasic scaffolds gelled by divalent ions with various components (e.g. hydroxyapatite in osseous layer) and embedding of living cells in chondral part.

Components which are dispersed in the alginate sol become integrated into the walls consisting of the alginate gel network during sol-gel transition (Fig. 6.1b), which holds for polymers as well as ceramic powders. Therefore, also composites with HAP and even ceramics with parallel aligned pores were developed and investigated as scaffolds for tissue engineering of bone by following the ceramic processing technology [45, 46, 52]. In those cases the ceramic slurry consisting of an alginate sol in which ceramic powder has been suspended, was gelled, dried, and finally the organic components were burnt out for ceramic processing. The temperature regime was chosen to impart a sufficient strength comparable to that of cancellous bone while conserving high porosity and nano-crystallinity, which is important for the tissue engineering approach. In this way, macroporosity is used for cell seeding, whereas micro-porosity can ensure nutrient supply and nano-crystallinity contributes for degradability of the scaffold.

However, scaffolds based on several layers of varying composition were envisioned for the treatment of osteochondral defects [16]. Besides components of the ECM of cartilage and bone like hyaluronic acid and HAP, respectively, the integration of living cells especially into the chondral layer of biphasic but monolithic scaffolds was evaluated [18] which should support healing of osteochondral defects by high cell seeding efficiency. Therefore, the entire process of ionotropic gelation needed to be translated to conditions fitting to the requirements belonging to the requirements of cell integration such as control of osmotic pressure, neutral pH conditions and last but not least sterility of all components.

## 6.2.2 Influence of Selected Process Parameters on Pore Channel Formation during Ionotropic Gelation

Some principal parameters influencing pore formation should be depicted here. First, monophasic scaffolds of excessive height (15 mm) were investigated, which is much larger than the 2–3 mm thickness needed for the chondral or osseous layer, but easier for evaluation of the processing parameters that effect pore formation, diameter and density as well as length of the pores. As more than one composition is suitable for pore formation by ionotropic gelation, the longer pore channels and more homogeneous pore arrangement should be observed.

The composition of the different scaffolds, described in the following, is given in mass percentage of the respective component (alginate, additional biopolymers or HAP powder) in the sol before gelation. Due to the fact that all components are integrated in the resulting hydrogels, the composition of the sol(s) is identical to that of the hydrogels, formed during ionotropic gelation.

The average pore diameter was unaffected by the concentration of the sol in an observation window of 0.5 to 2 wt.-% but pore density was diminished by increasing concentration (Fig. 6.2). This effect has also been observed already by Thiele and Hallich for solutions of copper, cadmium, lead and calcium nitrates as gelling agents [53]. Here 1 M $CaCl_2$ was used for alginate gelation.

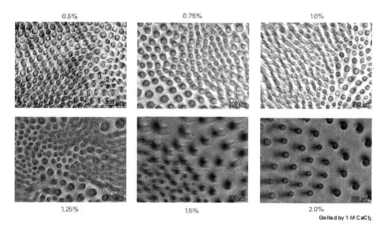

**Figure 6.2** Influence of polymer concentration on pore density in resulting hydrogel after gelation with 1 M $CaCl_2$: decrease in pore number with increasing concentration of alginate in a window of 0.5-2 wt.-%.

However, with increasing calcium chloride concentration, the average pore diameter and density were decreasing (Fig. 6.3). This finding is in line with the basic studies on pore formation of Thiele and Hallich where nitrates of calcium, copper, calcium-, copper-, cadmium and lead ions were used as gelling agents [53]. The toxic ions could not be used for the sol-gel process with the intention for application in tissue engineering and thus we studied the influence of various $CaCl_2$ concentrations aiming at embedding living cells [18] and for applications in the field of bone regeneration with incorporated gelatine and HAP [54]. For the structure formation 1 M $CaCl_2$ was found optimal, whereas for the embedding of living cells 400 mM was the compromise between structure formation and survival of the cells [53, 54]. In addition, Matyash et al. demonstrated that alginate hydrogels were more stable and less susceptible to swelling when 0.9 wt.-% NaCl was supplemented to the gelling agents [55]. However, in presence of physiological saline in the gelling solution, the pores were less homogenously arranged and exhibited a smaller pore diameter with increasing $Ca^{2+}$ ion concentration compared to gels that were prepared without sodium chloride (Fig. 6.3).

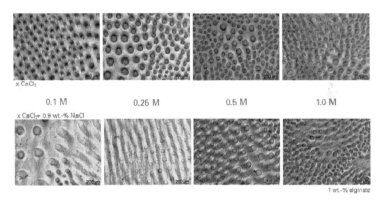

**Figure 6.3** Influence of electrolyte concentration and the addition of sodium chloride to the electrolyte on pore density: less homogenous arrangement of pores by addition of 0.9 wt.-% sodium chloride to the gelling agent solutions investigated at different $CaCl_2$ concentrations.

For embedding of cells into alginate, non-physiological osmotic pressure should be avoided. Therefore, structure formation of alginate suspended in different saline solutions, commonly used in cell culture, was evaluated using calcium chloride for gelation (Fig. 6.4). In order to ensure sterile processing, all raw powders were autoclaved. This sterilisation method was used since pore formation was less affected compared to gamma irradiation of alginate which resulted in formation of only short and small pores as well as a low number of pores [18].

In the present study, 0.2 wt.-% hyaluronic acid and 4 wt.-% hydroxyapatite were also integrated into the alginate (1 wt.-% alginate for the chondral and 1.25 wt.-% for the osseous composition). Parallel aligned pores were found in all cases independently of the saline buffer used. They were less homogeneously distributed when hydroxyethylpiperazineethanesulfonic acid

(HEPES) or tris(hydroxymethyl)aminomethane (TRIS) buffer were used as dispersion media for the alginate. In the case of phosphate buffered saline (PBS) some opaque regions were found which may correspond to precipitated calcium phosphates. This kind of precipitation has already been observed when phosphate buffer was used to strengthen alginate hydrogels and to adapt them to the composition of bone tissue, since $Ca^{2+}$ ions will react not only with alginate to form the gel but also with phosphate ions to calcium phosphate crystals as in the case of synchronous mineralisation [44]. However, the HAP precipitate was not intended in the chondral layer because no mineral phase is present in cartilage tissue.

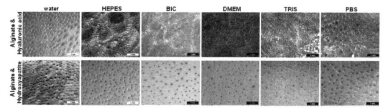

**Figure 6.4** Influence of different dispersing media (water and saline solutions (abbreviations see text)) on pore structure of the biphasic alginates in cross sections of respective layers (top: chondral layer with hyaluronic acid, bottom: bony layer containing HAP).

The most regular pore structure was found using water or Dulbecco's modified Eagle's medium (DMEM) as solvent. However, the stiffness of the resulting composites was highest for those prepared with water followed by DMEM and HEPES as dispersing medium (Fig. 6.5a). The softest scaffold was produced using bicarbonate buffered saline (BIC) which also exhibited lowest strength after 7 days of incubation in cell culture conditions (Fig. 6.5b). The ions of the saline solution seem to confine the molecule assembly in a way that softer hydrogels were generated maybe by hindering higher degree of ordered structure. The ions and salinity influence the conformation of alginate chains by shielding the negatively charged functional groups. The amino acids which are only present in the DMEM might strengthen the alginate-based structure by polyelectrolyte complexation leading to a stiffer biohybrid.

In order to further adapt the processing conditions to the embedding of cells, ionotropic gelation was carried out at different temperatures in a large range of alginate concentrations between 1 and 3 wt.-% (Fig. 6.6). For the very viscous 3 wt.-% alginate sol, there was no regular pore formation observed at 25°C but at 37°C some pores formed. However, body temperature hindered pore formation with a 1 wt.-% sol, whereas at room temperature homogeneous generation of parallel aligned pores was found. The 2 wt.-% alginate sol seemed to be less susceptible to changes in temperature. Temperature changes the viscosity, which is an important parameter for directed ionotropic gelation as also described by the model of dissipative structure formation [49, 50]. And therefore, high temperature and low concentration of alginate sol as well as low temperature and high concentration lead to too large or too small viscosities preventing structure formation.

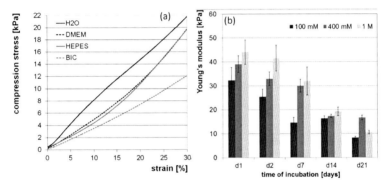

**Figure 6.5** Change in mechanical properties of alginate/hyaluronic acid composite due to preparation of biopolymer sols in different saline buffers. (a) Stiffness: slope of stress strain curve in elastic region. (b) Change in strength over an observation time of 7 days exposure to cell culture conditions (37°C, 5% $CO_2$, cell culture media with serum and antibiotics).

Interestingly, an adaption to in vivo conditions might not always be beneficial. The incorporation of living cells synchronous to the structure formation seems to demand for body temperature. In order to analyse the influence of different temperatures on the viability of embedded cells, human mesenchymal stem cells were dispersed in alginate/hyaluronate sol and ionotropic gelation was carried out with 1 M calcium chloride at 22 and 37°C. After 24 h, cells were imaged after live/dead staining with Calcein AM for living cells and Ethidium homodimer for dead cells (Fig. 6.7). More viable cells could be found inside the composite scaffolds that have been structured at room temperature compared to body temperature. Cells might bear the non-physiological high calcium ion concentration much better at a temperature where they are less metabolically active. Therefore, room temperature was chosen for embedding of living cells as being favourable for cell survival.

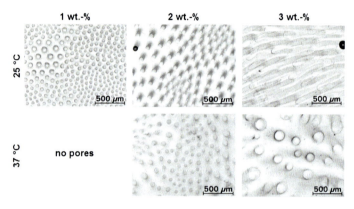

**Figure 6.6** Influence of temperature and alginate concentration on pore formation by ionotropic gelation: no parallel but radial pore formation for high concentration and low temperature as well as no channel-like pores at low concentration and high temperature.

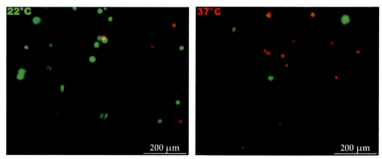

**Figure 6.7** Live/dead staining of human mesenchymal stem cells (hMSC) embedded into chondral layer: More viable hMSC in alginate/hyaluronic acid composite after structure formation by ionotropic gelation at room (22°C) compared to body temperature (37°C) imaged after 24 h (cLSM, green: living cells, red: dead cells, courtesy of Thomas Hanke (TU Dresden)).

## 6.3 Biphasic Alginate-Based Scaffolds with Channel-Like Pores

For the treatment of osteochondral defects, biphasic scaffolds should be developed that are structurally adapted to both tissues. Since the self-healing capacity of cartilage tissue is low, cells were embedded into the respective scaffold layer to enhance regeneration. The channel-like pores can help to guide cell migration from the blood or the underlying bone into the scaffold. Biphasic but monolithic scaffolds based on alginate were generated by superposing several alginate-based layers of different composition (Fig. 6.1).

The parallel aligned pores were generated by ionotropic gelation of alginate and entirely run through the whole length of biphasic scaffolds without being stopped or kinked at the interface (Fig. 6.8). Within the transparent chondral layer, pores are visible to the naked eye. The bony layer appears white because of the ceramic powder that is incorporated. In the cross section, the pores can easily be located. The distance between two pores is small enough that cells embedded in the matrix will be closer than 200 µm to the next channel which is the distance above cells might suffer from oxygen and nutrient shortage [56, 57]. Therefore, nutrient supply for the embedded cells should be facilitated even for the 2–3 mm thick chondral layer. The pore structure was generated by the optimised concentration of 0.4 M CaCl$_2$ solution.

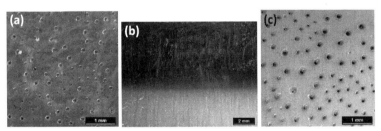

Figure 6.8 Macro-structure of biphasic but monolithic alginate-based hydrogel scaffolds with parallel aligned pore channels based on alginate/hyaluronate for the chondral and alginate/HAP for the osseous layer. (a) Chondral layer with circular entrance to the pore channels. (b) Longitudinal section showing perfect run of parallel pores passing interface unhindered. (c) Osseous layer with whitish appearance due to presence of hydroxyapatite.

The higher concentration of 1 M CaCl$_2$ will enable even denser pore arrangement; however, this was found less beneficial for cell viability and vice versa for 0.1 M CaCl$_2$ [18].

### 6.3.1 Components of the Biphasic Scaffolds beyond Alginate

The macro-structure of parallel aligned pores was generated by the biopolymer alginate (Fig. 6.1). In the present study, highly purified alginate especially suitable for cell embedding was applied compared to former studies [45, 54], in which food-grade alginate was used. Alginate molecules build a hydrogel, a network of molecules gelled by calcium ions (Fig. 6.9, left) even in low mass percentage. Likewise in natural tissues, fibrils that are embedded in a matrix will improve mechanical properties and might act as templates to govern tissue growth [58].

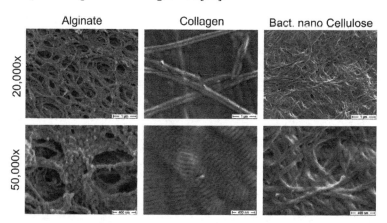

**Figure 6.9** Biopolymers used in the study as raw material (scanning electron microscopy).

The most abundant structural protein in vertebrates is collagen. The equine collagen type I (Opocrin, Italy) used here was delivered as a paste in acetic acid at pH 3.5. Thick collagen fibrils were found after rinsing and raising the pH to a neutral value (Fig. 6.9, centre). The fibrillogenesis of this type of collagen in acetic acid solution can also be controlled together with an in situ mineralisation [59]. It has been also processed to generate magnetic scaffolds [60] or multi-layered composite materials for osteochondral repair [61]. Its equine origin circumvents the risk of transmission of infectious agents causing bovine spongiform encephalopathy (BSA) from bovine or Creutzfeldt Jakob Disease (CJD) from ovine material and provide a greater acceptance compared to collagen of bovine or porcine origin due to some religious beliefs. Collagen was added to the chondral part of the biphasic alginate-based hydrogels in order to ameliorate mechanical properties and to act as binding site for living cells.

Hyaluronic acid (Fluka) was used as second component in the chondral part for this biomimetic approach because it is part of articular cartilage ECM and synovial fluid. It is capable to bind water and when squeezed out, the negatively charged functional groups generate repulsive forces which result in improved mechanical properties in compression.

Bacterial nano-cellulose (BNC) is a very versatile tool [62]. It was produced by Müller et al. as described in [63] and delivered as an autoclaved paste (Fig. 6.9, right) which has never been dried in any process step prior to scaffold fabrication (besides microstructural investigations by SEM). Those BNC had been also investigated as scaffold for cartilage tissue engineering after generating of pores of 20 to 30 µm in width and 50 to 70 µm in length by ice templating [64].

Bone ECM mainly consists of the protein collagen type I and calcium deficient carbonated hydroxyapatite. Since the calcium phosphate phase HAP resembles the mineral phase of natural bone, synthetic ceramic HAP powder (Merck, Germany) was used as particle reinforcement in the bony part. It exhibits an average particle size of 2.3 µm and a crystallite size of 22 nm [46].

In order to embed living cells, all components and processing had to be sterile. The components in form of powders (alginate, hyaluronic acid, HAP) were autoclaved by steam (121°C, 2 bar, 20 min). Bacterial nano-cellulose was delivered as already autoclaved paste. Collagen in soluble form was delivered in acetic acid which was rinsed out followed by disinfection with ethanol. The gelling agent calcium chloride was filtered through a sterile filter.

## 6.3.2 Macro- and Microstructure of Alginate Scaffolds Including Fibres

In order to understand the influence of the fibril components on structure formation and mechanical properties (stiffness), monophasic hydrogels composed of the individual layers likewise occurring in biphasic scaffold were produced first. The sterilely produced composites were based on 1.4 wt.-% of alginate. The sols were gelled by 1 M $CaCl_2$. Either collagen (chondral) or bacterial nano-cellulose (osseous part) were used as reinforcing fibrils.

Channel-like pores could only be generated by minor additions of fibrillar components to the predominant alginate which was up to 0.09 wt.-% of collagen and 0.05 wt.-% BNC, respectively. By using higher amounts of the fibril components, no macroscopic pores were found. The amount of collagen did not affect the diameter of the pores. All variants exhibited a mean pore diameter of 83 ± 31 μm (Fig. 6.10). However, pore density decreased with increasing collagen content. For the highest amount of collagen used here, pore density was only half as high as in the control without collagen addition, namely 19 compared to 38 pores/mm$^2$. The same trend holds for the incorporation of BNC into monophasic alginate/HAP scaffold designated for the use as bony part (1.4 and 4 wt.-% respectively, gelled by 1 M $CaCl_2$). Pore diameter was rarely affected by the presence of BNC but the density is decreasing with increasing fibril content. So 25 pores/mm$^2$ were found in gels without any BNC but only 10 pores/mm$^2$ in gels containing 0.03 wt.-% of BNC. However, in the application of biphasic scaffolds the pore pattern is determined by the upper part which gets first into contact with the gelling electrolyte. In our technology this is represented by the chondral part. Nevertheless, the length of the pores and their continuance depend on the composition of the gel.

The fibrils became incorporated inside the hydrogel network of alginate (Fig. 6.11, upper right). The long and thicker fibrils of collagen could be well distinguished in the fine entangled alginate network. The very tiny BNC fibrils were only indirectly detectable as elongated structures inside the alginate network. These structures presumably represent the coarser BNC fibrils which are well covered by alginate (Fig. 6.11, lower right).

*Biphasic Alginate-Based Scaffolds with Channel-Like Pores* | 161

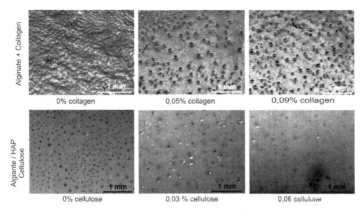

**Figure 6.10** Pore structure and arrangement for monophasic alginate composite hydrogels consisting of 1.4 wt.-% alginate and reinforcing components in different amounts (cross sections, light microscopy), top: alginate and collagen, bottom: alginate and HAP powder and cellulose.

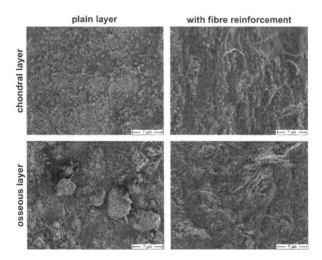

**Figure 6.11** Microstructure of chondral (top) and osseous (bottom) layers; plain (left) or with (right) fibrillar component collagen or BNC, respectively (SEM).

The long and stiff fibrils as well as the good interaction between the biopolymers might be the reason for the limited generation of channel-like pores during directed ionotropic gelation. They hinder the convection movement in front of the gelling zone and decelerate the contraction velocity of the alginate molecules as described by the model of dissipative structure formation developed by Kohler et al. [50].

### 6.3.3 Mechanical Strengthening by Fibre Reinforcement of Alginate Based Scaffolds

Compression tests were carried out with an Instron 5566 testing machine at a constant deformation rate of 3% per seconds to evaluate the influence of fibril content on stiffness. The addition of collagen as well as BNC leads to an increase of stiffness (Fig. 6.12)

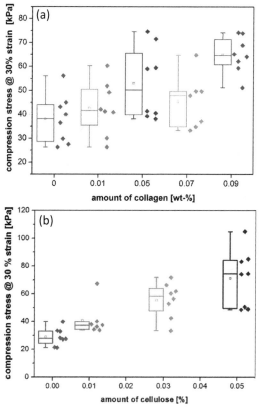

**Figure 6.12**  Compressive stress of chondral and bony layer depending on fibril content: Increase in strength due to incorporation of fibrils into respective layers based on alginate (1.4 wt.-%, gelled by 1 M $CaCl_2$): influence of incorporation of collagen into the chondral layer (top) and BNC into the osseous layer with HAP as mineral phase (bottom).

as measured by the compression stress at 30% strain. The change in stiffness of the alginate-based composites was twice as high if collagen and even slightly more when cellulose was incorporated as fibril component.

Schinagl et al. measured a gradual change in compressive modulus between 0.079 MPa and 2.1 MPa in articular cartilage from superficial to deep zone [4]. By incorporation of 0.09% collagen or 0.05% BNC, respectively, therefore, the lower range of the reported values was met. Collagen fibrils are hierarchically ordered in articular cartilage and thus a better arrangement of the fibrils in the alginate-based hydrogels would be beneficial. However, the average compression modulus of a full-thickness cartilage cylinder was reported to be 380 kPa. Therefore, the absolute value of our material even after fibril incorporation is still lower. Mauck et al. reported on 277 kPa for cartilage tissue [3]. Those authors found a doubling of Young's modulus within 2 weeks of cultivation of chondrocytes embedded in an agarose gel due to matrix production. Thus the embedding of cells into the alginate scaffolds followed by matrix production might also lead to an increase of stiffness over time.

## 6.3.4 Evaluation of Cytocompatibility

In a first approach, the suitability of the fibre-reinforced scaffolds should be evaluated by means of in vitro investigations. First, an indirect cytocompatibility test was performed with monophasic hydrogels of the respective layer: Cells that adhere to tissue culture plastic were cultivated in media which had been exposed to the material before for 1 or 7 days. In a second step, cells were embedded into the chondral part of the biphasic scaffold and cultivated for 3 weeks. In both cases, cell number was analysed by measurement of the activity of cytosolic lactate dehydrogenase (LDH).

### 6.3.4.1 Evaluation of cytocompatibility by indirect exposure

Monophasic scaffolds were prepared in saline buffer solution to adapt them to the physiologic environment and need of cells. Bicarbonate buffer or DMEM were used to ensure the right salinity; however, solutions did not contain any calcium ions to

**164** | *Fibre-Reinforced, Biphasic Composite Scaffolds*

avoid gelation of the alginate sol during preparation. Collagen and BNC were incorporated in the chondral or osseous part, respectively. The compositions are shown in Table 6.1.

**Table 6.1** Composition of monophasic scaffolds used for cytocompatibility testing, with or without additional fibrillar biopolymers

| | Chondral part | | | Osseous part | | | Electrolyte | Buffer |
|---|---|---|---|---|---|---|---|---|
| | Alginate wt.-% | Col | HYA | Alginate wt.-% | HAP | BNC | CaCl$_2$ | Dispersed in |
| Chondral with Col /buffer | 1.0 | 0.05 | 0.05 | | | | 0.1 M | BIC |
| Chondral with Col/ DMEM | 1.0 | 0.05 | 0.05 | | | | 0.1 M | DMEM |
| Chondral w/o Col | 1 | | 0.05 | | | | 0.1 M | DMEM |
| Osseous with BNC | | | | 1.0 | 4 | 0.05 | 0.1 M | DMEM |
| Osseous w/o BNC | | | | 1.0 | 4 | | 0.1 M | DMEM |

The increase in cell number from day 1 to day 7 indicated that all components were cytocompatible (Fig. 6.13), i.e. the composites did not release substances in sufficient amounts that negatively influence cell proliferation or bind or change essential components of cell culture media. Human MSC cultivated on tissue culture plastic with media which have been exposed to scaffolds of osseous composition with and without BNC showed a comparable cell number after 7 days of cultivation. Their behaviour was similar to cells which were cultivated in fresh medium (DMEM with 9% foetal calf serum (FCS) and 1% penicillin/streptomycin (P/S)). Higher increase in cell number was observed for cells which obtained media from preincubated scaffolds of chondral compositions. There was no difference whether or not the fibril components, i.e. collagen or bacterial nano-cellulose were present, thus no toxic effect was found by addition of those components.

The scaffolds of chondral composition basically consisted of alginate and hyaluronic acid but varied in the amount of added collagen. The beneficial effect on cell proliferation was observed for all chondral scaffold variants—independent of whether collagen was present or not. Thus, a possible explanation might be that hyaluronic acid has been partly leached out and has increased the proliferation of hMSC. Coates et al. reported on beneficial effects of hyaluronic acid on chondrocytes like binding via the CD44 receptor, enhanced proliferation as well as support of chondrogenic differentiation of MSC [65]. Kawasaki et al. showed an increase of proliferation by the factor of two of chondrocytes embedded in a collagen matrix when 0.1% hyaluronic acid was administered to the cell culture media [66].

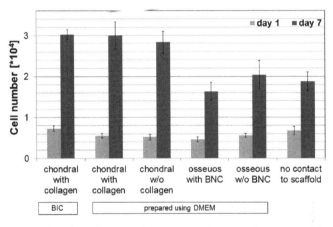

**Figure 6.13** Results of cytotoxicity assay: Increase in cell number for cells (analyzed by cytosolic LDH activity of hMSC) cultivated with media that has been exposed to differently composed scaffolds. Higher increase of cell number from day 1 to day 7 after contact to chondral (alginate and hyaluronic acid with or without collagen) compared to osseous (alginate and hydroxyapatite with or without BNC) composition or even with fresh media (without being in contact to scaffolds). One type of scaffold was prepared using bicarbonate buffered saline as dispersing media, and for all others DMEM was used.

The material designed for implantation into the bony part led to a similar behaviour like the reference, indicating that the ceramic material did not release any cytotoxic or absorb any substances essential for cell growth. Furthermore, cell growth studied in the indirect exposure test seemed not to be influenced by the different saline dispersing media used for the preparation of the alginate sol (BIC versus DMEM).

## 6.3.4.2 Generation of cell-laden scaffolds with embedded stem cells and long-term analysis of cell viability

As a compromise between pore structure formation, mechanical properties and considerations of cytocompatibility, four scaffold candidates were chosen for embedding of cells in combination with fibril components (Table 6.2). They must be biocompatible for cell embedding and all exhibit parallel pores running through the entire height of the scaffold.

**Table 6.2**  Composition of biphasic scaffolds for evaluation of behaviour of embedded hMSC over a period of 21 days

| | Chondral part (wt.-%) | | | Osseous part (wt.-%) | | | Electrolyte | Buffer |
|---|---|---|---|---|---|---|---|---|
| | Alginate | Col | HYA | Alginate | HAP | BNC | $CaCl_2$ | Dispersed in |
| **A** High conc. | 1.4 | 0.09 | 0.09 | 1.4 | 4 | 0.05 | 0.4 M | BIC |
| **B** Low conc. BIC | 1 | 0.05 | 0.05 | 1.0 | 4 | 0.05 | 0.1 M | BIC |
| **C** Low conc. DMEM | 1 | 0.05 | 0.05 | 1.0 | 4 | 0.05 | 0.1 M | DMEM |
| **D** No collagen | 1 | 0 | 0.05 | 1.0 | 4 | 0.05 | 0.1 M | DMEM |

Biphasic scaffolds consisted of alginate/hyaluronic acid and alginate/HAP for the chondral and the bony layer, respectively, in order to incorporate components of the target tissue type (composition depicted in Table 6.2). The composite scaffolds differed in concentration of components and electrolyte (low and high biopolymer and calcium chloride concentration) and dispersing media (BIC vs. DMEM) to generate looser or denser structures and softer or stiffer hydrogels. Collagen was chosen for the chondral and BNC for the osseous part of the scaffold as reinforcement, because BNC improved stiffness and collagen might additionally support adhesion and behaviour of embedded cells. Cytocompatibility of preparation conditions are to be assessed by the help of the four candidates as follows. Several tests have been carried out to find the best formulation in presence of fibre components where parallel aligned pores were still generated (Fig. 6.14) even using low calcium ion concentration, since usage of 1 M CaCl$_2$, most suitable, most suitable for structure formation, has been shown to hinder cell proliferation in another study [18].

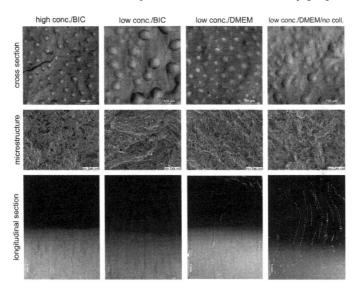

**Figure 6.14** Morphology of biphasic fibre-reinforced scaffolds chosen for cell embedding. Longitudinal sections of the entire height of the biphasic scaffolds exhibiting both parts (upper: chondral/transparent and lower: bony part/white due to the ceramic powder). Cross-sections as well as SEM images representing chondral layers. For information about composition of the different scaffolds please refer to Table 6.2.

Thus, all scaffold candidates were biphasic with pore channels running through the entire height of the biphasic scaffold. Their average pore diameters varied between 122 µm, > 231 µm, 118 µm to 169 µm (following the arrangement of the scaffolds in Fig. 6.14—from left to right; ca. 27% rel. error) and pore density was 13 ± 3 or 5 ± 3 pores/mm². These macropores should be supportive for nutrient supply to the cells.

Human MSC were suspended in the alginate-based sol of chondral composition and were embedded into the hydrogel during ionotropic gelation using optimised preparation conditions. The macro pore structure, mechanical properties and cytocompatibility were considered (see above). The embedded cells were metabolically active over the cultivation time of 21 days (Fig. 6.15). They could be stained by MTT where a yellow tetrazolium salt is converted into a dark blue/purple formazan derivative by mitochondrial dehydrogenases of living cells.

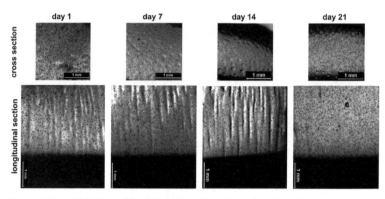

**Figure 6.15** Viability of hMSC embedded into the chondral part during long-term cultivation by means of MTT staining: Homogeneous distribution of cells (MTT stained living hMSC as dark dots in transparent layer) embedded in the chondral part of a biphasic scaffold (bony opaque layer at the bottom in longitudinal sections) and observed over a period of 3 weeks in vitro. Biphasic scaffolds were prepared from alginate and addition of 0.05% collagen as well as hyaluronic acid for the chondral layer and 4% HAP as well as 0.05% BNC for the bony layer dispersed in DMEM and gelled by 0.1 M CaCl$_2$ (according to type C in Table 6.2).

They were homogeneously distributed through the chondral part of the biphasic scaffolds as observed in cross (squared images on top) as well as in longitudinal (rectangular images at the bottom) sections. Besides the survival of cells and their uniform distribution in the alginate-based matrix, the images nicely prove the pore channel formation which had also occurred in presence of cells. The channel-like pores could be well distinguished as circles in cross sections and lines in longitudinal sections. The distance between pores is below 400 µm which is twice the 200 µm that Folkman and Hochberg reported being essential for oxygen supply to cells [56, 67].

During 21 days of cultivation, the number and density of viable cells observed by microscopy remained constant. However, biochemical analyses of the cell number provided different results, i.e. cell number decreased within the first week and remained on a constant level over the further time of cultivation (Fig. 6.16). Fedorovich et al. also described a decrease of cell viability between day 3 and 7 when MSC were embedded into solid, printed alginate scaffolds gelled by 102 mM $CaCl_2$ [68]. However, Duggal et al. reported on a constant cell number over cultivation time of 3 weeks at a level of 80% of the initially embedded hMSC in RGD-modified alginate [69]. We conducted experiments with embedding of hMSC but without fibre reinforcement and also found a decrease in cell number; however, cell number remained nearly constant when chondrogenic differentiation was induced by addition of supplements (ascorbic acid, dexamethasone, proline, transferrin, insulin, selenious acid, TGF-$\beta$) which resembled the behaviour of embedded human chondrocytes [18].

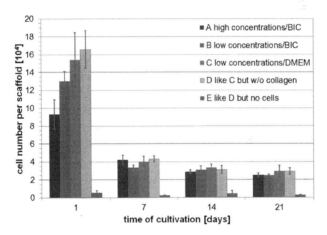

**Figure 6.16** Viability of embedded hMSC during cultivation for 3 weeks: decrease in cell number within first week; however, thereafter number remained constant up to third week independent of concentration of collagen (A–C vs. D) and bicarbonate buffered saline vs. DMEM (A, B vs. C, D).

Optical and biochemical analyses might be coupled to intrinsic variances that lead to discrepancies in observation. Slice thickness during cutting with a razor blade razor blade is hard to control and therefore number of stained cells might appear different in images derived from transmission microscopy. The activity of enzymes, known to be constantly expressed in 2D cell culture and used for quantification of cell number via a calibration curve, might also change when cells are embedded in a matrix and adapt themselves to the 3D environment. Finally, some assays tend to interfere with biopolymers or high salt concentration as it is still found at day 1 after scaffold generation with 400 mM compared to 2 mM as it is found in cell culture media. Thus interpretation needed to be carefully drawn.

In this light, the hMSC embedded into scaffolds of four different compositions exhibited a similar behaviour within the variation in cell number during cultivation for 21 days. The variance in pore diameter (118 to 231 µm) and density (5–13 pores/mm$^2$) did not seem to influence the behaviour of the cells under static cultivation conditions. The advantage of the embedding technology for tissue engineering is a high seeding efficiency. Here more than two third of the introduced cells (1.4 × 10$^5$ cells per scaffolds) were found viable in the scaffold after gelation and would be ready for implantation and thus, can be delivered for the treatment of an osteochondral defect.

## 6.4 Summary and Outlook

Biphasic, but monolithic scaffolds with parallel aligned pores were developed for the treatment of osteochondral defects. Besides the biopolymer alginate which gave rise to the fascinating anisotropic structure as well as the basic matrix properties, both layers additionally consisted of components of the respective tissue, i.e. hyaluronic acid and hydroxyapatite for the chondral and osseous part, respectively. Especially hyaluronic acid was found to be very beneficial for cell proliferation in a cytocompatibility assay. Fibrillar collagen and bacterial nano-cellulose were incorporated and the stiffness of the hydrogels was improved by this fibre reinforcement. The fibril content was limited, because the rigid fibres influence the gelation reaction and will stop formation of channel-like pores. Human mesenchymal stem cells were successfully embedded in the chondral layer to foster cartilage repair after their chondrogenic differentiation. The integration of fibrils and living cells was performed by translating the processing to fully sterile and cytocompatible conditions. The hMSC remained vital over three weeks of cultivation. The biocompatibility and performance of, first, the cell-free biphasic scaffolds with channel-like pores is now evaluated in an osteochondral defect model in sheep and histological analysis of explants is still ongoing. The advantage of the approach using this type of scaffolds by embedding of living cells and the incorporation of fibrillar components on the healing of osteochondral defects shall be evaluated in a future in vivo experiment.

## Acknowledgement

The authors want to thank Dr. Thomas Hanke for the characterisation of embedded hMSC via fluorescence imaging (cLSM). We would like to thank Marlen Eckert for preliminary experimental proof of principle in generating biphasic scaffolds. We gratefully acknowledge financial support received from the European Commission, project OPHIS (Grant no: FP7-NMP-2009-SMALL-3-246373).

## References

1. Park, S., Krishnan, R., Nicoll, S. B., and Ateshian, G. A. (2003). Cartilage interstitial fluid load support in unconfined compression. *J. Biomech.*, **36**, pp. 1785–1796.

2. Loparic, M., Wirz, D., Daniels, A. U., Raiteri, R., vanLandingham, M. R., Guex, G., Martin, I., Aebi, U., and Stolz, M. (2010). Micro- and nanomechanical analysis of articular cartilage by indentation-type atomic force microscopy: Validation with a gel-microfiber composite. *Biophys. J.*, **98**, pp. 2731–2740.

3. Mauck, R. L., Wang, C. C.-B., Oswald, E. S., Ateshian, G. A., and Hung, C. T. (2003). The role of cell seeding density and nutrient supply for articular cartilage tissue engineering with deformational loading. *Osteoarthritis Cartilage*, **11**, pp. 879–890.

4. Nooeaid, P., Salih, V., Beier, J. P., and Boccaccini, A. R. (2012). Osteochondral tissue engineering: Scaffolds, stem cells and applications. *J. Cell. Mol. Med.*, **16**, pp. 2247–2270.

5. Hunter, W. Of the structure and diseases of articulating cartilages (1742). *Philos. Trans. R. Soc. London*, **42**, pp. 514–521.

6. Getgood, A., Bhullar, T. P. S., and Rushton, N. (2009). Current concepts in articular cartilage repair. *Orthop. Trauma*, **23**, pp. 189–200.

7. Mano, J. F., and Reis, R. L. (2007). Osteochondral defects: Present situation and tissue engineering approaches. *J. Tissue Eng. Regen. Med.*, **1**, pp. 261–273.

8. Temenoff, J. S., and Mikos, A. G. (2000). Review: Tissue engineering for regeneration of articular cartilage. *Biomaterials*, **21**, pp. 431–440.

9. Pullig, O., Pfander, D., and Swoboda, B. (2001). Molekulare Grundlagen der Arthroseinduktion und -progression. *Orthopade*, **30**, pp. 825–833.

10. Schinagl, R. M., Gurskis, D., Chen, A. C., and Sah, R. L. (1997). Depth-dependent confined compression modulus of full-thickness bovine articular cartilage. *J. Orthop. Res.*, **15**, pp. 499–506.

11. Pullig, O. Zell- und molekularbiologische Grundlagen der humanen Arthrose (2003). *Akt. Rheumatol.*, **28**, pp. 308–315.

12. Khan, I. M., Gilbert, S. J., Singhrao, S. K., Duance, V. C. and Archer, C. W. (2008). Cartilage integration: Evaluation of the reasons for failure of integration during cartilage repair a review. *Eur. Cell. Mater.*, **16**, pp. 26–39.

13. Ahmed, T. A. E., and Hincke, M. T. (2009). Strategies for articular cartilage lesion repair and functional restoration. *Tissue Eng. Pt B Rev.*, **16**, pp. 305–329.

14. Mollon, B., Kandel, R., Chahal, J., and Theodoropoulos, J. (2013). The clinical status of cartilage tissue regeneration in humans. *Osteoarthritis Cartilage*, **21**, pp. 1824–1833.

15. Martin, I., Miot, S., Barbero, A., Jakob, M., and Wendt, D. (2007). Osteochondral tissue engineering. *J. Biomech.*, **40**, pp. 750–765.

16. Gelinsky, M., Eckert, M., and Despang, F. (2007). Biphasic, but monolithic scaffolds for the therapy of osteochondral defects. *Int. J. Mater. Res.*, **98**, pp. 749–755.

17. Tampieri, A., Sprio, S., Sandri, M., and Valentini, F. (2011). Mimicking natural bio-mineralization processes: A new tool for osteochondral scaffold development. *Trends Biotechnol.*, **29**, pp. 526–535.

18. Schütz, K., Despang, F., Lode, A., and Gelinsky, M. (2014). Cell-laden biphasic scaffolds with anisotropic structure mimic osteochondral tissue. *J. Tissue Eng. Regen. Med.* (in press, DOI:10.1002/term.1879).

19. Wenger, T. (1998). *Herstellung gerichtet-strukturierter Keramiken.* PhD thesis, Universität Regensburg.

20. Sabra, W., Zeng, A. P., and Deckwer, W. D. (2001). Bacterial alginate: Physiology, product quality and process aspects. *Appl. Microbiol. Biotechnol.*, **56**, pp. 315–325.

21. Zimmermann, H., Zimmermann, D., Reuss, R., Feilen, P. J., Manz, B., Katsen, A., Weber, M., Ihmig, F. R., Ehrhart, F., Gessner, P., Behringer, M., Steinbach, A. Wegner, L. H., Sukhorukov, V. L., Vasquez, J. A., Schneider, S., Weber, M. M., Volke, F., Wolf, R., and Zimmermann, U. (2005). Towards a medically approved technology for alginate-based

microcapsules allowing long-term immunoisolated transplantation. *J. Mater. Sci. Mater. Med.*, **16**, pp. 491–501.

22. Heinze, T., Klemm, D., Loth, F., and Philipp, B. (1990). Herstellung, Struktur und Anwendung von ionotropen Gelen aus carboxygruppenhaltigen Polysacchariden. Fortschrittsbericht. *Acta Polym.*, **41**, pp. 259–269.

23. Grasdalen, H., Larsen, B., and Smidsrød, O. (1979). A p.m.r. study of the composition and sequence of uronate residues in alginates. *Carbohydr. Res.*, **68**, pp. 23–31.

24. Rhim, J.-W., Lee, J.-H., and Hong, S.-I. (2006). Water resistance and mechanical properties of biopolymer (alginate and soy protein) coated paperboards. *LWT-Food Sci. Technol.*, **39**, pp. 806–813.

25. Andersson, C. (2008). New ways to enhance the functionality of paperboard by surface treatment: A review. *Packag. Technol. Sci.*, **21**, pp. 339–373.

26. Rinaudo, M. (2008). Main properties and current applications of some polysaccharides as biomaterials. *Polym. Int.*, **57**, pp. 397–430.

27. Orive, G., Carcaboso, A. M., Hernández, R. M., Gascón, A. R., and Pedraz, J. L. (2005). Biocompatibility evaluation of different alginates and alginate-based microcapsules. *Biomacromolecules*, **6**, pp. 927–931.

28. Zimmermann, H., Ehrhart, F., Zimmermann, D., Müller, K., Katsen-Globa, A., Behringer, M., Feilen, P. J., Gessner, P., Zimmermann, G., Shirley, S. G., Weber, M. M., Metze, J., and Zimmermann, U. (2007). Hydrogel-based encapsulation of biological, functional tissue: Fundamentals, technologies and applications. *Appl. Phys. A Mater. Sci.*, **89**, pp. 909–922.

29. Zimmermann, U., Klock, G., Federlin, K., Hannig, K., Kowalski, M., Bretzel, R. G., Horcher, A., Entenmann, H., Sieber, U., and Zekorn, T. (1992). Production of mitogen-contamination free alginates with variable ratios of mannuronic acid to guluronic acid by free flow electrophoresis. *Electrophoresis*, **13**, pp. 269–74.

30. Yamaoka, H., Asato, H., Ogasawara, T., Nishizawa, S., Takahashi, T., Nakatsuka, T., Koshima, I., Nakamura, K., Kawaguchi, H., Chung, U., Takato, T., and Hoshi, K. (2006). Cartilage tissue engineering using human auricular chondrocytes embedded in different hydrogel materials. *J. Biomed. Mater. Res. A*, **78**, pp. 1–11.

31. Gerard, C., Catuogno, C., Amargier-Huin, C., Grossin, L., Hubert, P., Gillet, P., Netter, P., Dellacherie, E., and Payan, E. (2005). The effect of alginate, hyaluronate and hyaluronate derivatives biomaterials on synthesis of non-articular chondrocyte extracellular matrix. *J. Mater. Sci. Mater. Med.*, **16**, pp. 541–551.

32. Balakrishnan, B., Mohanty, M., Fernandez, A. C., Mohanan, P. V., and Jayakrishnan, A. (2006). Evaluation of the effect of incorporation of dibutyryl cyclic adenosine monophosphate in an in situ-forming hydrogel wound dressing based on oxidized alginate and gelatin. *Biomaterials*, **27**, pp. 1355–1361.

33. Nakamura, S., Arai, Y., Takahashi, K. A., Terauchi, R., Ohashi, S., Mazda, O., Imanishi, J., Inoue, A., Tonomura, H., and Kubo, T. (2006). Hydrostatic pressure induces apoptosis of chondrocytes cultured in alginate beads. *J. Orthop. Res.*, **24**, pp. 733–739.

34. Wang, M., Childs, R. F., and Chang, P. I. (2005). A novel method to enhance the stability of alginate-poly-L-lysine-alginate microcapsules. *J. Biomater. Sci. Polym. Edn*, **16**, pp. 91–113.

35. Frampton, J. P., Hynd, M. R., Williams, J. C., Shuler, M. L., and Shain, W. (2007). Three-dimensional hydrogel cultures for modeling changes in tissue impedance around microfabricated neural probes. *J. Neural Eng.*, **4**, pp. 399–409.

36. Gombotz, W. R., and Wee, S.-F. (1998). Protein release from alginate matrices. *Adv. Drug Deliv. Rev.*, **31**, pp. 267–285.

37. Dai, C., Wang, B., Zhao, H., Li, B., and Wang, J. (2006). Preparation and characterization of liposomes-in-alginate (LIA) for protein delivery system. *Colloids Surf. B*, **47**, pp. 205–210.

38. Kim, D. H., and Martin, D. C. (2006). Sustained release of dexamethasone from hydrophilic matrices using PLGA nanoparticles for neural drug delivery. *Biomaterials*, **27**, pp. 3031–3037.

39. Freeman, I., and Cohen, S. (2009). The influence of the sequential delivery of angiogenic factors from affinity-binding alginate scaffolds on vascularization. *Biomaterials*, **30**, pp. 2122–2131.

40. Hashimoto, T., Suzuki, Y., Suzuki, K., Nakashima, T., Tanihara, M., and Ide, C. (2005). Review Peripheral nerve regeneration using non-tubular alginate gel crosslinked with covalent bonds. *J. Mater. Sci. Mater. Med.*, **16**, pp. 503–509.

41. Prang, P., Müller, R., Eljaouhari, A., Heckmann, K., Kunz, W., Weber, T., Faber, C., Vroemen, M., Bogdahn, U., and Weidner, N. (2006). The promotion of oriented axonal regrowth in the injured spinal cord by alginate-based anisotropic capillary hydrogels. *Biomaterials*, **27**, pp. 3560–3569.

42. Pawar, K., Müller, R., Caioni, M., Prang, P., Bogdahn, U., Kunz, W., and Weidner, N. (2011). Increasing capillary diameter and the incorporation of gelatin enhance axon outgrowth in alginate-based anisotropic hydrogels. *Acta Biomater.*, **7**, pp. 2826–2834.

43. Yamamoto, M., James, D., Li, H., Butler, J., Rafii, S., and Rabbany, S. Y. (2010). Generation of stable co-cultures of vascular cells in a honeycomb alginate scaffold. *Tissue Eng. Part A*, **16**, pp. 299–308.

44. Despang, F., Börner, A., Dittrich, R., Tomandl, G., Pompe, W., and Gelinsky, M. (2005). Alginate/calcium phosphate scaffolds with oriented, tube-like pores. *Materwiss. Werksttech.*, **36**, pp. 761–767.

45. Bernhardt, A., Despang, F., Lode, A. Demmler, A., Hanke, T., and Gelinsky, M. (2009). Proliferation and osteogenic differentiation of human bone marrow stromal cells on alginate-gelatine-hydroxyapatite scaffolds with anisotropic pore structure. *J. Tissue Eng. Regen. Med.*, **3**, pp. 54–62.

46. Despang, F., Bernhardt, A. Lode, A., Dittrich, R., Hanke, T., Shenoy, S. J., Mani, S., and Gelinsky, M. (2013). Synthesis, physico-chemical and in vitro/vivo evaluation of an anisotropic, nano-crystalline hydroxyapatite bisque scaffold with parallel aligned pores mimicking the microstructure of cortical bone. *J. Tissue Eng. Regen. Med.*, (DOI: 10.1002/term.1729).

47. Khairou, K. S., Al-Gethami, W. M., and Hassan, R. M. (2002). Kinetics and mechanism of sol-gel transformation between sodium alginate polyelectrolyte and some heavy divalent metal ions with formation of capillary structure polymembranes ionotropic gels. *J. Membr. Sci.*, **209**, pp. 445–456.

48. Thiele, H. (1964). Ordnen von Fadenmolekülen durch Ionendiffusion-ein Prinzip der Strukturbildung. *Protoplasma*, **58**, pp. 318–341.

49. Kohler, H.-H., and Thumbs, J. (1995). Wo kommen die Kapillaren im Alginatgel her? *Chem. Ing. Tech.*, **67**, pp. 489–492.

50. Treml, H., Woelki, S., and Kohler, H.-H. (2003). Theory of capillary formation in alginate gels. *Chem. Phys.*, **293**, pp. 341–353.

51. Maneval, J. E., Bernin, D., Fabich, H. T., Seymour, J. D., and Codd, S. L. (2011). Magnetic resonance analysis of capillary formation reaction front dynamics in alginate gels. *Magn. Reson. Chem.*, **49**, pp. 627–640.

52. Despang, F., Dittrich, R., and Gelinsky, M. (2011). Novel biomaterials with parallel aligned pore channels by directed ionotropic gelation of alginate: Mimicking the anisotropic structure of bone tissue, in *Advances in Biomimetics*, Chapter 17 (InTech, Rijeka, Croatia), pp. 349–372.

53. Thiele, H., and Hallich, K. (1957). Kapillarstrukturen in ionotropen Gelen. *Colloid Polym. Sci.*, **151**, pp. 1–12.

54. Dittrich, R., Despang, F., Bernhardt, A., Hanke, T., Tomandl, G., Pompe, W., and Gelinsky, M. (2007). Scaffolds for hard tissue engineering

by ionotropic gelation of alginate-influence of selected preparation parameters. *J. Am. Ceram. Soc.*, **90**, pp. 1703–1708.

55. Matyash, M., Despang, F., Ikonomidou, C., and Gelinsky, M. (2014). Swelling and mechanical properties of alginate hydrogels with respect to promotion of neural growth. *Tissue Eng. Pt C Meth.*, **20**, pp. 401–411.

56. Folkman, J., and Hochberg, M. (1973). Self-regulation of growth in three dimensions. *J. Exp. Med.*, **138**, pp. 745–753.

57. Carmeliet, P., and Jain, R. K. (2000). Angiogenesis in cancer and other diseases. *Nature*, **407**, pp. 249–257.

58. Bar-On, B., and Wagner, H. D. (2012). Elastic modulus of hard tissues. *J. Biomech.*, **45**, pp. 672–678.

59. Tampieri, A., Celotti, G., Landi, E., Sandri, M., Roveri, N., and Falini, G. (2003). Biologically inspired synthesis of bone-like composite: Self-assembled collagen fibers/hydroxyapatite nanocrystals. *J. Biomed. Mater. Res. A*, **67**, pp. 618–625.

60. Bock, N., Riminucci, A., Dionigi, C., Russo, A., Tampieri, A., Landi, E., Goranov, V. A., Marcacci, M., and Dediu, V. (2010). A novel route in bone tissue engineering: Magnetic biomimetic scaffolds. *Acta Biomater.*, **6**, pp. 786–796.

61. Tampieri, A., Sandri, M., Landi, E., Pressato, D., Francioli, S., Quarto, R., and Martin, I. (2008). Design of graded biomimetic osteochondral composite scaffolds. *Biomaterials*, **29**, pp. 3539–3546.

62. Klemm, D., Heublein, B., Fink, H.-P., and Bohn, A. (2005). Cellulose: Fascinating biopolymer and sustainable raw material. *Angew. Chem. Int. Ed.*, **44**, pp. 3358–3393.

63. Wesarg, F., Schlott, F., Grabow, J., Kurland, H.-D., Hessler, N., Kralisch, D., and Müller, F. A. (2012). In situ synthesis of photocatalytically active hybrids consisting of bacterial nanocellulose and anatase nanoparticles. *Langmuir*, **28**, pp. 13518–13525.

64. Flauder, S., Heinze, T., and Müller, F. A. (2014). Cellulose scaffolds with an aligned and open porosity fabricated via ice-templating. *Cellulose*, **21**, pp. 97–103.

65. Coates, E. E., Riggin, C. N., and Fisher, J. P. (2013). Photocrosslinked alginate with hyaluronic acid hydrogels as vehicles for mesenchymal stem cell encapsulation and chondrogenesis. *J. Biomed. Mater. Res. Pt A*, **101**, pp. 1962–1970.

66. Kawasaki, K., Ochi, M., Uchio, Y., Adachi, N., and Matsusaki, M. (1999). Hyaluronic acid enhances proliferation and chondroitin sulfate

synthesis in cultured chondrocytes embedded in collagen gels. *J. Cell Physiol.*, **179**, pp. 142–148.

67. Laschke, M. W., Harder, Y., Amon, M., Martin, I., Farhadi, J., Ring, A., Torio-Padron, N., Schramm, R., Rücker, M., Junker, D., Häufel, J. M., Carvalho, C., Heberer, M., Germann, G., Vollmar, B., and Menger, M. D. (2006). Angiogenesis in tissue engineering: Breathing life into constructed tissue substitutes. *Tissue Eng.*, **12**, pp. 2093–2104.

68. Fedorovich, N. E., Kuipers, E., Gawlitta, D., Dhert, W. J. A., and Alblas, J. (2011). Scaffold porosity and oxygenation of printed hydrogel constructs affect functionality of embedded osteogenic progenitors. *Tissue Eng. Pt A*, **17**, pp. 2473–2486.

69. Duggal, S., Fronsdal, K. B., Szöke, K., Shahdadfar, A., Melvik, J. E., and Brinchmann, J. E. (2009). Phenotype and gene expression of human mesenchymal stem cells in alginate scaffolds. *Tissue Eng. Pt A*, **15**, pp. 1763–1773.

# Chapter 7

# Hybrid Nanocomposites with Magnetic Activation for Advanced Bone Tissue Engineering

Ugo D'Amora,[a] Teresa Russo,[a] Roberto De Santis,[a] Antonio Gloria,[a] and Luigi Ambrosio[a,b]

[a]Institute of Polymers, Composites and Biomaterials,
National Research Council of Italy,
Viale J. F. Kennedy 54, Mostra d'Oltremare, Pad. 20, 80125 Naples, Italy
[b]Department of Chemical Science and Materials Technology,
National Research Council of Italy,
Piazzale A. Moro 7, 00185 Rome, Italy

rosantis@unina.it

This chapter deals with recent and innovative approaches in the field of bone tissue regeneration. After a brief introduction on tissue engineering, bone biology and on the traditional strategies currently adopted in the field of bone repair, the chapter focuses on the applications of hybrid magnetic nanocomposite materials in bioengineering and regenerative medicine, as well as on the design, preparation and characterization of three-dimensional (3D) magnetic scaffolds obtained through innovative rapid prototyping technologies such as 3D fiber deposition

---

*Bio-Inspired Regenerative Medicine: Materials, Processes, and Clinical Applications*
Edited by Simone Sprio and Anna Tampieri
Copyright © 2016 Pan Stanford Publishing Pte. Ltd.
ISBN 978-981-4669-14-6 (Hardcover), 978-981-4669-15-3 (eBook)
www.panstanford.com

technique, which offers the fascinating opportunity to develop morphologically controlled structures with tailored mechanical and mass transport properties.

Over the past years, the basic principles of magnetism and magnetic materials have been widely used in many interesting medical applications such as drug and gene delivery, hyperthermia treatment of tumors and radionuclide therapy, magneto-mechanical stimulation or activation of cell-constructs and mechanosensitive ion channels, magnetic cell-seeding procedures and controlled cell proliferation and differentiation. The possibility to extend these concepts to tissue engineering has opened an exciting wide research area of interest. Magnetic scaffolds should be considered as a potential alternative to bone graft substitutes with attractive new performances; they can be manipulated by means of magnetic force gradients in order to attract magnetized cells, increasing scaffold-cell loading efficiency, or bioaggregates (i.e., vascular endothelial growth factor, VEGF), stimulating angiogenesis and bone regeneration, they can also be employed as hyperthermia agents able to deliver thermal energy to targeted bodies (i.e., tumors) or as devices in chemotherapy or radiotherapy. Finally, the possibility to employ magnetic forces for achieving an efficient scaffold fixation is also briefly discussed.

## 7.1  Introduction

Tissue engineering and regenerative medicine is a rapidly expanding field of research that aims to create tissue substitutes of blood vessels, heart, nerves, muscle, cartilage, bone, and other organs for the replacement of damaged tissues. A fascinating aspect of this multidisciplinary field is the fundamental need to employ principles from biology, chemistry, materials science, medicine, clinical research, and mechanical engineering in the design and development of new analogs with the goal of creating new tissues and organs that can grow with the patient, without causing adverse reactions [1, 2].

In the last two decades, researchers focused on scaffolds as natural and synthetic porous structures that can temporarily support cell growth and release biological factors. In these terms, a scaffold may act as a temporary extracellular matrix (ECM) during the process of new tissue growth [3, 4].

Two important strategies are usually adopted in tissue engineering. A first approach is based on the in vitro use of a synthetic three-dimensional (3D) cell-seeded scaffold, which acts as a template and stimulus for tissue regeneration, and on the implantation of this cell-construct into the patient. In vivo degradation mechanisms lead to the formation of nontoxic products, consequently allowing cells to produce their own ECM. On the other hand, the in situ implantation of a bioresorbable scaffold into the defect site is the key feature of a second strategy, in which the body is used as its own bioreactor [5, 6].

Therefore, the design of scaffolds able to guide cells and tissue growth represents one of the most challenging goals of tissue engineering. An ideal scaffold should be characterized by suitable chemical, biochemical and biophysical cues and it should be able to promote specific events at cellular level; it should be possible to manufacture a scaffold into different shapes and size, finally it should not induce adverse reactions. Excellent biocompatibility, tailored biodegradability and/or bioresorbability, interconnected porous network and pore scale to promote tissue integration and/or vascularization, appropriate mechanical properties, adequate morphology and surface chemistry are important features that an ideal scaffold should necessarily exhibit [3, 7–10].

## 7.2 Bone Tissue Engineering

Bone and cartilage build up the skeletal system that provides mechanical support, protection of vital organs and a site of muscle attachment for locomotion. Bone is a dynamic, highly vascular, and mineralized connective tissue that ensures also as a mineral reservoir of calcium and phosphate. Bone behaves as a complex composite with unique remodeling properties that allows it to adapt its own microstructure to the external mechanical loads [7, 11, 12].

In the adult skeleton, bone tissue is arranged in two architectural forms: compact or cortical bone, and trabecular or cancellous bone (also called spongy bone). Compact bone, almost solid, can be found in long bones (i.e., femur and tibia), short bones (i.e., wrist and ankle), and flat bones (i.e., skull vault and irregular bones) [13–16]. On the other hand, spongy bone appears as a sponge-like, with a honeycomb of branching bars, plates and rods of various sizes called *trabeculae*. It is commonly found in metaphysis of long bones, covered by cortical bone, and in the vertebral bodies. If compared to cortical bone, it shows a higher porosity, modulus and ultimate compressive strength about 20 times lower [13–17].

Even though properties and structure of the bone can change according to the anatomical location, it is still possible to observe some similarities between bone types: Bone represents a hybrid hierarchical nanostructured composite wherein hydroxyapatite nanocrystals, the lowest mineral component at the nanoscale, are dispersed in an organic matrix predominantly composed of oriented collagen fibers. Furthermore, bone tissue needs the highest demand for tissue reconstruction and replacement [7, 11, 12], and elaboration, maintenance and resorption of bone tissue depend on the mutual interaction of three cell types: osteoblasts, osteocytes, and osteoclasts each one characterized by defined tasks and essential for the maintenance of a healthy bone tissue [18–22].

Over the past years, bone tissue engineering has attempted to mimic the natural process of bone repair by means of scaffolds suitably functionalized in order to release inductive growth and differentiation factors to support cell attachment, migration and proliferation [23].

The guiding process of bone regeneration is gaining extraordinary importance as an alternative treatment of bone defects, as an innovative strategy that employs neither synthetic prostheses nor bone grafts, the aim being to overcome the limitations of the current approaches. Synthetic prostheses partially restore large defects for a relatively short useful life. On the other hand, autologous bone graft is not always available in sufficient amounts. Bone allografts are expensive and present well-known risks of bacterial contamination, viral transmission and immunogenicity if compared to autologous bone grafts.

An ideal bone scaffold should possess all the above-mentioned properties, but the biomechanical environment introduces another level of complexity. The scaffold needs to be able to withstand external forces, and it is known that during bone regeneration, the remodeling is mediated by mechanical stimuli known as mechanotransduction. Through tissue engineering approaches, it would be possible to re-establish the full functionality of damaged tissues, with a relatively long regeneration time. Moreover, the temporal control of the various aspects of the tissue growth is very important to allow optimal clinical outcomes. In order to obtain a histomorphologically mature tissue, as bone, the restoration of the mechanical resistance to physiological stresses should be followed by *angiogenesis*, which is a crucial feature in the regenerative medicine approaches, since the vascularization of tissue-engineered structures is rapidly required.

Several biodegradable/bioresorbable polymers in combination with other materials as well as different fabrication methods (both conventional and nonconventional techniques) have been considered to make scaffolds for tissue engineering.

Synthetic polymers are characterized by higher flexibility and processability, as well as by tailored physicochemical, mechanical and degradation properties if compared to ceramic materials. Among all the biodegradable polymers, poly(lactic acid) (PLA), poly(glycolic acid) (PGA), their copolymer poly(lactic-co-glycolic acid) (PLGA), and poly($\varepsilon$-caprolactone) (PCL) are the most commonly used polymers in the field of tissue engineering. Conversely, if compared to polymeric materials, ceramic ones tended to be too brittle [7, 24, 25].

As a consequence, none of these materials used on their own can satisfy all the required goals, such as suitable fracture strength, toughness, stiffness, osteoinductivity/osteoconductivity, and in vitro and in vivo controlled rate of degradation [3].

To this aim, research attention has been focused on composite materials consisting of polymers reinforced with inorganic ceramic fillers. Therefore, the tailored combination of biomaterials to form "biocomposites" is being increasingly considered for the development of optimal scaffolds [3, 7, 26–29]. Typical biomaterials adopted in the field of bone tissue engineering include bioactive glasses, hydroxyapatite (HA), calcium phosphates such as tricalcium phosphate (TCP) and biphasic calcium phosphate (BCP) and calcium carbonates. Showing better osteoconductivity, they can be considered the inorganic reinforcing phase of the composite scaffold, wherein polymers (i.e., PCL, PLA, PGA, PLGA) represent the organic matrix [7]. In the recent years, much research has been driven towards the design and development of hybrid materials for bone and osteochondral tissue engineering, using different approaches [30–43].

Highly porous composite scaffolds consisting of PCL and stoichiometric HA particles have been developed through phase inversion and salt leaching techniques [44]. Results from mechanical tests highlighted that the presence of HA particles improves mechanical properties contemporarily enhancing the scaffold bioactivity and human osteoblast cell response, evidencing their role as "bioactive solid signals" in promoting surface mineralization and, consequently, suitable cell-material interactions [45].

3D porous PCL-based composite scaffolds were also manufactured through the combination of a filament winding technique and phase inversion/salt leaching process, using $\beta$-TCP particles and PLA fibers as two reinforcement systems. The effective synergistic influence of $\beta$-TCP bioactive particles and PLA fibers on the morphology and mechanical behavior of the composite scaffold as well as the interaction between the ceramic phase and the highly organized fiber-reinforced polymeric structure were assessed [46]. The mechanical performances ideal to maintain spaces required for cellular in-growth and extracellular matrix production were obtained through the inclusion of biodegradable PLA fibers into the PCL matrix. The addition of bioactive $\beta$-TCP particles, through a hardening reaction, generates needle-like crystals of calcium-deficient hydroxyapatite similar to natural bone apatite, interacting with the fiber-reinforced polymer. This interaction strongly enhances the mechanical response in compression by up to an order of magnitude [46].

Another interesting approach to design biomimetic HA/PCL composite scaffolds was to involve a wet chemical method at room temperature. The response of bone marrow–derived mesenchymal stem cells (BMSCs) in terms of cell proliferation and differentiation to the osteoblastic phenotype was assessed using the Alamar Blue assay and alkaline phosphatase (ALP) activity. The results from biological analyses suggested that HA/PCL composite scaffolds should be suitable for bone regeneration, supporting osteogenesis after 15 days from cell seeding [47].

Furthermore, suspensions of type I collagen, the main constituent of tendon and bone tissue [48, 49], were also investigated [32, 36, 39–42] in order to strictly reproduce the chemical–physical–morphological characteristics of newly formed bone, as a template for biomimetic mineralization. Tampieri et al.

(2011) exploited the ability of the negatively charged carboxylate groups of collagen to bind the calcium ions of HA, by nucleating bone-like hydroxyapatite nanocrystals directly on self-assembling collagen fibers [43]. Similarly, Du et al. (1998) designed and manufactured HA/collagen nanocomposite scaffolds that promoted the deposition of bone matrix at the interface of bone fragments and the composite [50], also highlighting that the porous HA/collagen nanocomposite scaffold provides a microenvironment similar to that observed in vivo with osteoblasts within the composite, eventually showing a 3D polygonal shape [51].

Titania/PLGA nanocomposites were also obtained by using several ultrasonic powers to ensure a homogeneous dispersion of ceramic nanoparticles into the polymer matrix, since nanoparticle agglomeration in polymers represents a common problem, sometimes solved through the sonication techniques [52–54]. Osteoblast adhesion and long-term functions were enhanced on titania/PLGA nanocomposites prepared with greater sonication powers. In particular, the greatest osteoblast adhesion was achieved on nanocomposite scaffolds with surface roughness values closer to natural bone [52, 55] and, in particular, up to 3 times more osteoblasts adhered to titania/PLGA nanocomposites than the conventional titania/PLGA composites at the same values of weight ratio and porosity [52, 54].

On the other hand, McManus et al. (2005) reported an improvement in terms of mechanical properties of polymer/ceramic composites with nanometer particle size if compared to micro-sized ones [52, 56]. Composites made of PLA reinforced with 40 and 50 wt% nanophase (i.e., alumina, titania, and HA) showed bending moduli values closer to bone and greater than that of composites with conventional coarser-grained ceramics [56].

Furthermore, considering the excellent mechanical properties of carbon nanotubes (CNTs) and carbon nanofibers (CNFs), interesting approaches were proposed to use them as reinforcing agents in polymer-based composite materials, especially in scaffolds for bone tissue engineering [57–59]. Compared to other ceramic-based scaffolds for bone, the use of single-walled carbon nanotubes (SWCNTs) ensures the fabrication of lighter scaffolds with very high strength, since SWCNTs are less dense and highly flexible with a very high Young's modulus [59, 60]. CNTs/CNFs can be also functionalized with different side groups, thus improving the biocompatibility and/or mechanical strength of tube/fiber-reinforced composite scaffolds [59]. The amount of CNFs in a polymer-based composite influences mechanical performances and surface-free energies, and, hence, cell adhesion and proliferation [59, 60]. It is also possible to obtain nanocomposites that may selectively enhance the functions of a specific cell type and decrease the functions of the other ones. In this context, Price et al. (2003) studied the in vitro adhesion of different cell types (osteoblasts, fibroblasts, chondrocytes, and smooth muscle cells) on polycarbonate urethane/CNF (PCU/CNF) nanocomposites obtained through the dispersion of CNFs in PCU [61]. Results showed that composites with smaller scale (i.e., nano-sized) carbon fibers just promoted osteoblast adhesion [59, 61]. Other works highlighted that ALP activity and the deposition of extracellular calcium were higher for osteoblasts in the presence of CNFs [62]. Moreover, the size of CNFs plays an important role in increasing osteoblast functions [62].

PCL reinforced with sol-gel synthesized organic-inorganic hybrid fillers (PCL/TiO$_2$ and PCL/ZrO$_2$) as composite substrates and 3D rapid prototyped scaffolds for hard tissue engineering were suitably developed benefiting from the bioactivity of PCL/TiO$_2$ and PCL/ZrO$_2$ fillers, highlighted by the formation of a hydroxyapatite layer on the surfaces of samples soaked in a fluid simulating the composition of human blood plasma (SBF) [63–65]. Results from small punch tests and Alamar Blue assay performed on these advanced nanocomposite substrates showed that hybrid fillers provided better mechanical and biological performances while compression tests performed on the 3D scaffolds highlighted that the inclusion of hybrid fillers also improves the compressive modulus of rapid prototyped structures [63, 66].

However, using traditional approaches wherein scaffolds are loaded with growth factors before the implantation, a temporal control of the various aspects of the tissue growth is hardly achievable. Anyway, pre-loading affects a localized and temporally controlled delivery of growth factors, reducing the scaffold tissue regeneration potential. The possibility of developing innovative scaffolds, able to modify on-demand intrinsic properties, should offer new perspectives and possibilities to control bone regeneration process.

Accordingly, recent works have been focused on the design and development of novel bioactive scaffolds able to be manipulated in situ by means of magnetic force gradients [67], the aim being to repair large bone defects and osteochondral lesions. The rationale may be summarized in the fascinating opportunity to obtain magnetic structures also capable of tailoring specific processes at cell level through the release of biomolecules and bioactive factors, in turn linked to magnetic nanocarriers, benefiting from external magnetic fields [67, 68].

## 7.3 Magnetism in Biomedicine: Basic Principles in the Design of Magnetic Scaffolds

Over the past years, magnetism and magnetic materials have revolutionized different aspects of health care, suggesting new interesting opportunities in drug and gene delivery, magneto-mechanical stimulation or activation of cell-constructs and mechanosensitive ion channels, hyperthermia treatment of tumors and radionuclide therapy, magnetic cell-seeding procedures, controlled cell proliferation and differentiation, and tissue engineering [43, 67–88]. In the latter case, the use of magnetic materials in biological environment for implantation or for replacement of a part or a function of the body in a reliable and physiologically satisfactory way is a great and stimulating challenge.

Therefore, in the field of biology and biomaterials, magnetic nanoparticles (MNPs) either alone or in combination with other materials have been found useful in complex biomedical applications.

Due to their interesting and peculiar physical features such as their dimensions, ranging from a few nanometers up to tens of nanometers, which make them comparable to several biological entities, magnetic nanoparticles have been widely used. They show sizes that are close to or smaller than those of a protein (5–50 nm), a cell (10–100 µm), a gene (10–100 nm) or a virus (20–450 nm). Anyway, among all the physical properties that make magnetic materials as attractive tools for biomedical applications, it appears clear to take into account their intrinsic magnetic features.

Magnetic properties dramatically change when particle size reduces beyond a critical limit and goes to single domain and sub-domain regions. Below a critical size (i.e., 30 nm in size) MNPs show superparamagnetic properties, stressing their capability to be magnetized by applying an external magnetic field without remanence once the field is turned off [67, 68, 72, 89]. Due to the absence of remanence, with regard to biomedical applications, superparamagnetic nanoparticles are much more used than respective ferro/ferri-magnetic particles [90].

Therefore, they can be manipulated by an external magnetic field gradient; this suggests that it would be possible to transport MNPs and magnetically tagged biological units towards specific sites and through a switch on/switch off command scheme, it would be possible to allow them to release bound cells, molecules, and growth factors to a selected region of the body. They can be also heated up allowing their use as hyperthermia agents able to deliver thermal energy to targeted bodies (i.e., tumors) or as elements capable of improving chemotherapy or radiotherapy by providing a degree of tissue warming suitable for the destruction of cancerous cells [68, 72]. Superparamagnetic nanoparticles would not exhibit hysteresis losses; however, Néel relaxation is equally useful in generating and dissipating heat.

Magnetic materials involve also magneto-mechanical stimulation as an innovative technique for bone tissue in-growth. The use of bonded networks of ferromagnetic fibers (i.e., nickel-free ferritic stainless steel) in a nonmagnetic matrix located in inter-fiber space has been proposed by Markaki and Clyne (2004 and 2005) to improve implant fixation. When the network is subjected to an external magnetic field, the alignment of the fibers imposes mechanical strains to in-growing bone tissue [68, 75, 76].

In a similar way, Mannix et al. (2008) developed a revolutionary magnetic nanoparticles technology, which activates a biochemical signaling mechanism normally switched-on by binding of multivalent chemical ligands [68, 77]. Magnetic nanoparticles were used as nanomagnetic actuators of receptor-mediated signal transduction. Mannix et al. (2008) elegantly demonstrated the power of nanoparticles for immune receptors, but the technique could be extended to physically manipulate other receptor types.

Taking into account that most cells respond to mechanical cues, Hughes et al. (2008) focused their attention on novel techniques, which use magnetic micro/nanoparticles coupled to external applied magnetic fields for activating and investigating mechano-sensitive ion channels and cytoskeletal mechanics. This technique should permit the direct manipulation of ion channels in real time without the need for pharmacological drugs and should be potentially considered as a tool for the treatment of human diseases ascribed to ion-channel dysfunction [68, 78].

Recently, the influence of static or time-dependent magnetic fields on biological systems has become a topic of considerable interest. It was generally found that, static moderate-intensity fields (SMFs) and extremely low frequency (ELF) magnetic fields are capable of affecting a number of biological phenomena such as cell proliferation [91, 92], migration [91, 93] and orientation [91, 94] stimulating angiogenesis and osteogenic precursor proliferation [95].

Interestingly, Kanczler et al. (2010) studied the controlled differentiation of human bone marrow stromal cells using remote magnetic field activation and MNPs [68, 79].

Among other biomedical applications, magnetic nanoparticles and magnetic materials are widely considered in tissue engineering and regenerative medicine. When introduced into cells, MNPs allow cells to be positioned by means of magnets, in order to create more complex tissue structures than those usually achieved by conventional culture methods [96]. In this scenario, Ito et al. (2005) proposed novel methodologies, defined as "magnetic force-based tissue engineering," and techniques for designing tissue-engineered tubular and sheet-like constructs using MNPs and magnetic force [68, 80, 81]. It has also been demonstrated that magnetic forces enable rapid endothelialization of a knitted Dacron graft externally covered by a magnetic sheet, benefiting from biophysical forces able to attach blood-derived endothelial outgrowth cells (EOCs) to the surface of prosthetic vascular grafts, since EOCs endocytose magnetic particles and result attracted to the magnetized graft surfaces [68, 82].

Dobson et al. (2006) proposed the basic principles in designing a novel magnetic force mechanical conditioning bioreactor for tissue engineering [68, 83, 84]. Furthermore, by binding MNPs to the surface of cells, the possibility to manipulate and control cell function through the application of an external magnetic field has been studied, providing information on cellular mechanics and ion channel activation [68, 85]. This technique has been proposed as an investigative potential tool for actively controlling cellular function and processes with a special focus toward tissue engineering and regenerative medicine [68, 85].

Magnetically actuable tubular scaffolds for smooth muscle tissue engineering were first fabricated from sheets of electrospun fibrils of biocompatible and biodegradable polymers containing uniform dispersions of $Fe_2O_3$ NPs and then wound into tubes for cell seeding from the inner layer to the outer one [68, 86]. As a consequence of the magnetic field application, the induced deformation produces strains in the tube walls and fluid pumping through the walls, which should promote cell proliferation and differentiation. The design of these tubular scaffolds was optimized through a model used to predict the deformation and fluid flow for specific magnetic field strength, material properties and geometrical parameters [68, 86]. Furthermore, involving direct magnetic cell-seeding procedures and MNPs, novel strategies for vascular tissue engineering were proposed by Perea et al. (2006) [68, 87] and Shimizu et al. (2007) [68, 88].

The idea to develop magnetic scaffolds in order to control in vivo angiogenesis was first considered by Bock et al. (2010) [67]. In their research, magnetic scaffolds were manufactured through dip-coating of scaffolds in aqueous ferrofluids that contained iron oxide nanoparticles coated with different polymers for biomedical applications [67]. The magnetization of Hydroxyapatite/Collagen scaffold, achieved by attaching MNPs to the structures using the impregnation with ferrofluids showed some limitations; the magnetic particles are feebly linked to the scaffold with all the possible drawbacks for both in vitro and in vivo applications.

A relevant breakthrough is represented by the development of bio-hybrid HA/collagen magnetic scaffolds prepared by a biologically inspired mineralization process [38] that incorporates magnetic nanoparticles directly during the stage of HA nucleation [97]. Thus, MNPs become an intrinsic component of the scaffold improving considerably the biocompatibility expectations [43].

Taking into consideration a superparamagnetic material, the resulting magnetic scaffold acts as a local field amplificator; its relatively powerful internal magnetization can be aligned in the same direction by a relatively weak external field, but it may also be magnetically "turned off" by removing the applied magnetic field [67, 68]. The magnetic scaffold modifies the magnetic flux distribution and leads to much higher intensification of magnetic "lines" near/inside the scaffold. This point results crucial as these magnetization values can generate magnetic gradients, and via magnetic driving, scaffolds may attract and take up cells or other bioagents (i.e., in vivo growth factors) bound to MNPs. In particular, MNPs may play as shuttles that can transport these bioagents in the direction of a static scaffold. As a consequence, a magnetic scaffold can be viewed as a fixed "station" that ensures a long-living support to implanted tissue-engineered constructs, providing the fascinating chance to tailor the scaffold activity taking into account the personal needs of the patient [67]. By this point of view, the scaffold is no longer just considered as a guide for tissue growth, but it actively participates in the process also acting as a controlled delivery device.

In addition to the reloading function, magnetic scaffolds should be able to play further significant roles. Magnetic scaffolds and MNPs should be used as delivery systems triggered by a temperature switch due to the possibility to control their temperature through the use of an external time-dependent magnetic field. Benefiting from this approach, it should be possible to investigate the effect of a prolonged localized temperature increase on angiogenesis during tissue regeneration process. It is well known that the application of magnetic fields stimulates angiogenesis and osteogenic precursor proliferation and can also promote bone formation [95].

Magnetic scaffolds should be also employed to achieve efficient scaffold fixation via magnetic forces providing a very smart solution to the clinical problems of fixation that many traditional scaffolds meet. Today, regarding the treatment of small osteochondral lesions, most surgeons do not use any fixation system, while in the treatment of wide bone defects, fixation is ensured through the use of external systems, such as intramedullary nails, screws, and plates, which require continuous control and often multiple surgical interventions. To this aim, Russo et al. (2012) proposed an innovative magnetic fixation approach based on the application of a magnetic scaffold highlighting a saturation value of 17 emu/g. In their study, different configurations were proposed and a finite element modeling (FEM) was exploited to investigate the fixation efficiency. It was found that for most appropriate magnetic materials and optimized magnet-scaffold positioning, all the considered configurations should provide an interesting solution in terms of scaffold fixation [98].

## 7.4 Magnetic Scaffolds for Advanced Bone Tissue Engineering

The introduction of rapid prototyping technologies into the biomedical field has allowed to obtain tissue-engineered scaffolds characterized by a continuous, uninterrupted pore structure, with a reproducible internal morphology, a higher degree of micromacro architectural control. This point is really important because these features enable cells to assemble into an ordered matrix and to allow adequate mass transport of oxygen and nutrients throughout the scaffold [2, 99, 100]. Among all the rapid prototyping techniques, 3D fiber deposition has emerged as a powerful tool for the manufacture of well-defined scaffolds with 100% interconnected pores, also due to its flexibility in processing a wide range of materials.

Benefiting from the theoretical knowledge of polymer-solvent thermodynamics and material chemistry, a suitable solvent should be considered to dissolve a selected polymer for a specific application, according to the solubility parameters ($\delta$) defined as follows:

$$\delta = \left| \frac{\Delta E}{V} \right|^{1/2},\qquad(7.1)$$

where $\Delta E/V$ represents the energy of vaporization per cm$^3$, which is also called the cohesive energy density.

In particular, tetrahydrofuran (THF) was chosen to dissolve PCL pellets. Afterwards, magnetic nanoparticles were added to the PCL/THF solution during stirring, also optimizing their dispersion in the polymer solution.

Nanocomposite magnetic scaffolds with a fully interconnected pore network were successfully manufactured through 3D fiber deposition technique (Fig. 7.1).

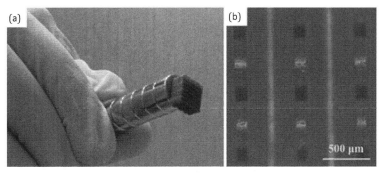

**Figure 7.1** (a) Image of a 3D fiber-deposited nanocomposite magnetic scaffold attracted by a neodymium magnet; (b) optical microscopy image of a magnetic scaffold showing that fibers were very well aligned and regularly spaced along each layer. Both images are adapted from De Santis et al. (2011) [102, 103].

In a first step, 3D fiber-deposited PCL/iron oxide (PCL/Fe$_3$O$_4$) magnetic scaffolds were designed. The effect of 10 wt% of Fe$_3$O$_4$ nanoparticle amount on the mechanical, magnetic, and biological performances was also investigated [101–103]. Mechanical analysis suggested that the inclusion of Fe$_3$O$_4$ nanoparticles improves the tensile modulus and the yield stress of the fibers composing the scaffold if compared to those of neat PCL and reduces the maximum strain. Moreover, values of the tensile modulus obtained for nanocomposite fibers match those of trabecular bone [104]; consequently each fiber may be seen as a "basic element" of the 3D fiber-deposited scaffold. On the other hand, compression tests highlighted a mechanical behavior very similar to that of flexible foams with a stress–strain curve characterized by three different stiff zones. First, a linear region at low values of strain suggests an initial stiff mechanical response. This zone is followed by a region with a lower stiffness. Finally, it is possible to observe a third stiff zone of the stress–strain curve. According to previous works [99, 105], in contrast to the typical behavior of the flexible foams [105] and 3D scaffolds obtained through fused deposition modeling [106] the central region of the stress–strain curve does not present a plateau. However, it shows a lower stiffness compared with the other two regions of the curve.

The increase of stiffness and strength observed for PCL/Fe$_3$O$_4$ suggested that the use of 10 wt% magnetic nanoparticles is still an effective reinforcement (Fig. 7.2).

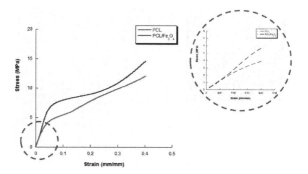

**Figure 7.2** Typical stress–strain curve obtained from compression tests performed on 3D fiber-deposited scaffolds up to a strain level of 0.4 mm/mm and stress–strain curve reported up to a strain level of 0.04 mm/mm in order to better highlight the initial mechanical behavior.

Magnetic analyses performed at 37°C have highlighted magnetization curves that are not hysteretic as expected in the superparamagnetic regime with values of saturation magnetization of about 3.9 emu/g. In vitro biological investigations suggested an increase in the adhered number and a marked spreading of human mesenchymal stem cells (hMSCs).

Even though iron oxide-based phases such as maghemite or magnetite have been widely considered in biomedical applications, their long-term effects in the human body remain still unknown [68, 107, 108]. Consequently, the development of suitably surface-modified magnetic nanoparticles through the design of specific biocompatible layers consisting of polymers, inorganic phases or metals deposited on their surface could avoid dangerous problems related to their eventual toxicity, such as to leave, inside the repaired tissue, nonbioresorbable magnetic inclusion (i.e., magnetite) [68, 89, 109]. To this aim, research attention has been focused on the synthesis of innovative biocompatible and fully biodegradable materials such as iron-doped hydroxyapatite (FeHA) nanoparticles, which can be potentially employed to develop new magnetic ceramic scaffolds with enhanced regenerative properties for bone surgery [89, 110, 111].

Chemical modifications as well as the engineering of hydroxyapatite have been well investigated in order to produce new biomimetic nonstoichiometric apatites, which would better resemble the chemical composition and structure of the mineral phase in bones, providing higher rate of biodegradability and bioactivity compared to stoichiometric apatites or to improve HA mechanical properties by optimizing the process and the synthesis conditions [109, 112–114].

The ionic substitutions can modify the surface structure and electrical charge of HA. Among the substituents of the calcium ion ($Ca^{2+}$), $Mg^{2+}$ is of great interest. As reported in literature, Mg ion substitution accelerates the nucleation kinetics of HA, inhibits its crystallization, producing a synthetic apatite more similar to natural one [109, 112–114]. Mg-doped hydroxyapatite is more solubile and absorbable than unmodified apatites, but there is a limit to the introduction of Mg ion into the apatite network without altering the reticular structure. The introduction of carbonate ions ($CO_3^{2-}$) into the apatite structure may allow to increase Mg ion substitution. The carbonate ion can partially substitute the $OH^-$ sites (site A), leading to an apatite characterized by less affinity to osteoblast cell, and/or the $PO_4^{3-}$ (site B) leading to an apatite less crystalline and more soluble if compared to stoichiometric apatites. However, Mg ions are bivalent as Ca ions; thus carbonate ion is not forced to substitute in the site B [110, 112, 113]. Consequently, the co-substitution of Mg and $CO_3$ ions into HA structure has allowed to obtain a biomimetic apatite.

In the last years, great efforts have been devoted to the synthesis of FeHA nanoparticles. By stressing the importance of having nontoxic MNPs, Tampieri et al. (2012) synthesized a novel biocompatible and bioresorbable superparamagnetic-like phase by doping hydroxyapatite with $Fe^{3+}/Fe^{2+}$ ions, minimizing the formation of magnetite as secondary phase [89, 115]. Microstructural, physico-chemical and magnetic analyses were carried out on the nanoparticles, highlighting their intrinsic magnetization and suggesting new perspectives in bone tissue engineering and anti-cancer therapies [89].

PCL/FeHA nanocomposite substrates were designed and characterized using different polymer-to-particle weight ratios, spanning from 10 to 30 wt% of FeHA nanoparticles. The effect of FeHA nanoparticle inclusion on morphological, mechanical, magnetic, and biological performances was assessed.

Scanning electron microscopy (SEM) analysis allowed to evaluate morphological features of the substrates. In particular, all of the substrates have the same structure and morphology except for 90/10 PCL/FeHA nanocomposite, which is characterized by the presence of several pores, randomly distributed, due to solvent extraction. Just as an example, in Fig. 7.3 SEM and micro-computed tomography (Micro-CT) images of 90/10 PCL/FeHA and 70/30 PCL/FeHA are reported.

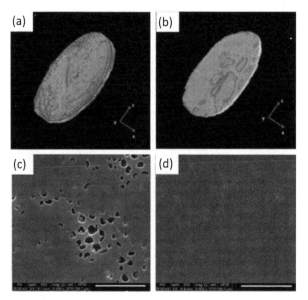

**Figure 7.3** Representative images obtained from Micro-CT and SEM analyses performed on nanocomposite magnetic PCL/FeHA substrates: 90/10 (a, c, respectively) and 70/30 (b, d, respectively). Scale bar for SEM images: 20 µm. Micro-CT images are adapted from Gloria et al. (2013) [69].

The synergistic contribution of both surface chemistry and topography influence the overall features of the substrates, thus allowing to enhance not only the hydrophilic character, but also cell attachment and proliferation, as shown by confocal laser scanning microscopy (CLSM, Fig. 7.4) and cell viability assays.

The inclusion of a specifically modified hydroxyapatite into the polymer matrix is able to improve the mechanical properties, in terms of higher maximum load if compared to neat PCL substrates, as shown by small punch tests. However, beyond a specific limit of nanoparticle amount, by further increasing the nanoparticle concentration, mechanical performances of nanocomposite substrates should decrease since the nanoparticles play as "weak points" instead of a reinforcement for the polymer matrix. It is worth noting that weakness in a structure may be due to discontinuities in the stress transfer and generation of stress concentration at the nanoparticle/matrix interface. This effect may be ascribed to the difference in ductility between the polymer matrix and the inorganic nanofillers.

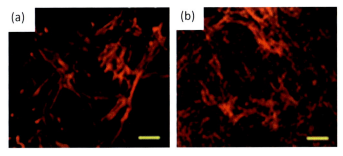

**Figure 7.4** CLSM images of (a) PCL and (b) 80/20 PCL/FeHA substrates at 14 days after cell seeding. Scale Bar: 100 μm. Both images are adapted from Gloria et al. (2013) [69].

From a biological point of view, FeHA nanoparticles enhance scaffold bioactivity and cell response also evidencing the role of the HA in promoting surface mineralization as expressed by the increase of ALP activity [69].

Benefiting from the intrinsic magnetism of FeHA nanoparticles, nanocomposite PCL/FeHA substrates have shown a superparamagnetic character at body temperature with a saturation value spanning from 0.3 to 0.9 emu/g, strictly proportional to the FeHA content. Even though the values of saturation magnetization value obtained for FeHA nanocomposites are lower than those reported in literature for dip-coated scaffolds [67] or those shown by PCL/$Fe_3O_4$ nanocomposites with the smallest nanoparticle amount [101–103], these results are very promising since it would be possible to obtain magnetic field gradients able to attract bioaggregates into the fully interconnected pore network of the completely biodegradable scaffolds.

With regard to magnetic hyperthermia, the application of a radio-frequency magnetic field to the samples has suggested their potential use in the treatment of tumors, since significant temperature increases between 2 and 10°C were achieved after 5 min of exposition by strictly varying the substrate composition.

These multidisciplinary studies on hybrid PCL/FeHA nanocomposite magnetic substrates allowed to choose the optimal polymer-to-particle weight ratio, embedding a nanoparticle amount of 20 wt% into the polymer matrix. Taking into account all of these results, 3D morphologically controlled fully biodegradable PCL/FeHA nanocomposite magnetic scaffolds were manufactured through 3D fiber deposition technique.

The performances of these novel 3D PCL/FeHA scaffolds were assessed through different experimental analyses. Tensile and compression tests highlighted results consistent with those obtained from PCL/Fe$_3$O$_4$. The inclusion of magnetic nanoparticles into the polymer matrix increases mechanical performances in terms of tensile modulus and yield stress, compression modulus and maximum strain, respectively. Furthermore, an indirect tensile test performed on 3D cylindrically shaped specimens (the Brasilian Test) highlighted the different ductility of the designed PCL and PCL/FeHA scaffolds. Benefiting from magnetically charged cells and magnetic scaffolds, further analyses were also performed, the aim being to assess the possibility to increase scaffold cell loading efficiency. The in vitro results showed that the cell growth in the magnetized scaffolds is greater than that in nonmagnetized ones. Preliminary in vivo experiments, performed on a rabbit animal model, suggested the use of a 3D nanocomposite magnetic scaffold as potential alternative to autologous bone implantation, eventually benefiting from the application of an external magnetic field [116–118].

For this reason, further in vitro experiments will be performed on the designed 3D magnetic scaffolds, to study the influence of a static or a time-dependent magnetic field on cell adhesion, proliferation, and differentiation.

## 7.5 Conclusions and Future Trends

Over the past years, many efforts have been made in designing nanocomposite scaffolds for advanced bone tissue engineering.

Hybrid nanocomposite scaffolds with magnetic activation could be considered as a suitable candidate for bone tissue regeneration and could open new perspectives for the application of magnetic fields in a clinical setting.

Customized nanocomposite magnetic scaffolds could also be designed and manufactured benefiting from reverse engineering approach, specifically by integrating different techniques such as 3D scanning, 3D modeling and rapid prototyping, with those related to the preparation of nanocomposite material for scaffold processing.

Furthermore, the possibility to manufacture 3D heterogeneous bilayered scaffolds, composed of two distinct but integrated polymeric and nanocomposite magnetic layers, for the cartilage and bone regions, should be also taken into account for the regeneration of osteochondral defects. To this aim, it is worth noting that in order to generate a smooth transition between such different tissues, material and porosity gradients should be considered when moving from the bone side to the joint surface.

Finally, further important features of the magnetic scaffolds could be also studied. In a first analysis, it would be interesting to demonstrate the effect of a static or a dynamic magnetic field on cell adhesion, proliferation and differentiation, trying to find the optimal conditions for stimulating bone tissue growth.

## Acknowledgments

The research leading to these results has received funding from the European Community's seventh Framework Programme under grant agreement no. NMP3-LA-2008-214685 project MAGISTER (www.magister-project.eu).

## References

1. Lavik, E., and Langer, R. (2004). Tissue engineering: Current state and perspectives, *Appl. Microbiol. Biotechnol.*, **65**, pp. 1–8.
2. Sachlos, E., and Czernuske, J. T. (2003). Making tissue engineering scaffold work: Review on the application of SFF technology to the production of tissue engineering scaffolds, *Eur. Cell Mater.*, **5**, pp. 29–40.

3. Meng, D., and Boccaccini, A. R. (2010). Nanostructured biocomposites for tissue engineering scaffolds, in *Biomedical Composites* (ed. Ambrosio, L.), Chapter 20, Woodhead Publishing Limited, CRC Press, Cambridge, UK, pp. 509–546.

4. Atala, A., and Lanza, R. P. (2001). *Methods of Tissue Engineering.* (Academic Press, San Diego).

5. Langer, R., and Vacanti, J. (1993). Tissue engineering, *Science,* **260**, pp. 920–926.

6. Ohgushi, H., and Caplan, A. I. (1999) Stem cell technology and bioceramics: From cell to gene engineering, *J. Biomed. Mater. Res.,* **48**, pp. 913–27.

7. Gloria, A., De Santis, R., and Ambrosio, L. (2010). Polymer-based composite scaffolds for tissue engineering, *J. Appl. Biomater. Biomech.,* **8**(2), pp. 57–67.

8. Guarino, V., Causa, F., and Ambrosio, L. (2007). Bioactive scaffolds for bone and ligament tissue, *Expert. Rev. Med. Devices.,* **4**(3), pp. 405–418.

9. Causa, F., Netti, P. A., and Ambrosio, L. (2007). A multi-functional scaffold for tissue regeneration: The need to engineer a tissue analogue, *Biomaterials,* **28**, pp. 5093–5099.

10. Chaikof, E. L., Matthew, H., Kohn, J., Mikos, A. G., Prestwich, G. D., and Yip, C. M. (2002). Biomaterials and scaffolds in reparative medicine, *Ann. N. Y. Acad. Sci.,* **961**, pp. 96–105.

11. Park, J. B. (1984). *Biomaterial Science and Engineering.* (New York: Plenum Press).

12. Rogel, M. R., Qiu, H., and Ameer, G. A. (2008). The role of nanocomposites in bone regeneration, *J. Mater. Chem.,* **18**, pp. 4233–4241.

13. Sikavitsas, V. I., Temenoff, J. S., and Mikos, A. G. (2001). Biomaterials and bone mechanotransduction, *Biomaterials,* **22**(19), pp. 2581–2593.

14. Hill, P. A., and Orth, M. (1998). Bone remodelling, *Br. J. Orthod.,* **25**, pp. 101–107.

15. Baron, R. (1999). Primer *on the Metabolic Bone Diseases and Disorders of Mineral Metabolism,* 2nd ed. (Raven Press, New York).

16. Salgado, A. J., Coutinho, O. P., and Reis, R. L. (2004). Bone tissue engineering: State of the art and future trends, *Macromol. Biosci.,* **4**, pp. 743–765.

17. Temenoff, J. S., Lu, L., and Mikos, A. G. (1999) *Bone Engineering,* 1st ed. (Em squared, Toronto).

18. Aubin, J. E., and Liau, F. (1996) *Principles of Bone Biology*, 1st ed. (Academic Press, San Diego).

19. Ducy, P., Schinke, T., and Karsenty, G. (2000). The osteoblast: A sophisticated fibroblast under central surveillance, *Science*, **289**, pp. 5484, 1501–1504.

20. Mackie, E. J. (2003). Osteoblasts: Novel roles in orchestration of skeletal architecture, *Int. J. Cell Biochem. Cell Biol.*, **35**(9), pp. 1301–1305.

21. Nijweide, P. J., Burger, E. H., Nulend, J. K., Van der Plas, A. (1996). *Principles of Bone Biology*, 1st ed. (Academic Press, San Diego).

22. Vaananen, K. (1996). *Principles of Bone Biology*, 1st ed. (Academic Press, San Diego).

23. Bruder, S. P., and Fox, B. S. (1999). Tissue engineering of bone: Cell based strategies, *Clin. Orthop. Relat. Res.*, **367**, pp. S68–S83.

24. Mathieu, L. M., Mueller, T. L. Bourban, P. E., Pioletti, D. P., Muller, R., and Manson, J. A. E. (2006). Architecture and properties of anisotropic polymer composite scaffolds for bone tissue engineering, *Biomaterials,* **27**, pp. 905–916.

25. Devin, J. E., Attawia, M. A., and Laurencin, C. T. (1996). Three-dimensional degradable porous polymer-ceramic matrices for use in bone repair, *J. Biomater. Sci. Polymer Ed.*, **7**, pp. 661–669.

26. Nicolais, L., Gloria, A., and Ambrosio, L. (2010). The mechanics of biocomposites, in *Biomedical Composites* (ed. Ambrosio, L.), Chapter 17, Woodhead Publishing Limited, CRC Press, Cambridge, UK, pp. 411–440.

27. Ramakrishna, S., Mayer, J., Wintermantel, E., and Leong, K. W. (2001). Biomedical applications of polymer-composite materials: A review, *Comp. Sci. Tech.*, **61**, pp. 1189–1224.

28. Rezwan, K., Chen, Q. Z., Blaker, J. J., and Boccaccini, A. R. (2006). Biodegradable and bioactive porous polymer/inorganic composite scaffolds for bone tissue engineering, *Biomaterials,* **27**, pp. 3143–3431.

29. Zhang, K., Wang, Y., Hillmayer, M. A., and Francis, L. F. (2004). Processing and properties of porous poly(L-lactide)/ bioactive glass composites, *Biomaterials*, **25**, pp. 2489–2500.

30. Bernhardt, A., Lode, A., Boxberger, S., Pompe, W., and Gelinsky, M. (2007). Mineralised collagen-an artificial, extracellular bone matrix-improves osteogenic differentiation of bone marrow stromal cells, *J. Mater. Sci. Mater. Med.*, **19**, pp. 269–275.

31. Domaschke, H., Gelinsky, M., Burmeister, B., Fleig, R., Hanke, T., Reinstorf, A., Pompe, W., and Rösen-Wolff, A. (2006). In vitro ossification and remodeling of mineralized collagen I scaffolds, *Tissue Eng.*, **12**, pp. 949–958.

32. Gelinsky, M., Welzel, P. B., Simon, P., Bernhardt, A., and König, U. (2007). Porous three-dimensional scaffolds made of mineralized collagen: Preparation and properties of a biomimetic nanocomposite material for tissue engineering of bone, *Chem. Eng. J.*, **137**, pp. 84–96.

33. Martin, I., Miot, S., Barbero, A., Jakob, M., and Wendt, D. (2007). Osteochondral tissue engineering, *J. Biomech.*, **40**, pp. 750–765.

34. Yokoyama, A., Gelinsky, M., Kawasaki, T., Kohgo, T., König, U., Pompe, W., and Watari, F. (2005). Biomimetic porous scaffolds with high elasticity made from mineralized collagen-an animal study, *J. Biomed. Mater. Res. Part B: Appl. Biomater.*, **75B**, pp. 464–472.

35. Newman, A. P. (1998). Articular cartilage repair, *Am. J. Sports Med.*, **26**, pp. 309–324.

36. Tampieri, A., Celotti, G., Landi, E., Sandri, M., Roveri, N., and Falini, G. (2003). Biologically inspired synthesis of one like composite: Self assembled collagen fibres/hydroxyapatite nanocrystals, *J. Biomed. Mater. Res.*, **67A**, pp. 618–625.

37. Rhee, S. H, Lee, J. D., and Tanaka, J. (2000). Nucleation of hydroxyapatite crystal through chemical interaction with collagen, *J. Am. Ceram. Soc.*, **83**, 2890–2892.

38. Tampieri, A., Sandri, M., Landi, E., Sprio, S., Valentini, F., and Boskey, A. (2008). Synthetic bio-mineralization yielding HA/ collagen hybrid composite, *Adv. Appl. Ceram.*, **107**, pp. 298–302.

39. Kikuchi, M., Itoh, S., Ichinose, S., Shinomiya, K., and Tanaka, J. (2001). Self-organization mechanism in a bone-like hydroxyapatite/collagen nanocomposite synthesized in vitro and its biological reaction in vivo, *Biomaterials*, **22**, pp. 1705–1711.

40. Goissis, G., Maginador, S. V. D., and Martins, V. D. A. (2003). Biomimetic mineralization of charged collagen matrices: In vitro and in vivo study, *Artif. Organs*, **27**, pp. 437–443.

41. Bradt, J. H., Mertig, M., Teresiak, A., and Pompe, W. (1999). Biomimetic mineralization of collagen by combined fibril assembly and calcium phosphate formation, *Chem. Mater.*, **11**, pp. 2694–2701.

42. Chen, J., Burger, C., Krishnan, C. V., Chu, B., Hsiao, B. S., and Glimcher, M. J. (2005). In vitro mineralization of collagen in demineralized fish bone, *Macromol. Chem. Phys.*, **206**, pp. 43–51.

43. Tampieri, A., Sprio, S., Sandri, M., and Valentini, F. (2011). Mimicking natural bio-mineralization processes: A new tool for osteochondral scaffold development, *Trends Biotechnol.*, **29**(10), pp. 526–535.

44. Guarino, V., Causa, F., Netti, P. A., Ciapetti, G., Pagani, S., Martini, D., Baldini, N., and Ambrosio, L. (2008). The role of hydroxyapatite as solid signal on performance of PCL porous scaffolds for bone tissue regeneration, *J. Biomed. Mater. Res. B Appl. Biomater.*, **86**, pp. 548–557.

45. Guarino, V., Taddei, P., Di Foggia, M., Fagnano, C., Ciapetti, G., and Ambrosio, L. (2009). The Influence of hydroxyapatite particles on in vitro degradation behavior of poly $\varepsilon$-caprolactone-based composite scaffolds, *Tissue Eng. Part A*, **15**, pp. 3655–3668.

46. Guarino, V., and Ambrosio, L. (2008). The synergic effect of polylactid fiber and calcium phosphate particle reinforcement in poly $\varepsilon$-caprolactone-based composite scaffolds, *Acta Biomater.*, **4**, pp. 1778–1787.

47. Raucci, M. G., D'Antò, V., Guarino, V., Sardella, E., Zeppetelli, S., Favia, P., and Ambrosio, L. (2010). Biomineralized porous composite scaffolds prepared by chemical synthesis for bone tissue regeneration, *Acta Biomater.*, **10**, pp. 4090–4099.

48. Lin, H., Clegg, D. O., and Lal, R. (1999). Imaging real-time proteolysis of single collagen I molecules with an atomic force microscope, *Biochemistry*, **38**, pp. 9956–9963.

49. Nimni, M. E. (ed.) (1988). *Collagen*, CRC Press.

50. Du, C., Cui, F. Z., Feng, Q. L., Zhu, X. D., and de Groot, K. (1998). Tissue response to nano-hydroxyapatite/collagen composite implants in marrow cavity, *J. Biomed. Mater. Res.*, **42**, pp. 540–548.

51. Du, C., Cui, F. Z., Zhu, X. D., and de Groot, K. (1999). Three-dimensional nano-HAP/collagen matrix loading with osteogenic cells in organ culture, *J. Biomed. Mater. Res.*, **44**, pp. 407–415.

52. Tran, N., and Webster, T. J. (2009). Nanotechnology for bone materials, *WIREs Nanomed. Nanobiotechnol.*, **1**, pp. 336–351.

53. Liu, H., Slamovich, E. B., and Webster, T. J. (2005). Increased osteoblast functions on nanophase titania dispersed in poly-lactic-co-glycolic acid composites, *Nanotechnology*, **16**, pp. S601–S608.

54. Smith, T. A., and Webster, T. J. (2005). Increased osteoblast function on PLGA composites containing nanophase titania, *J. Biomed. Mater. Res. A*, **74**, pp. 677–686.

55. Christensen, E. M., Anseth, K. S., van den Beucken, J. J., Chan, C. K., Ercan, B., Jansen, J. A., Laurencin, C. T., Li, W. J., Murugan, R., Nair, L. S., Ramakrishna, S., Tuan, R. S., Webster, T. J., and Mikos, A. G. (2007). Nanobiomaterial applications in orthopedics, *J. Orthop. Res.*, **25**, pp. 11–22.

56. McManus, A. J., Doremus, R. H., Siegel, R. W., and Bizios, R. (2005). Evaluation of cytocompatibility and bending modulus of nanoceramic/ polymer composites, *J. Biomed. Mater. Res. A*, **72**, pp. 98–106.

57. Qian, D., Dickey, E. C., Andrews, R., and Rantell, R. (2000). Load transfer and deformation mechanisms in carbon nanotube-polystyrene composites, *Appl. Phys. Lett.*, **76**, pp. 2868–2870.

58. Cadek, M., Coleman, J. N., Barron, V., Hedicke, K., and Blau, W. J. (2002). Morphological and mechanical properties of carbonnanotube-reinforced semicrystalline and amorphous polymer composites, *Appl. Phys. Lett.*, **81**, pp. 5123–5125.

59. Tran, P. A., Zhang, L., and Webster, T. J. (2009). Carbon nanofibers and carbon nanotubes in regenerative medicine, *Adv. Drug Deliv. Rev.*, **61**, pp. 1097–1014.

60. Iijima, S., Brabec, C., Maiti, A., and Bernholc, J. (1996). Structural flexibility of carbon nanotubes, *J. Chem. Phys.*, **104**, pp. 2089–2092.

61. Price, R. L., Waid, M. C., Haberstroh, K. M., and Webster, T. J. (2003). Selective bone cell adhesion on formulations containing carbon nanofibers, *Biomaterials*, **24**, pp. 1877–1887.

62. Elias, K. L., Price, R. L., and Webster, T. J. (2002). Enhanced functions of osteoblasts on nanometer diameter carbon fibers, *Biomaterials*, **23**, pp. 3279–3287.

63. Russo, T., Gloria, A., D'Antò, V., D'Amora, U., Ametrano, G., Bollino, F., De Santis, R., Ausanio, G., Catauro, M., Rengo, S., and Ambrosio, L. (2010). Poly($\varepsilon$-caprolactone) reinforced with sol-gel synthesized organic-inorganic hybrid fillers as composite substrates for tissue engineering, *J. Appl. Biomater. Biomech.*, **8**(3), pp. 146–152.

64. Catauro, M., Raucci, M. G., De Marco, D., and Ambrosio, L. (2006). Release kinetics of ampicillin, characterization and bioactivity of $TiO_2$/PCL hybrid materials synthesized by sol–gel processing, *J. Biomed. Mater. Res. A*, **77A**, pp. 340–350.

65. Catauro, M., Raucci, M. G., and Ausanio, G. (2008). Sol–gel processing of drug delivery zirconia/polycaprolactone hybrid materials, *J. Mater. Sci. Mater. Med.*, **19**, pp. 531–540.

66. De Santis, R., Gloria, A., Russo, T., D'Amora, U., D'Antò, V., Bollino, F., Catauro, M., Mollica, F., Rengo, S., and Ambrosio, L. (2013). Advanced composites for hard-tissue engineering based on PCL/organic–inorganic hybrid fillers: From the design of 2D substrates to 3D rapid prototyped scaffolds, *Polym. Compos.*, DOI: 10.1002/pc.22446.

67. Bock, N., Riminucci, A., Dionigi, C., Russo, A., Tampieri, A., Landi, E., Goranov, V. A., Marcacci, M., and Dediu, V. (2010). A novel route in bone tissue engineering: Magnetic biomimetic scaffold, *Acta Biomater.*, **6**, pp. 786–796.

68. Schieker, M., Seitz, H., Drosse, I., Seitz, S., and Mutschler, W. (2006). Biomaterials as scaffold for bone tissue engineering, *Eur. J. Trauma*, **32**, pp. 114–124.

69. Gloria, A., Russo, T., D'Amora, U., Zeppetelli, S., D'Alessandro, T., Sandri, M., Bañobre-Lopez, M., Piñeiro-Redondo, Y., Uhlarz, M., Tampieri, A., Rivas, J., Herrmannsdörfer, T., Dediu, V. A., Ambrosio, L., and De Santis, R. (2013). Magnetic poly($\varepsilon$-caprolactone)/iron-doped hydroxyapatite nanocomposite substrates for advanced bone tissue engineering, *J. R. Soc. Interface*, **80**(10), pp. 1–11.

70. Patel, Z. S., Young, S., Tabata, Y., Jansen, J. A., Wong, M. E., and Mikos, A. G. (2008). Dual delivery of an angiogenic and osteogenic growth factor for bone regeneration enhances in a critical size defect model, *Bone*, **43**, pp. 931–940.

71. Laschke, M. W., Harder, Y., Amon, M., Martin, I., Farhadi, J., Ring, A., Torio-Padron, N., Schramm, R., Rücker, M., Junker, D., Häufel, J. M., Carvalho, C., Heberer, M., Germann, G., Vollmar, B., and Menger, M. D. (2006). Angiogenesis in tissue engineering: Breathing life into constructed tissue substitutes, *Tissue Eng.*, **12**, pp. 2093–2104.

72. Pankhurst, Q. A., Connolly, J., Jones, S. K., and Dobson, J. (2003). Applications of magnetic nanoparticles in biomedicine, *J. Phys. D: Appl. Phys.*, **36**, pp. R167–R181.

73. Barry, S. E. (2008). Challenges in the development of magnetic particles for therapeutic applications, *Int. J. Hyperthermia*, **24**, pp. 451–66.

74. Muthana, M., Scott, S. D., Farrow, N., Morrow, F., Murdoch, C., Grubb, S., Brown, N., Dobson, J., and Lewis, C. E. (2008). A novel magnetic approach to enhance the efficacy of cell-based gene therapies, *Gene Ther.*, **15**, pp. 902–910.

75. Markaki, A. E., and Clyne, W. T. (2005). Magneto-mechanical actuation of bonded ferromagnetic fibre arrays, *Acta Mater.*, **53**, pp. 877–889.

76. Markaki, A. E., and Clyne, T. W. (2004). Magneto-mechanical stimulation of bone growth in a bonded array of ferromagnetic fibres, *Biomaterials*, **25**, pp. 4805–4815.

77. Mannix, R. J., Kumar, S., Cassiola, F., Montoya-Zavala, M., Feinstein, E., Prentiss, M., and Ingber, D. E. (2008). Nanomagnetic actuation of receptor-mediated signal transduction, *Nat. Nanotech.*, **3**, pp. 36–40.

78. Hughes, S., McBain, S., Dobson, J., and El Haj, A. J. (2008). Selective activation of mechanosensitive ion channels using magnetic particles, *J. R. Soc. Interface*, **5**, pp. 855–863.

79. Kanczler, J. M., Sura, H. S., Magnay, J., Attridge, K., Green, D., Oreffo, R. O. C., Dobson, J. P., and El Haj, A. J. (2010). Controlled differentiation of human bone marrow stromal cells using magnetic nanoparticle technology, *Tissue Eng.*, **16**, pp. 3241–3250.

80. Ito, A., Hibino, E., Kobayashi, C., Terasaki, H., Kagami, H., Ueda, M., Kobayashi, T., and Honda, H. (2005). Construction and delivery of tissue-engineered human retinal pigment epithelial cell sheets, using magnetite nanoparticles and magnetic force, *Tissue Eng.*, **11**, pp. 489–496.

81. Ito, A., Ino, K., Hayashida, M., Kobayashi, T., Matsunuma, H., Kagami, H., Ueda, M., and Honda, H. (2005). Novel methodology for fabrication of tissue-engineered tubular constructs using magnetite nanoparticles and magnetic force, *Tissue Eng.*, **11**, pp. 1553–1561.

82. Pislaru, S. V., Harbuzariu, A., Agarwal, G., Witt, T., Gulati, R., Sandhu, N. P., Mueske, C., Kalra, M., Simari, R. D., and Sandhu, G. S. (2006). Magnetic forces enable rapid endothelialization of synthetic vascular grafts, *Circulation*, **114**, pp. I314–I318.

83. Dobson, J. (2006). Magnetic nanoparticles for drug delivery, *Drug Dev. Res.*, **67**, 55–60.

84. Dobson, J., Cartmell, S. H., Keramane, A., and El Haj, A. J. (2006). Principles and design of a novel magnetic force mechanical conditioning bioreactor for tissue engineering, stem cell conditioning, and dynamic in vitro screening IEEE trans, *NanoBiosci.*, **5**, pp. 173–177.

85. Dobson, J. (2008). Remote control of cellular behaviour with magnetic nanoparticles, *Nat. Nanotech.*, **3**, pp. 139–143.

86. Mack, J. J., Cox, B. N., Sudre, O., Corrin, A. A., dos Santos, S. L., Lucato, Ma, C., and Andrew, J. S. (2009). Achieving nutrient pumping and strain stimulus by magnetic actuation of tubular scaffolds, *Smart Mater. Struct.*, **18**, pp. 104025–104040.

87. Perea, H., Aigner, J., Hopfner, U., and Wintermantel, E. (2006). Direct magnetic tubular cell seeding: A novel approach for vascular tissue engineering, *Cells Tiss. Org.* **183**, pp. 156–165.

88. Shimizu, K., Ito, A., Arinobe, M., Murase, Y., Iwata, Y., Narita, Y., Kagami, H., Ueda, M., and Honda, H. (2007). Effective cell-seeding technique using magnetite nanoparticles and magnetic force onto decellularized blood vessels for vascular tissue engineering, *J. Biosci. Bioeng.*, **103**, pp. 472–478.

89. Tampieri, A., D'Alessandro, T., Sandri, M., Sprio, S., Landi, E., Bertinetti, L., Panseri, S., Pepponi, G., Goettlicher, J., Bañobre-López, M., and Rivas, J. (2012). Intrinsic magnetism and hyperthermia in bioactive Fe-doped hydroxyapatite, *Acta Biomater.*, **8**, pp. 843–851

90. Bahadur, D., and Jyotsnendu, G. (2003). Biomaterials and magnetism, *Sadhana—Acad. P. Eng. Sci.*, **28**, pp. 639–656.

91. Xiaolan, B., Hadjiargyrou, M., Di Masi, E., Meng, Y., Simon, M., Tan, Z., and Rafailovich, M. H. (2011). The role of moderate static magnetic fields on biomineralization of osteoblasts on sulfonated polystyrene films, *Biomaterials*, **32**, pp. 7831–7838.

92. Ross, S. M. (1990). Combined DC and ELF magnetic fields can alter cell proliferation, *Bioelectromagnetics,* **11**, pp. 27–36.

93. Hashimoto, Y., Kawasumi, M., and Saito, M. (2007). Effect of static magnetic field on cell migration, *Electr. Eng. Jpn.*, **160**, pp. 46–52.

94. Kotani, H., Kawaguchi, H., Shimoaka, T., Iwasaka, M., Ueno, S., Ozawa, H., Nakamura, K., and Hoshi, K. (2002). Strong static magnetic field stimulates bone formation to a definite orientation in vitro and in vivo, *J. Bone Miner. Res.*, **17**, pp. 1814–1821.

95. Nakajima, T., Ishiguro, A., and Wakatsuki, Y. (2001). Formation of super wires of clusters by self-assembly of transition metal cluster anions with metal cations, *Angew. Chem. Int. Ed.,* **40**(6), pp. 1066–1068.

96. Castro, E., and Mano, J. F. (2013). Magnetic force-based tissue engineering and regenerative medicine, *J. Biomed. Nanotech.*, **9**(7), pp. 1129–1136.

97. Tampieri, A., Landi, E., Valentini, F., Sandri, M., D'Alessandro, T., Dediu, V., and Marcacci, M. (2011). Conceptually new type of bio-hybrid scaffold for bone regeneration, *Nanotechnology*, **22**(1), pp. 1–8.

98. Russo, A., Shelyakova, T., Casino, D., Lopomo, N., Strazzari, A., Ortolani, A., Visani, A., Dediu, V., and Marcacci, M. (2012). A new approach to scaffold fixation by magnetic forces: Application to large osteochondral defects, *Med. Eng. Phys.,* **34**, pp. 1287–1293.

99. Gloria, A., Russo, T., De Santis, R., and Ambrosio, L. (2009). 3D fiber deposition technique to make multifunctional and tailor-made scaffolds for tissue engineering applications, *J. Appl. Biomater. Biomech.*, **7**(3), pp. 141–152.

100. Peltola, S. M., Melchels, F. P. W., Grijpma, D. K., and Kellomäki, M. (2008). A review of rapid prototyping techniques for tissue engineering purposes, *Ann. Med.*, **40**, pp. 268–280.

101. De Santis, R., Gloria, A., Russo, T., D'Amora, U., Zeppetelli, S., and Ambrosio, L. (2010). An approach in developing 3D fiber-deposited magnetic scaffolds for tissue engineering, in $V^{th}$ *International Conference on Times of Polymers (TOP) and Composites* (eds. D'Amore, A., Acierno, D., and Grassia, L.), pp. 420–422, American Institute of Physics, Melville, New York.

102. De Santis, R., Gloria, A., Russo, T., D'Amora, U., Zeppetelli, S., Dionigi, C., Sytcheva, A., Herrmannsdörfer, T., Dediu, V. A., and Ambrosio, L. (2011). A basic approach toward the development of nanocomposite magnetic scaffolds for advanced bone tissue engineering, *J. Appl. Pol. Sci.*, **122**, pp. 3599–3605.

103. De Santis, R., Gloria, A., Russo, T., D'Amora, U., Zeppetelli, S., Tampieri, A., Herrmannsdörfer, T., and Ambrosio, L. (2011). A route toward the development of 3D magnetic scaffolds with tailored mechanical and morphological properties for hard tissue regeneration: Preliminary study, *Virt. Phys. Prototyp.*, **6**(4), pp. 189–195.

104. De Santis, R., Ambrosio, L., Mollica, F., Netti, P., and Nicolais, L. (2007). Mechanical properties of human mineralised connective tissues, in *Modeling of Biological Materials* (eds. Mollica, F., Preziosi, L., and Rajagopal, K. R.), Birkhauser, Boston.

105. Kyriakidou, K., Lucarini, G., Zizzi, A., Salvolini, E., Mattioli Belmonte, M., Mollica, F., Gloria, A., and Ambrosio, L. (2008). Dynamic co-seeding of osteoblast and endothelial cells on 3D polycaprolactone scaffolds for enhanced bone Tissue Engineering, *J. Bioact. Compat. Polym.*, **23**, pp. 227–243.

106. Hutmacher, D. W., Schantz, T., Zein, I., Ng, K. W., Teoh, S. H., and Tan, K. C. (2001). Mechanical properties and cell cultural response of polycaprolactone scaffolds designed and fabricated via fused deposition modelling, *J. Biomed. Mater. Res.*, **55**, pp. 203–216.

107. Singh, N., Jenkins, G. J. S., Asadi, R., and Doak, S. H. (2010). Potential toxicity of superparamagnetic iron oxide nanoparticles (SPION), *Nano Rev.*, **1**, pp. 53–58.

108. Lewinski, N., Colvin, V., and Drezek, R. (2008). Cytotoxicity of nanoparticles, *Small*, **4**, pp. 26–49.

References | 209

109. Berry, C. C., and Curtis, A. S. G. (2003). Functionalisation of magnetic nanoparticles for applications in biomedicine, *J. Phys. D. Appl. Phys.*, **36**, pp. 198–206.

110. Pon-On, W., Meejoo, S., and Tang, I. M. (2007). Incorporation of iron into nano hydroxyapatite particles synthesized by the microwave process, *Int. J. Nanosci.*, **6**(1), pp. 9–16.

111. Jiang, M., Terra, J., Rossi, A. M., Morales, M. A., Baggio Saitovitch, E. M., and Ellis, D. E. (2002). $Fe^{2+}/Fe^{3+}$substitution in hydroxyapatite: Theory and experiment, *Phys. Rev. B*, **66**, p. 224107.

112. Landi, E., Tampieri, A., Mattioli-Belmonte, M., Celotti, G., Sandri, M., Gigante, A., Fava, P., and Biagini, G. (2006). Biomimetic-Mg- and $Mg,CO_3$- substituted hydroxyapatites: Synthesis characterization and in vitro behaviour, *J. Eur. Ceram. Soc.*, **26**, pp. 2593–2601.

113. Barinov, S. M., Rau, J. V., Fadeeva, I. V., Nunziante Cesaro, S., Ferro, D., Trionfetti, G., Komlev, V. S., and Bibikov, V. Y. (2006). Carbonate loss from two magnesium-substituted carbonated apatites prepared by different synthesis techniques, *Mater. Res. Bull.*, **41**, pp. 485–494.

114. Gervaso, F., Scalera, F., Padmanabhan, S. K., Sannino, A., and Licciulli, A. (2012). High-performance hydroxyapatite scaffolds for bone tissue engineering applications, *Int. J. Appl. Ceram. Technol.*, **9**(3), pp. 507–516.

115. Tampieri, A., Landi, E., Sandri, M., Pressato, D., Rivas, J. R., Bañobre López, M., and Marcacci, M. (2010). Idrossiapatite intrinsecamente magnetica. Italian Patent No. MI2010A001420.

116. De Santis, R., Gloria, A., Russo, T., D'Amora, U., Zeppetelli, S., Tampieri, A., Herrmannsdörfer, T., and Ambrosio, L. (2011). A route toward the development of 3D magnetic scaffolds with tailored mechanical and morphological properties for hard tissue regeneration: Preliminary study. *Virtual Phys. Prototyp.*, **4**, pp. 189–195.

117. Russo, T., D'Amora, U., Gloria, A., Tunesi, M., Sandri, M., Rodilossi, S., Albani, D., Forloni, G., Giordano, C., Cigada, A., Tampieri, A., De Santis, R., and Ambrosio, L. (2013). Systematic analysis of injectable materials and 3D rapid prototyped magnetic scaffolds: From CNS applications to soft and hard tissue repair/regeneration. *Procedia Eng.*, **59**, pp. 233–239.

118. De Santis, R., Russo, A., Gloria, A., D'Amora, U., Russo, T., Panseri, S., Sandri, M., Tampieri, A., Marcacci, M., Dediu, V. A., Wilde, C. J., and Ambrosio, L. (2015). Towards the design of 3D fiber-deposited poly($\varepsilon$-caprolactone)/iron-doped hydroxyapatite nanocomposite magnetic scaffolds for bone regeneration, *J. Biomed. Nanotech.*, **11**, pp. 1236–1246.

**Chapter 8**

# Bio-Inspired Organized Structures Guiding Nerve Regeneration

Rahmat Cholas, Marta Madaghiele, Luca Salvatore, and Alessandro Sannino

*Department of Engineering for Innovation, University of Salento, Via per Monteroni, Lecce, 73100, Italy*

alessandro.sannino@unisalento.it

Autologous nerve grafting is the current gold standard treatment for peripheral nerve injury in cases where direct suturing of nerve ends is not possible. Even though the functional restoration achieved by the autograft is not optimal, autologous nerve tissues still show higher regenerative capability than several synthetic conduits available in the clinical setting, the latter used only for gaps that do not exceed 3 cm in length. The aim of this chapter is to highlight how bio-mimicry, inspired by nerve development, structure, and spontaneous regeneration following mild nerve injury, can help in the design of synthetic templates with optimized bioactivity for nerve regeneration.

## 8.1 Introduction

The peripheral nervous system is an extensive network of nerve fibers encompassing the entire body outside of the brain and

---

*Bio-Inspired Regenerative Medicine: Materials, Processes, and Clinical Applications*
Edited by Simone Sprio and Anna Tampieri
Copyright © 2016 Pan Stanford Publishing Pte. Ltd.
ISBN 978-981-4669-14-6 (Hardcover), 978-981-4669-15-3 (eBook)
www.panstanford.com

spinal cord, which enables the transmission of sensory and motor signals to and from the brain. Understanding the formation of this network during development, the structural organization of the fully mature tissue, and the spontaneous regeneration that occurs following limited nerve damage, provides valuable insight into strategies for facilitating restoration of peripheral nerve structure and function following extensive nerve injury.

Although peripheral nerves have the capacity to regenerate following injury, this capacity is only present in cases for which the nerve is not completely severed and continuity of the connective tissue of the nerve is at least partially maintained. In cases of complete severing of the nerve, surgical tension-free suturing is required, or when tension-free suturing is not possible, a bridging method between the nerve stumps is needed for reinnervation of the distal nerve segment to occur. The current best approach to bridging nerve gaps is the use of a nerve autograft, containing viable Schwann cells and an intact nerve structure. However, even when a nerve autograft is available, the functional outcome of the repaired nerve is often significantly lacking. As such, many alternative bridging techniques have been and continue to be explored including the use of muscle and vein autografts, and many different types of natural and synthetic materials in the form of tubular and cylindrical structures. Although many of these techniques have shown promise in their ability to facilitate nerve regeneration, none have yet been able to surpass the efficacy of the nerve autograft. However, identification and optimization of key structural and biochemical properties of engineered constructs for nerve regeneration have the potential to greatly enhance the efficacy of these devices. To this aim, the design and the optimization of scaffolds for nerve regeneration are inspired by Nature, with focus on the formation of the peripheral nervous system during embryonic and fetal development, the structural organization of the fully mature tissue, and the spontaneous regeneration that occurs following minor nerve damage—specifically considering the roles and interdependence of the four main cell types in nerve: neurons (axons), Schwann cells, endothelial cells, and fibroblasts. Additionally, understanding how to modulate the body's default response to tissue damage— to rapidly perform wound closure by scar formation and tissue contraction—is necessary to direct a regenerative response leading to restoration of function, rather than tissue repair through fibrous scar formation.

## 8.1.1 Key Aspects of Peripheral Nerve Development, Regeneration, and Structure

Proper functioning of a peripheral nerve depends on a close partnership among four different cell types: neurons, Schwann cells, endothelial cells, and fibroblasts. These cells work in coordination to permit the transmission of action potentials across substantial distances. The initial formation of the peripheral nervous system involves the growth and appropriate guidance of axons, the proliferation, migration, and maturation of Schwann cells, and the organization of the vascular network and connective tissue sheaths.

Axonal growth during embryonic development involves the processes of path finding and target selection carried out by the growth cone at the tip of the advancing axon, which is guided by gradients of both attractive and repulsive signals which are soluble, substrate or cell membrane-bound. Appropriate growth cone signaling is required up until the axon reaches its final target of innervation. Precise guidance of extending axons to distant synaptic targets relies on intermediate target points presented by glial cells and other axons [1]. Molecules known to be involved in axonal guidance include netrins, slits, semaphorins, ephrins, cell adhesion molecules (CAMs), bone morphogenetic proteins (BMPs), Wnts, Hedgehog, growth factors such as fibroblast growth factor (FGF) and nerve growth factor (NGF), extracellular matrix (ECM) adhesion molecules such as laminin, fibronectin, and tenascins, and proteoglycans. Studies have shown that in addition to molecular cues, the geometric features of the extracellular environment provide contact guidance to axons [2].

In coordination with the process of axonal growth is the proliferation and migration of Schwann cells. Schwann cells are derived from the neural crest and undergo three main transitional points during their development: (1) Neural crest cells produce Schwann precursor cells; (2) Schwann precursor cells differentiate into immature Schwann cells; (3) Beginning postnatally, immature Schwann cells transition into mature myelinating or non-myelinating Schwann cells [3]. Schwann precursor cells present starting at day E14/15 in rat embryos and by E17 most have differentiated into immature Schwann cells. Beginning early in embryonic development and thereafter, there is crosstalk between neurons and Schwann cells. Interestingly, Schwann cell precursor survival and function depend on axonal signaling of which the expression of neuregulin-1 (NRG1) by axons plays an important role [4]. This dependence facilitates the matching of Schwann cell number to axon number during development. Of importance, mature Schwann cells are able to survive temporarily in the absence of axons following nerve injury and axon degradation, due to autocrine signaling including insulin-like growth factor 2 (IGF-2), platelet derived growth factor-BB (PDGF-BB), and Neurotrophin 3 (NT3), in combination with laminin [5]. However, following prolonged periods of denervation (i.e., greater than 4 weeks) Schwann cells in distal segments of severed nerves progressively reduce in number leading to substantial decrease in the number of regenerating axons reaching their distal targets. Nonetheless, the Schwann cells that do survive prolonged denervation retain their capacity to remyelinated the few axons that do succeed to reinnervate their target tissue [6]. Conversely, axons depend on Schwann cell signaling for long-term survival. For example, somatic motor neurons whose cell bodies are located in the spinal cord depend on trophic support in the form of secreted growth factors by Schwann cells, astrocytes or target muscle tissue [7]. Furthermore, Schwann cells regulate axonal caliber and neuronal numbers during development, and the distribution of ion channels and neurofilament phosphorylation in myelinated axons [5]. As such, the role of Schwann cells in properly functioning peripheral nerves extends well beyond their most well-known function of myelinating axons.

Although myelination is essential for enabling rapid action potential propagation along the length of the axon, it is surprising to know that the majority of peripheral nerve fibers are unmyelinated [8]. In fact, non-myelinated axons outnumber myelinated axons by approximately 4 fold, and as such, non-myelinating Schwann cells greatly outnumber myelin-forming Schwann cells [9]. Mature Schwann cells are not permanently restricted to their myelinating or non-myelinating phenotype, but instead depend on axonal signaling. Specifically, the expression level of neuregulin-1 (NRG1) type III by axons (which remains bound to the axon surface) determines whether the axon will be myelinated or not. High expression levels of NRG1 type III result in myelination whereas low expression levels result in ensheathment but not myelination of axons [10–12]. NRG1 expression and thus myelin thickness correlates with axon diameter, with myelination generally occurring for axons with a diameter of 1 μm or larger. Axons with diameters smaller than 1 μm are typically unmyelinated, with Schwann cells ensheathing multiple axons together in a bundle. Following nerve transection or cell plating, myelinating and non-myelinating Schwann cells dedifferentiate into immature Schwann cells, and can then again differentiate into myelinating and non-myelinating Schwann cells during nerve regeneration. Interestingly, following peripheral nerve injury, NRG1 type III expression is required for axon regeneration and remyelination [10].

Another key aspect of peripheral nerve development and regeneration is the vascularization process. Peripheral nerve and vascular networks have strikingly similar complex arborization throughout the body, and there is a close association, even in development, of blood vessels and nerves [13]. Similar to the leading role the growth cone plays for axonal elongation and guidance, the specialized endothelial cells at the tip of developing blood vessels respond to environmental cues in the process of new vessel formation. The guidance of endothelial tip cells is controlled in part by growth factor signaling, among which vascular endothelial growth factor (VEGF) plays a major role [14]. Interestingly, endothelial tip cells have been shown to also respond to neural guidance signals including Netrins, Slits, Semaphorins, and Ephrins [15, 16]. In fact, in zebra fish it has been shown that axons of motor neurons directly contribute to vascular path finding during development [17]. Conversely, there is evidence that VEGF, which induces the formation of new blood vessels by endothelial cells, plays a role in neuron migration and axonal guidance [14].

The fourth main cell type found in peripheral nerves, after neurons (axons), Schwann cells, and endothelial cells, are the fibroblasts of the epineurium, perineurium, and endoneurium. The connective tissue comprising these three nerve sheaths serves to mechanically protect, form a barrier to surrounding tissue and cells, and provide structural support to the nerve. The epineurium contains the blood supply of the nerve and connects with the vascular network within the endoneurium. It forms the outermost barrier and mechanical support structure for the nerve. The perineurium is structured as alternating layers of cell sheets and collagen, which surround individual fascicles, or nerve bundles, that comprise nerve fibers that typically have a common origin and destination. The layers of the perineurium contain longitudinally oriented blood vessels and each layer is separated by a basal lamina. The endoneurium is the connective tissue surrounding individual Schwann cell-axon units, and contains the supporting vasculature (Fig. 8.1). Interestingly, it is suggested that endoneurial fibroblast, like Schwann cells, are derived from neural crest stem cells [18]. Another important example of signaling between different cell types in peripheral nerve is the evidence that Schwann cells control the formation of the connective tissue sheaths through Desert Hedgehog signaling [19, 20].

## 8.2 Spontaneous Nerve Regeneration

Spontaneous capacity of peripheral nerves to regenerate following injury is limited to cases in which the nerve is not completely severed and continuity of the connective tissue of the nerve is maintained. Mild injuries, such as nerve crush, result in complete and rapid recovery. When an axon is interrupted but its basement membrane is intact, regeneration is still possible and takes place only after proper degeneration does occur. Following axonotmesis, the distal segment undergoes anterograde or Wallerian degeneration, while an intense and unusual proliferation of Schwann cells occurs both in the proximal and distal segments. The final outcome of Wallerian degeneration is the formation of an endoneurial tube (i.e., the cylindrical basement membrane free of axon and myelin), along which Schwann cells can align to form peculiar structures (bands of Büngner). Schwann cells secrete growth factors to attract nerve sprouts that are sent out by the proximal end. When a sprout reaches the endoneurial tube, it can penetrate the distal segment and finally reinnervate the target tissue.

When the damage is extended to the connective tissues of the nerve, as in the case of nerve transection or neurotmesis, the spontaneous response to injury is tissue repair or wound closure attained through fibrous scar formation (i.e., neuroma), instead of regeneration. Surgical intervention is thus required in an attempt to limit scarring and stimulate nerve regeneration.

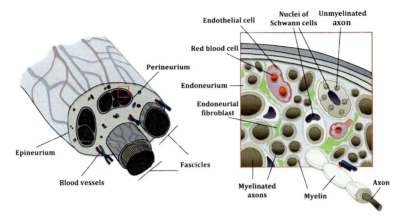

**Figure 8.1**  Schematic view of a peripheral nerve, showing the spatial arrangement of the four cell types playing key roles in nerve function, i.e., neurons (axons), Schwann cells, endothelial cells and fibroblasts: nerve cross section (left); zoom within a fascicle (right).

## 8.3  Surgical Approaches to Neurotmesis

### 8.3.1  Direct Repair (Neurorrhaphy)

Direct repair of injured peripheral nerves consists of the coaptation of two separate nerve stumps, in order to allow proximal axons to reach the endoneurial tubes resulting from the Wallerian degeneration of the distal stump. Good clinical results are particularly obtained for purely motor or purely sensory nerves.

Direct repair can be performed when the tissue loss is not significant (i.e., for small gaps, <5 mm) and the nerve ends can be approximated with minimal tension. Excessive nerve stretching is indeed detrimental, as the resulting decrease in blood flow might lead to nerve ischemia and scar formation [21]. Following neurotmesis, the amount of retraction of the nerve ends, which affects the nerve tension induced by the surgery, is time-dependent. Acute repair or primary surgery, performed up to 7 days after injury, corresponds to a nerve retraction that is about 4% of the original length, thus making direct, mostly tension-free suturing a possible option of intervention [22]. Conversely, secondary or delayed repair may likely require nerve grafting, since nerve retraction could be too high for direct tension-free suturing. The retraction of the nerve ends may reach 8% value in the first three weeks post-injury and is reported to further increase with time [23, 24].

Among direct repair techniques, end-to-end repair comprises several surgical techniques including epineural, group-fascicular and fascicular repair [22]. Proper fascicle alignment is fundamental for nerve regeneration and should be surgically obtained by minimizing the tissue damage, in order to reduce intraneural scarring. In epineural repair, the nerve stumps are approximated by means of 4–8 sutures passing through the epineurium. In this case, fascicle alignment is confirmed during the surgery by the continuity of the blood vessels within the epineurium (Fig. 8.2a). Group-fascicular repair provides precise fascicle alignment as bundles of fascicles are approximated with 2–3 sutures passing through the interfascicular epineurium. However, the higher number of sutures required, compared to epineural repair, might lead to increased scarring (Fig. 8.2b). For the same reason, fascicular repair, where single fascicles are approximated with 2–3 sutures placed within the perineurium, is not widely used anymore. Fibrin glue used instead of standard sutures has been recently suggested as a less traumatic surgical tool for nerve coaptation [25].

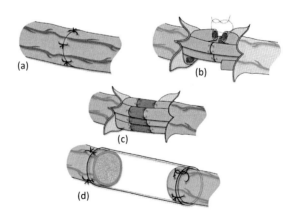

**Figure 8.2** Surgical approaches to neurotmesis. (a) Epineurial and (b) group-fascicular repair (direct repair); (c) autograft by means of standard cable grafting; (d) tubulization or entubulation.

End-to-side repair is another technique of direct repair, particularly used in brachial plexus and facial nerve injuries. In this case, the proximal stump is not available for end-to-end repair, thus the distal end is approximated to a donor nerve from which sensory and motor axons can sprout.

## 8.3.2 Autologous Nerve Graft (Autograft)

Nerve autograft is the current gold standard for peripheral nerve surgery, in cases where direct coaptation is not feasible. An autologous nerve graft, commonly harvested from a donor sensory cutaneous nerve, is interposed between two resected nerve stumps and used as an ideal biological chamber where nerve regeneration can occur. The donor nerve graft undergoes Wallerian degeneration and works as a native ECM scaffold permissive for Schwann cell migration and axonal elongation. Both topographical and biochemical cues of nerve ECM, e.g., basal lamina endoneurial tubes, are retained in the graft and provide optimal guidance and support to ingrowing axons.

The cellular components of the donor nerve also play a key role in promoting axonal regeneration. Grafted Schwann cells are an invaluable source of ECM adhesion molecules and neurotrophic factors, while stromal tissues in the graft help in preserving the structural integrity of the regenerating nerve and facilitating nerve re-vascularization. Successful vascularization of the graft allows for proper axonal elongation through the graft length and across its whole diameter, leading to improved outcomes. Small caliber grafts work thus better than large caliber grafts, due to higher and faster re-vascularization and reduced risk of central necrosis. Among currently used donor nerves, the sural nerve, which supplies sensation to the posterior and lateral lower third of the leg and lateral foot, is likely the most commonly chosen by surgeons, due to its small diameter (2–4 mm) and high available length (up to 50 cm) [22, 26]. In spite of representing the gold standard to treat peripheral nerve injuries over relatively long gaps, nerve autograft is yet far from being an optimal clinical approach, as complete recovery of nerve function is rare. Moreover, donor site morbidity is a major drawback of the autograft procedure. Undesired complications at the harvesting site, including neuroma and chronic pain, might occur.

Depending on the diameter and length of the nerve gap to be bridged, different grafting techniques might be adopted, provided a sufficient amount of donor nerve is available. The standard cable grafting technique (Fig. 8.2c) aims at maximizing the coverage of the cross-sectional area of the nerve to be repaired, by suturing multiple graft segments to the groups of fascicles of the proximal and distal stumps, similarly to what is performed in group-fascicular repair [22]. An alternative surgical technique, known as single-fascicle method, has been also proposed to reduce the donor site morbidity [27]. A relatively small portion of the cross-sectional area of the severed nerve (up to about 60%) is covered by a single fascicle harvested from the donor nerve. The single graft is aligned centrally with respect to the cross section of the injured nerve and coaptated to the proximal and distal stumps by means of single pullout sutures, in order to minimize the formation of fibrotic scar tissue. Studies performed on rat sciatic nerves seem to suggest a faster regeneration and better functional outcome when performing the single-fascicle graft compared to the standard grafting technique [27].

It is worth mentioning that, when a sufficient amount of autologous nerve is not available, nerve allografts harvested from cadaver donors represent a valid clinical option. With regard to immunosuppression, decellularized nerve allografts show the advantage of retaining most of the topographical and chemical cues of the native ECM, while reducing the risk of undesired immunological rejection.

### 8.3.3 Tubulization

Several "off the shelf" conduits (also called neural guides), based either on natural or synthetic biomaterials, are currently available in the clinical practice to bridge gaps in nerve tissues that usually do not exceed 3 cm in length [28–32]. Instead of using a donor nerve, surgeons may choose to suture the proximal and distal stumps of the resected nerve to the ends of a tubular chamber, which is usually filled with saline solution. Such a technique is often referred to as tubulization or entubulation (Fig. 8.2d). In the past, the use of autologous vein grafts to bridge peripheral nerve defects was an example of entubulation yielded by means of biological conduits [33, 34]. However, such biological conduits require harvesting from donor sites, show poor clinical outcomes, and often kink and collapse, thus impeding nerve regeneration. Conversely, synthetic tubular chambers can be designed to provide a suitable environment with appropriate stiffness, where a fibrin-based matrix can form and work as a temporary scaffold to support Schwann cell migration and direct axons from the proximal to the distal end. Moreover, the chamber is required to retain the growth factors released by injured nerve cells at the defect site, while preventing the infiltration of surrounding soft tissues. Its tubular wall is also envisaged to host myofibroblasts, thus limiting their contractile activity, in order to reduce the undesired formation of scar tissue [35, 36]. In the ideal case, the tubular matrix degrades progressively as the nerve regenerates, with a perfect matching between the rates of material degradation and tissue regeneration. A non-degradable nerve conduit would indeed cause nerve compression in the long-term, requiring surgical removal [32].

Compared to the grafting of autologous nerves, the tubulization by means of synthetic conduits appears particularly advantageous to avoid the problems related to donor site morbidity. However, the regenerative capability of currently available neural guides significantly decreases as the length and/or the diameter of the nerve gap to be bridged increase. Even when encouraging animal data have been provided, results on relatively large human nerves, such as the ulnar and median nerves (which have a diameter of approximately 3–4 mm), have been rarely successful [30, 31, 37, 38]. This is why neural guides have a limited use, finding application only in the treatment of short defects in small calibre nerves (e.g., digital and radial sensory nerves). Several types of conduits, mainly differing for the biomaterial used, the microstructure and the degradation rate, are approved for clinical use and are comprehensively reviewed in the literature [29–32, 39]. Among them, the Neuragen® tube, a collagen-based guide with a random, cell impermeable porosity, is the one with the largest number of prospective and retrospective clinical studies and is reported to perform as well as the autograft for gaps up to 20 mm [29].

## 8.4 Bio-Inspired Design of Nerve Regenerative Templates

### 8.4.1 Mimicking Native Nerve ECM Topography

Although the autograft represents the gold standard for nerve repair, its limitations related to donor site morbidity and weak functional recovery (not to mention the possible unavailability of nerve grafts with suitable length for some patients) boost the research in the fields of regenerative medicine and tissue engineering towards the development of bio-engineered constructs, which might perform as well as or better than the nerve autograft. Neural guides can be considered as first-generation devices conceived by bio-engineers to avoid the formation of neuromas and to facilitate the regeneration of thin peripheral nerves over short gaps. The current challenge is to increase the gap length and the diameter bridgeable by a synthetic graft.

In order to explain the failure, i.e., poor regenerative capability, of empty tubes over long nerve gaps and/or for large nerves, the existence of a critical chamber volume has been postulated [31]. The traditional idea of a critically sized defect length, below which the entubulation performs quite well regardless of the specific device used, is being replaced by the idea of a critically sized defect volume. Several interrelated factors might justify the existence of such a volume. First of all, a tubular chamber alone, used to bridge a large defect, might not be able to provide a crossing fibrin cable, which is necessary to support initial cell migration into the defect. Schwann cell migration along linearly oriented structures is essential and preliminary to axonal regrowth, whose speed should be then high enough to avoid chronic degeneration and denervation of the distal stump (i.e., the disruption of the basement membrane of the distal endoneurial tubes) [40]. In clinical practice, the distal endoneurial tubes should be in contact with the regrowing axons within 18–24 months after injury [22]. An additional reason why the entubulation fails over large defects might be a too low concentration of neurotrophic factors into the conduit, which is thus unable to provide an efficiently regenerative environment. Furthermore, the difficult vascularization of large grafts is a key factor to consider. As discussed above for autografts, the success of any grafting procedure is affected by the volume of the tissue to be replaced and vascularized. Appropriate formation of blood vessels in the stromal tissues of peripheral nerves (i.e., endoneurium, perineurium, and epineurium) is fundamental for cell survival, especially in the center of large grafts, and for fast nerve regeneration.

In an attempt to replicate the native structure of nerves, which might be the reason for the regenerative (although limited) success of nerve autografts compared to synthetic conduits, bio-engineers have been working on the development of luminal fillers, characterized by a preferential orientation along the longitudinal axis, to be implanted within the chamber. Such cylindrical fillers, in either sponge or fibrous form, can potentially improve nerve regeneration by providing prompt contact guidance to Schwann cells and axons, which is extremely important to accelerate axonal regrowth in large defects. At the same time, the filler may act as a scaffold facilitating vascularization and retention of endogenous growth factors at the defect site. The combined use of oriented muscle tissue within a vein graft, explored in the past with some success [41], is the biological analogue of what bio-engineers are trying to pursue by designing anisotropic matrices filling tubular guides (and the related fabrication methods), in order to enhance nerve regeneration.

As also shown for neural guides, whose regenerative potential can be increased by adjusting the microstructure and surface alignment [42–44], the design of porous luminal fillers should be focused on the optimization of the true surface area and contact guidance available for cell-material interactions, with the aim of closely mimicking the function performed by the endoneurial tubes in spontaneous nerve regeneration. Oriented, sponge-like collagen matrices, inserted into a collagen tube, were found to provide optimal results in an animal model, comparable to the ones achieved by the nerve autograft, when possessing a pore size of approximately 20 μm [35, 45, 46]. Pore orientation along the direction of Schwann cell migration, i.e., the contact guidance, is clearly essential to nerve regeneration [47]. A few studies show that non-oriented fillers might be deleterious, as they seem to obstruct axonal elongation [48, 49]. However, the chemical composition and the degradation rate of the luminal filler should also be carefully addressed, as both these variables may affect not only the rate of cell infiltration, but also the inflammatory response and, more in general, the response of cells to the implanted biomaterial. For instance, recent studies on keratin-based hydrogel fillers show that such structures are able to perform as well as the autograft in some animal models [50, 51], and that this success might be ascribed to a stronger activation of Schwann cells in the distal stump, for a more efficient debris clearance and ECM remodeling [52]. With regard to the degradation rate, it is worth highlighting that the optimal residence time in vivo of a scaffold for nerve regeneration has not been quantified yet. While in a rat model the optimal half-life of collagen chambers seems to be approximately 2–3 weeks [53], the neural guides currently available for clinical use have quite different residence times, mostly in the range of 3–16 months, with the exception of the Neuragen® tube, which is reported to require 36–48 months to fully degrade [29]. Interestingly, a recent clinical investigation showed that, in cases where Neuragen® implants were failing, the tubes were also resorbed within 6–17 months [54]. This seems to suggest that a close correlation exists between the in vivo residence time and the performance of nerve conduits. Also for luminal fillers, the identification of an optimal degradation rate is very likely necessary for a proper design of the devices, thus definitely deserving further exploration. The understanding of the kinetic of initial nerve regeneration in a rat model, with innervation of the distal stump requiring about 10–12 weeks to occur [55], might provide the basis for the identification of an optimal time frame for a biomaterial's degradation.

A number of oriented, sponge-like matrices have been developed, mostly based on collagen [46, 56–59] and/or other natural polymers, e.g., chitosan and agarose [60, 61]. With the aim of further mimicking the structure of the basement membrane making up the endoneurial tubes, laminin, and fibronectin are often adopted to modify the surface of aligned pore channels or fibers [62, 63].

Oriented fibrous matrices, instead of sponge-like ones, have been indeed explored as alternative luminal fillers. Fibers or filaments of collagen [62, 64], polyesters [65–67] and silk [68, 69] have been used to enhance nerve regeneration in animal models. A higher number of filaments within the lumen of the neural guide were found to enhance the number of regenerated axons [70], likely due to increased surface area and contact guidance. However, the packing density of fibers and their spatial distribution within the conduit are also important for nerve regeneration [71]. If bio-mimicry inspires the design of scaffolds, it can be observed that fibers are difficult to align over macro-scale distances, thus are not likely to provide continuous channels that closely mimic the morphology of the crossing fibrin cable and/or the endoneurial tubes accommodating Schwann cells. This suggests that sponge-like matrices, possessing aligned micro-channels over their entire length, might be more successful for nerve regeneration than fibrous scaffolds [72]. However, the combined use of a hydrogel matrix might help in supporting the fibers within the tube lumen, thus maintaining their longitudinal orientation [66].

In addition to the development of aligned luminal fillers, several studies focused on the synthesis of multi-channeled nerve guides, i.e., cylindrical nerve guides with a selected number of oriented channels throughout their length. Fabrication methods such as fiber templating and porogen leaching [73, 74] are useful to control both the macro- and microstructure of the devices, which are usually based on synthetic polymers. Although bio-inspired, this tissue engineering approach denotes a low degree of mimicry of both structural and biochemical features of native nerve ECM.

## 8.4.2 Mimicking Native Nerve ECM Biochemistry

Beyond providing aligned topography, which facilitates optimal contact guidance of regenerating axons, the appropriate biochemical signals must be presented in the correct temporal and spatial pattern to direct and sustain the regenerative process until complete reinnervation of motor and sensory targets is achieved. These biochemical signals come in the form of both soluble factors or ECM- or cell membrane-bound molecules and receptors. Regenerating neurons up-regulate integrins and other adhesion molecules which are able to bind to ECM proteins such as laminin, collagen, and fribronectin, and interact with cell adhesion proteins on Schwann cell membranes [75]. In vitro experiments of explanted dorsal root ganglia (DRG) have shown significant increases in the degree of Schwann cell migration, and axonal outgrowth when the DRG were cultured on surfaces coated with various adhesion proteins. Considering that peripheral nerve ECM contains abundant amounts of collagen I, collagen IV, and laminin, the affinity of growing axons and migrating Schwann cells for these molecules is not surprising. Conversely, Schwann cells express collagen V during peripheral nerve development at the period during which myelination occurs, and may serve as an inhibitory signal used in the process of axonal fascicular organization [76]. An in vitro study by Chernousov et al. demonstrated robust Schwann cell migration and axonal outgrowth from embryonic rat DRG on surfaces coated with collagen IV, laminin, or collagen I, whereas collagen V coated surfaces supported equivalent Schwann cell migration but inhibited axonal outgrowth [76]. A different study by Hammarback et al. showed that DRG grown on laminin coated surfaces had significantly increased axonal outgrowth, and demonstrated that laminin guides the growth of axons in a concentration dependent manner [77]. Indeed, ECM proteins such as laminin and collagen I are often used in combination with synthetic materials as a way to functionalize scaffolds designed with controlled mechanical and structural properties but lacking cell binding sites [78–80]. ECM proteins are often used as luminal fillers of nerve conduits to serve as bioactive substrates for migrating Schwann cells, endothelial cells, macrophages and axons [81].

In addition to bioactive substrates, appropriate neurotrophic support is essential for achieving substantial functional recovery following nerve injury. During nerve development, neurotrophic factors play an important role in Schwann cell proliferation and migration, axonal growth, and in neuronal and Schwann cell survival. Numerous studies have shown the beneficial effects of including neurotrophic factors as part of nerve regeneration strategies [82–85]. The addition of glial cell line derived neurotrophic factor (GDNF) and NGF within a tubular collagen nerve conduit was found to stimulate increased Schwann cell migration and axonal outgrowth in a rat sciatic nerve injury model at an early (2 week) time point compared to the collagen conduits not containing the neurotrophic factors [86]. Similarly, GDNF added to a synthetic nerve conduit was reported to facilitate significant motor axon regeneration 6 weeks after injury in the rat facial nerve, whereas neurotrophin-3 (NT-3) induced a much smaller degree of axon regeneration [87]. These results are consistent with in vitro studies which have shown increased neurite outgrowth from rat DRG explants through the addition, individually and in combination, of GDNF, NGF, and ciliary neurotrophic factor (CNTF) to the cell culture medium [88]. Basic fibroblast growth factor (bFGF) has also been demonstrated to improve the efficacy of a polymeric nerve conduit when incorporated in a gelatin hydrogel delivered within the conduit lumen [89]. Highlighting the importance of vascularization, Hobson et al. reported that VEGF delivered in a gel within a silicone nerve conduit in the rat sciatic nerve, not only lead to increased numbers of blood vessels within the tube lumen, but also enhanced Schwann cell migration and axonal growth compared to the gel alone [90].

Inclusion of neurotrophic factors within a matrix allows for more sustained localized delivery than direct injection of a neurotrophic factor suspension, and many studies have reported on improved axon regeneration when factors are incorporated within the conduit wall or within a luminal matrix [83, 84, 91]. Other delivery methods include polymeric microencapsulation to better preserve the structure and release profile of the therapeutic agent [92–95], and affinity binding of factors directly to a biomaterial matrix [96]. However, further optimization of growth factor encapsulation delivery systems can be made, as resulting in vivo improvements in functional recovery are not always seen [97]. Several in vitro studies have highlighted the importance of the distribution of guidance molecules in gradients, rather than at constant concentrations [98–100]. Dodla et al. reported that laminin and NGF gradients within an agarose hydrogel filling a polysulfone nerve conduit in a rat sciatic nerve gap supported axon regeneration and functional recovery comparable to a nerve graft, whereas when laminin and NGF were instead presented at constant concentrations along the nerve conduit this regenerative response was not seen [101].

An effective alternative to the delivery of neurotrophic factors is the delivery of autologous or allogenic Schwann cells within a nerve conduit. This approach takes advantage of the supportive role Schwann cells play in the proper formation and maintenance of peripheral nerves, as well as their therapeutic role following nerve injury. Schwann cells secrete numerous neurotrophic factors, express cell adhesion molecules (which positively interact with growing axons), synthesize the basal lamina, and myelinate regenerating axons. The delivery of exogenous Schwann cells within a nerve conduit augments the numbers of locally proliferating and migrating Schwann cells within the nerve stumps and may be particularly important for large diameter nerve or long gap defects [28]. Not surprisingly, the inclusion of exogenous Schwann cells in therapies to treat nerve injury has been demonstrated to lead to significantly improved histological and functional outcomes. Various theories have been suggested to explain the therapeutic effect of implanted Schwann cells, including assisting in debris clearance, providing trophic support to axons, modulating the inflammatory response, synthesizing an extracellular matrix to serve as a scaffold, and inducing an appropriate vascular response. These are many of the same activities performed by endogenous Schwann cells found at the site of injury and within the distal segment of an injured nerve. In short nerve gaps (i.e., less than 10 mm), it has been shown that proliferating Schwann cells are able to migrate into a nerve bridge from the proximal and distal nerve segments. But in cases of injuries resulting in long gaps in a nerve (>10 mm), the ability of the Schwann cells to migrate from the adjacent nerve stumps is limited and slow. Factors that accelerate endogenous Schwann cell migration and proliferation within a nerve bridge may be able to augment the limited cell infiltration seen in large nerve gaps, and negate the need for exogenous Schwann cells, which in clinical practice are not easily obtained. Stem cells, such as bone marrow derived mesenchymal stem cells (MSCs) are a potentially more accessible source of cells for implantation, and can be genetically modified to over express a desired factor to positively modulate the injury environment in a sustained fashion.

A significant challenge that remains is providing optimal temporal delivery of therapeutic agents. At the acute stage of injury, it is likely that factors that support neuronal survival and reduce inflammation would be desirable, whereas at the sub-acute stage factors that support Schwann cell proliferation and migration as well as vascularization would be ideal. Finally, during the chronic stage of nerve regeneration emphasis should be on factors that stimulate axonal growth and myelination.

### 8.4.3 Multi-Faceted Approaches

In spite of the myriad of efforts made to produce biomimetic "off the shelf" devices potentially able to enhance nerve regeneration, none of the devices have yet been shown to perform better than the nerve autograft. This finding seems to suggest that multi-modal approaches, targeting different aspects of nerve tissue engineering, are more likely to succeed. Luminal fillers, which attempt to replicate the topography and the biochemistry of nerve ECM, are thus often exploited as delivery vehicles for exogenous cells (regarded as efficient factories of biomolecules) and/or growth factors. The supply and the prolonged release of selected growth factors, used either singularly or in cocktail mixtures, are well known to promote nerve regeneration [66, 82]. Among the most effective growth factors, it is worth citing nerve growth factor (NGF) [102], neurotrophin-3 (NT3) [66], brain-derived neurotrophic factor (BDNF) [62], ciliary neurotrophic factor (CNTF) [62], glial growth factor (GGF) [103], leukemia inhibitory factor (LIF) [66, 104], vascular endothelial growth factor (VEGF) and platelet-derived growth factor (PDGF) [105, 106]. Since such molecules are highly instable in the physiological environment, due to denaturation and degradation, it is essential to use suitable delivery vehicles able to preserve the biological activity of the molecules, while providing their sustained release over specific time windows. Several biodegradable drug delivery devices have thus been investigated to efficiently supply exogenous growth factors to injured peripheral nerves, including microcapsules or microspheres [107–109], hydrogel matrices [66] and core-shell nanofibers produced by means of coaxial electrospinning [110].

Modern and recent approaches to nerve regeneration are also focused on the electrical conductivity of nerves, which is very important for functional recovery but is often neglected in the design of nerve conduits and luminal fillers. Interesting studies have highlighted the regenerative potential of conductive nerve chambers, made up of conducting polymers (e.g., polypyrrole) [111] or doped with carbon nanotubes [63, 112]. Furthermore, it is worth underscoring that a more comprehensive view of nerve regeneration encompasses the understanding of the effects of various stimulation techniques, commonly adopted in physiotherapy, on the regenerative potential of nerve scaffolds [113]. Electrical, ultrasound, and low-level laser stimulation have been demonstrated to yield positive outcomes on functional recovery and might also act in synergy with selected biomimetic devices to enhance nerve regeneration.

## 8.5 Conclusion

Nerve development and structure, as well as spontaneous regeneration occurring after mild injury, are significant sources of inspiration for the design of biomimetic, anisotropic scaffolds able to promote the regeneration of peripheral nerves over critically sized defects. The careful modulation of both topography and biochemistry of nerve scaffolds, in an attempt to replicate the properties of the gold standard autograft, can lead to the development of "off the shelf" devices ready for clinical use and much more effective than currently available neural guides. Such engineered constructs would be extremely advantageous compared to autografts, as there would be no concerns regarding donor site morbidity and availability of tissue. However, the experimental findings reported so far seem to suggest that the potential of these devices to surpass the regenerative capability of autograft is poor. Further improvement of functional outcome (which is very limited, even in the case of autografts) is thus likely to require a multi-faceted tissue engineering approach, where exogenous cells and/or growth factors are incorporated in the device in order to accelerate nerve regeneration and avoid chronic denervation of the target tissue. Several physiotherapy stimulation techniques might also concur to enhance the functional recovery induced by a given device. While the translation of novel biomaterial-based devices from lab benches to clinics seems achievable in the near future, the implementation of complex cell-based or growth factor-based devices in the clinical practice is pursued as a long-term goal.

### References

1. Chotard, C., and Salecker, I. (2004). Neurons and glia: Team players in axon guidance, *Trends Neurosci.*, **27**, pp. 655–661.

2. Smeal, R. M., Rabbitt, R., Biran, R., and Tresco, P. A. (2005). Substrate curvature influences the direction of nerve outgrowth, *Ann. Biomed. Eng.*, **33**, pp. 376–382.

3. Jessen, K. R., and Mirsky, R. (1997). Embryonic Schwann cell development: The biology of Schwann cell precursors and early Schwann cells, *J. Anat.*, **191** (Pt 4), pp. 501–505.

4. Woodhoo, A., and Sommer, L. (2008). Development of the Schwann cell lineage: From the neural crest to the myelinated nerve, *Glia*, **56**, pp. 1481–1490.

5. Mirsky, R., Jessen, K. R., Brennan, A., Parkinson, D., Dong, Z., Meier, C., Parmantier, E., and Lawson, D. (2002). Schwann cells as regulators of nerve development, *J. Physiol. Paris*, **96**, pp. 17–24.

6. Sulaiman, O. A., and Gordon, T. (2000). Effects of short- and long-term Schwann cell denervation on peripheral nerve regeneration, myelination, and size, *Glia*, **32**, pp. 234–246.

7. Kilpatrick, T. J., and Soilu-Hanninen, M. (1999). Molecular mechanisms regulating motor neuron development and degeneration, *Mol. Neurobiol.*, **19**, pp. 205–228.

8. Armati, P. J., and Mathey, E. K. (2013). An update on Schwann cell biology: Immunomodulation, neural regulation and other surprises, *J. Neurol. Sci.*, **333**, pp. 68–72.

9. Griffin, J. W., and Thompson, W. J. (2008). Biology and pathology of nonmyelinating Schwann cells, *Glia*, **56**, pp. 1518–1531.

10. Fricker, F. R., and Bennett, D. L. (2011). The role of neuregulin-1 in the response to nerve injury, *Future Neurol.*, **6**, pp. 809–822.

11. Quintes, S., Goebbels, S., Saher, G., Schwab, M. H., and Nave, K. A. (2010). Neuron-glia signaling and the protection of axon function by Schwann cells, *J. Peripher. Nerv. Syst.*, **15**, pp. 10–16.

12. Taveggia, C., Zanazzi, G., Petrylak, A., Yano, H., Rosenbluth, J., Einheber, S., Xu, X., Esper, R. M., Loeb, J. A., Shrager, P., Chao, M. V., Falls, D. L., Role, L., and Salzer, J. L. (2005). Neuregulin-1 type III determines the ensheathment fate of axons, *Neuron*, **47**, pp. 681–694.

13. Zacchigna, S., Ruiz de Almodovar, C., and Carmeliet, P. (2008). Similarities between angiogenesis and neural development: What small animal models can tell us, *Curr. Top. Dev. Biol.*, **80**, pp. 1–55.

14. Chauvet, S., Burk, K., and Mann, F. (2013). Navigation rules for vessels and neurons: Cooperative signaling between VEGF and neural guidance cues, *Cell. Mol. Life Sci.*, **70**, pp. 1685–1703.

15. Carmeliet, P., and Tessier-Lavigne, M. (2005). Common mechanisms of nerve and blood vessel wiring, *Nature*, **436**, pp. 193–200.

16. Eichmann, A., Le Noble, F., Autiero, M., and Carmeliet, P. (2005). Guidance of vascular and neural network formation, *Curr. Opin. Neurobiol.*, **15**, pp. 108–115.

17. Lim, A. H., Suli, A., Yaniv, K., Weinstein, B., Li, D. Y., and Chien, C. B. (2011). Motoneurons are essential for vascular pathfinding, *Development,* **138**, pp. 3847–3857.

18. Joseph, N. M., Mukouyama, Y. S., Mosher, J. T., Jaegle, M., Crone, S. A., Dormand, E. L., Lee, K. F., Meijer, D., Anderson, D. J., and Morrison, S. J. (2004). Neural crest stem cells undergo multilineage differentiation in developing peripheral nerves to generate endoneurial fibroblasts in addition to Schwann cells, *Development,* **131**, pp. 5599–5612.

19. Jessen, K. R., and Mirsky, R. (2002). Signals that determine Schwann cell identity, *J. Anat.,* **200**, pp. 367–376.

20. Parmantier, E., Lynn, B., Lawson, D., Turmaine, M., Namini, S. S., Chakrabarti, L., McMahon, A. P., Jessen, K. R., and Mirsky, R. (1999). Schwann cell-derived Desert hedgehog controls the development of peripheral nerve sheaths, *Neuron,* **23**, pp. 713–724.

21. Millesi, H. (1991). Indications and techniques of nerve grafting, in *Operative Nerve Repair and Reconstruction,* vol. **1** (ed. Gelberman, R. H.), (JB Lippincot, Philadelphia) pp. 525–543.

22. Siemionow, M., and Brzezicki, G. (2009). Current techniques and concepts in peripheral nerve repair, *Int. Rev. Neurobiol.,* **87**, pp. 141–172.

23. Trumble, T. E. (1999). Peripheral nerve injury: Pathophysiology and repair, in *Trauma* (eds. Feliciano, D. V., Moore, E. E., and Mattox, K. L.), McGraw-Hill, New York, pp. 2048–2053.

24. Trumble, T. E., and Shon, F. G. (2000). The physiology of nerve transplantation, *Hand Clin.,* **16**, pp. 105–122.

25. Sameem, M., Wood, T. J., and Bain, J. R. (2011). A systematic review on the use of fibrin glue for peripheral nerve repair, *Plast. Reconstr. Surg.,* **127**, pp. 2381–2390.

26. Ortiguela, M. E., Wood, M. B., and Cahill, D. R. (1987). Anatomy of the sural nerve complex, *J. Hand Surg. Am.,* **12**, pp. 1119–1123.

27. Siemionow, M., Zielinski, M., and Meirer, R. (2004). The single-fascicle method of nerve grafting, *Ann. Plast. Surg.,* **52**, pp. 72–79.

28. Daly, W., Yao, L., Zeugolis, D., Windebank, A., and Pandit, A. (2012). A biomaterials approach to peripheral nerve regeneration: Bridging the peripheral nerve gap and enhancing functional recovery, *J. R. Soc. Interface,* **9**, pp. 202–221.

29. Kehoe, S., Zhang, X. F., and Boyd, D. (2012). FDA approved guidance conduits and wraps for peripheral nerve injury: A review of materials and efficacy, *Injury,* **43**, pp. 553–572.

30. Meek, M. F., and Coert, J. H. (2008). US FOOD and Drug Administration/ Conformit Europe-approved absorbable nerve conduits for clinical repair of peripheral and cranial nerves, *Ann. Plast. Surg.,* **60**, pp. 466–472.

31. Moore, A. M., Kasukurthi, R., Magill, C. K., Farhadi, H. F., Borschel, G. H., and Mackinnon, S. E. (2009). Limitations of conduits in peripheral nerve repairs, *Hand,* **4**, pp. 180–186.

32. Schlosshauer, B., Dreesmann, L., Schaller, H. E., and Sinis, N. (2006). Synthetic nerve guide implants in humans: A comprehensive survey, *Neurosurgery,* **59**, pp. 740–747; discussion 747–748.

33. Kelleher, M. O., Al-Abri, R. K., Eleuterio, M. L., Myles, L. M., Lenihan, D. V., and Glasby, M. A. (2001). The use of conventional and invaginated autologous vein grafts for nerve repair by means of entubulation, *Br. J. Plast. Surg.,* **54**, pp. 53–57.

34. Stahl, S., and Goldberg, J. A. (1999). The use of vein grafts in upper extremity nerve surgery, *Eur. J. Plast. Surg.,* **22**, pp. 255–259.

35. Chamberlain, L. J., Yannas, I. V., Arrizabalaga, A., Hsu, H. P., Norregaard, T. V., and Spector, M. (1998). Early peripheral nerve healing in collagen and silicone tube implants: Myofibroblasts and the cellular response, *Biomaterials,* **19**, pp. 1393–1403.

36. Chamberlain, L. J., Yannas, I. V., Hsu, H. P., and Spector, M. (2000). Connective tissue response to tubular implants for peripheral nerve regeneration: The role of myofibroblasts, *J. Comp. Neurol.,* **417**, pp. 415–430.

37. Stanec, S., and Stanec, Z. (1998). Ulnar nerve reconstruction with an expanded polytetrafluoroethylene conduit, *Br. J. Plast. Surg.,* **51**, pp. 637–639.

38. Weber, R. A., Breidenbach, W. C., Brown, R. E., Jabaley, M. E., and Mass, D. P. (2000). A randomized prospective study of polyglycolic acid conduits for digital nerve reconstruction in humans, *Plast. Reconstr. Surg.,* **106**, pp. 1036–1045; discussion 1046–1038.

39. Nectow, A. R., Marra, K. G., and Kaplan, D. L. (2012). Biomaterials for the development of peripheral nerve guidance conduits, *Tissue Eng. Part B Rev.,* **18**, pp. 40–50.

40. Hoke, A. (2006). Mechanisms of Disease: What factors limit the success of peripheral nerve regeneration in humans?, *Nat. Clin. Pract. Neurol.,* **2**, pp. 448–454.

41. Battiston, B., Tos, P., Cushway, T. R., and Geuna, S. (2000). Nerve repair by means of vein filled with muscle grafts I. Clinical results, *Microsurgery,* **20**, pp. 32–36.

42. Chew, S. Y., Mi, R., Hoke, A., and Leong, K. W. (2007). Aligned protein-polymer composite fibers enhance nerve regeneration: A potential tissue-engineering platform, *Adv. Funct. Mater.*, **17**, pp. 1288–1296.

43. Hsu, S. H., Su, C. H., and Chiu, I. M. (2009). A novel approach to align adult neural stem cells on micropatterned conduits for peripheral nerve regeneration: A feasibility study, *Artif. Organs*, **33**, pp. 26–35.

44. Wang, W., Itoh, S., Matsuda, A., Ichinose, S., Shinomiya, K., Hata, Y., and Tanaka, J. (2008). Influences of mechanical properties and permeability on chitosan nano/microfiber mesh tubes as a scaffold for nerve regeneration, *J. Biomed. Mater. Res. A*, **84**, pp. 557–566.

45. Chang, A. S., Yannas, I. V., Krarup, C., Sethi, R. R., Norregaard, T. V., and Zervas, N. T. (1988). Polymeric templates for peripheral nerve regeneration. Electrophysiological study of functional recovery, *Proc. ACS Div. Polym. Mater. Sci. Eng.*, **59**, pp. 906–910.

46. Chang, A. S., Yannas, I. V., Perutz, S., Loree, H., Sethi, R. R., Krarup, C., Norregaard, T. V., Zervas, N. T., and Silver, J. (1990). Electrophysiological study of recovery of peripheral nerves regenerated by a collagen-glycosaminoglycan copolymer matrix, in *Progress in Biomedical Polymers* (ed. Gebelein, C. G.), Plenum, New York.

47. Yao, L., Billiar, K. L., Windebank, A. J., and Pandit, A. (2010). Multichanneled collagen conduits for peripheral nerve regeneration: Design, fabrication, and characterization, *Tissue Eng. Part C Methods*, **16**, pp. 1585–1596.

48. Evans, G. R., Brandt, K., Katz, S., Chauvin, P., Otto, L., Bogle, M., Wang, B., Meszlenyi, R. K., Lu, L., Mikos, A. G., and Patrick, C. W., Jr. (2002). Bioactive poly(L-lactic acid) conduits seeded with Schwann cells for peripheral nerve regeneration, *Biomaterials*, **23**, pp. 841–848.

49. Stang, F., Fansa, H., Wolf, G., Reppin, M., and Keilhoff, G. (2005). Structural parameters of collagen nerve grafts influence peripheral nerve regeneration, *Biomaterials*, **26**, pp. 3083–3091.

50. Apel, P. J., Garrett, J. P., Sierpinski, P., Ma, J., Atala, A., Smith, T. L., Koman, L. A., and Van Dyke, M. E. (2008). Peripheral nerve regeneration using a keratin-based scaffold: Long-term functional and histological outcomes in a mouse model, *J. Hand. Surg. Am.*, **33**, pp. 1541–1547.

51. Sierpinski, P., Garrett, J., Ma, J., Apel, P., Klorig, D., Smith, T., Koman, L. A., Atala, A., and Van Dyke, M. (2008). The use of keratin biomaterials derived from human hair for the promotion of rapid regeneration of peripheral nerves, *Biomaterials*, **29**, pp. 118–128.

52. Pace, L. A., Plate, J. F., Smith, T. L., and Van Dyke, M. E. (2013). The effect of human hair keratin hydrogel on early cellular response to sciatic nerve injury in a rat model, *Biomaterials*, **34**, pp. 5907–5914.

53. Harley, B. A., Spilker, M. H., Wu, J. W., Asano, K., Hsu, H. P., Spector, M., and Yannas, I. V. (2004). Optimal degradation rate for collagen chambers used for regeneration of peripheral nerves over long gaps, *Cells Tissues Organs,* **176**, pp. 153–165.

54. Liodaki, E., Bos, I., Lohmeyer, J. A., Senyaman, O., Mauss, K. L., Siemers, F., Mailaender, P., and Stang, F. (2013). Removal of collagen nerve conduits (NeuraGen) after unsuccessful implantation: Focus on histological findings, *J. Reconstr. Microsurg.,* **29**, pp. 517–522.

55. Williams, L. R., Longo, F. M., Powell, H. C., Lundborg, G., and Varon, S. (1983). Spatial-temporal progress of peripheral nerve regeneration within a silicone chamber: Parameters for a bioassay, *J. Comp. Neurol.,* **218**, pp. 460–470.

56. Kuberka, M., von Heimburg, D., Schoof, H., Heschel, I., and Rau, G. (2002). Magnification of the pore size in biodegradable collagen sponges, *Int. J. Artif. Organs,* **25**, pp. 67–73.

57. Madaghiele, M., Sannino, A., Yannas, I. V., and Spector, M. (2008). Collagen-based matrices with axially oriented pores, *J. Biomed. Mater. Res. A,* **85**, pp. 757–767.

58. Schoof, H., Bruns, L., Fischer, A., Heschel, I., and Rau, G. (2000). Dendritic ice morphology in unidirectionally solidified collagen suspensions, *J. Cryst. Growth,* **209**, pp. 122–129.

59. Schoof, H., Apel, J., Heschel, I., and Rau, G. (2001). Control of pore structure and size in freeze-dried collagen sponges, *J. Biomed. Mater. Res.,* **58**, pp. 352–357.

60. Stokols, S., and Tuszynski, M. H. (2004). The fabrication and characterization of linearly oriented nerve guidance scaffolds for spinal cord injury, *Biomaterials,* **25**, pp. 5839–5846.

61. Xiao, W., Hu, X. Y., Zeng, W., Huang, J. H., Zhang, Y. G., and Luo, Z. J. (2013). Rapid sciatic nerve regeneration of rats by a surface modified collagen-chitosan scaffold, *Injury,* **44**, pp. 941–946.

62. Cao, J., Xiao, Z., Jin, W., Chen, B., Meng, D., Ding, W., Han, S., Hou, X., Zhu, T., Yuan, B., Wang, J., Liang, W., and Dai, J. (2013). Induction of rat facial nerve regeneration by functional collagen scaffolds, *Biomaterials,* **34**, pp. 1302–1310.

63. Mottaghitalab, F., Farokhi, M., Zaminy, A., Kokabi, M., Soleimani, M., Mirahmadi, F., Shokrgozar, M. A., and Sadeghizadeh, M. (2013). A biosynthetic nerve guide conduit based on silk/SWNT/fibronectin nanocomposite for peripheral nerve regeneration, *PLoS ONE,* **8**, p. e74417.

64. Okamoto, H., Hata, K., Kagami, H., Okada, K., Ito, Y., Narita, Y., Hirata, H., Sekiya, I., Otsuka, T., and Ueda, M. (2010). Recovery process of sciatic nerve defect with novel bioabsorbable collagen tubes packed with collagen filaments in dogs, *J. Biomed. Mater. Res. A*, **92**, pp. 859–868.

65. Hu, W., Gu, J., Deng, A., and Gu, X. (2008). Polyglycolic acid filaments guide Schwann cell migration in vitro and in vivo, *Biotechnol. Lett.*, **30**, pp. 1937–1942.

66. Quigley, A. F., Bulluss, K. J., Kyratzis, I. L., Gilmore, K., Mysore, T., Schirmer, K. S., Kennedy, E. L., O'Shea, M., Truong, Y. B., Edwards, S. L., Peeters, G., Herwig, P., Razal, J. M., Campbell, T. E., Lowes, K. N., Higgins, M. J., Moulton, S. E., Murphy, M. A., Cook, M. J., Clark, G. M., Wallace, G. G., and Kapsa, R. M. (2013). Engineering a multimodal nerve conduit for repair of injured peripheral nerve, *J. Neural Eng.*, **10**, p. 016008.

67. Wang, X., Hu, W., Cao, Y., Yao, J., Wu, J., and Gu, X. (2005). Dog sciatic nerve regeneration across a 30-mm defect bridged by a chitosan/PGA artificial nerve graft, *Brain*, **128**, pp. 1897–1910.

68. Radtke, C., Allmeling, C., Waldmann, K. H., Reimers, K., Thies, K., Schenk, H. C., Hillmer, A., Guggenheim, M., Brandes, G., and Vogt, P. M. (2011). Spider silk constructs enhance axonal regeneration and remyelination in long nerve defects in sheep, *PLoS ONE*, **6**, p. e16990.

69. Yang, Y., Ding, F., Wu, J., Hu, W., Liu, W., Liu, J., and Gu, X. (2007). Development and evaluation of silk fibroin-based nerve grafts used for peripheral nerve regeneration, *Biomaterials*, **28**, pp. 5526–5535.

70. Yoshii, S., Oka, M., Shima, M., Taniguchi, A., and Akagi, M. (2003). Bridging a 30-mm nerve defect using collagen filaments, *J. Biomed. Mater. Res. A*, **67**, pp. 467–474.

71. Ngo, T. T., Waggoner, P. J., Romero, A. A., Nelson, K. D., Eberhart, R. C., and Smith, G. M. (2003). Poly(L-Lactide) microfilaments enhance peripheral nerve regeneration across extended nerve lesions, *J. Neurosci. Res.*, **72**, pp. 227–238.

72. Spivey, E. C., Khaing, Z. Z., Shear, J. B., and Schmidt, C. E. (2012). The fundamental role of subcellular topography in peripheral nerve repair therapies, *Biomaterials*, **33**, pp. 4264–4276.

73. Flynn, L., Dalton, P. D., and Shoichet, M. S. (2003). Fiber templating of poly(2-hydroxyethyl methacrylate) for neural tissue engineering, *Biomaterials*, **24**, pp. 4265–4272.

74. Tran, R. T., Choy, W. M., Cao, H., Qattan, I., Chiao, J. C., Ip, W. Y., Yeung, K. W., and Yang, J. (2013). Fabrication and characterization of biomimetic multichanneled crosslinked-urethane-doped polyester tissue engineered nerve guides, *J. Biomed. Mater. Res. A*.

75. Patodia, S., and Raivich, G. (2012). Downstream effector molecules in successful peripheral nerve regeneration, *Cell Tissue Res.*, **349**, pp. 15–26.

76. Chernousov, M. A., Stahl, R. C., and Carey, D. J. (2001). Schwann cell type V collagen inhibits axonal outgrowth and promotes Schwann cell migration via distinct adhesive activities of the collagen and noncollagen domains, *J. Neurosci.*, **21**, pp. 6125–6135.

77. Hammarback, J. A., McCarthy, J. B., Palm, S. L., Furcht, L. T., and Letourneau, P. C. (1988). Growth cone guidance by substrate-bound laminin pathways is correlated with neuron-to-pathway adhesivity, *Dev. Biol.*, **126**, pp. 29–39.

78. Koh, H. S., Yong, T., Chan, C. K., and Ramakrishna, S. (2008). Enhancement of neurite outgrowth using nano-structured scaffolds coupled with laminin, *Biomaterials*, **29**, pp. 3574–3582.

79. Rangappa, N., Romero, A., Nelson, K. D., Eberhart, R. C., and Smith, G. M. (2000). Laminin-coated poly(L-lactide) filaments induce robust neurite growth while providing directional orientation, *J. Biomed. Mater. Res.*, **51**, pp. 625–634.

80. Schnell, E., Klinkhammer, K., Balzer, S., Brook, G., Klee, D., Dalton, P., and Mey, J. (2007). Guidance of glial cell migration and axonal growth on electrospun nanofibers of poly-epsilon-caprolactone and a collagen/poly-epsilon-caprolactone blend, *Biomaterials*, **28**, pp. 3012–3025.

81. Matsumoto, K., Ohnishi, K., Kiyotani, T., Sekine, T., Ueda, H., Nakamura, T., Endo, K., and Shimizu, Y. (2000). Peripheral nerve regeneration across an 80-mm gap bridged by a polyglycolic acid (PGA)-collagen tube filled with laminin-coated collagen fibers: A histological and electrophysiological evaluation of regenerated nerves, *Brain Res.*, **868**, pp. 315–328.

82. Fine, E. G., Decosterd, I., Papaloizos, M., Zurn, A. D., and Aebischer, P. (2002). GDNF and NGF released by synthetic guidance channels support sciatic nerve regeneration across a long gap, *Eur. J. Neurosci.*, **15**, pp. 589–601.

83. Midha, R., Munro, C. A., Dalton, P. D., Tator, C. H., and Shoichet, M. S. (2003). Growth factor enhancement of peripheral nerve regeneration through a novel synthetic hydrogel tube, *J. Neurosurg.*, **99**, pp. 555–565.

84. Moore, A. M., Wood, M. D., Chenard, K., Hunter, D. A., Mackinnon, S. E., Sakiyama-Elbert, S. E., and Borschel, G. H. (2010). Controlled delivery of glial cell line-derived neurotrophic factor enhances motor nerve regeneration, *J. Hand. Surg. Am.*, **35**, pp. 2008–2017.

85. Sterne, G. D., Brown, R. A., Green, C. J., and Terenghi, G. (1997). Neurotrophin-3 delivered locally via fibronectin mats enhances peripheral nerve regeneration, *Eur. J. Neurosci.,* **9**, pp. 1388–1396.

86. Madduri, S., di Summa, P., Papaloizos, M., Kalbermatten, D., and Gander, B. (2010). Effect of controlled co-delivery of synergistic neurotrophic factors on early nerve regeneration in rats, *Biomaterials,* **31**, pp. 8402–8409.

87. Barras, F. M., Pasche, P., Bouche, N., Aebischer, P., and Zurn, A. D. (2002). Glial cell line-derived neurotrophic factor released by synthetic guidance channels promotes facial nerve regeneration in the rat, *J. Neurosci. Res.,* **70**, pp. 746–755.

88. Deister, C., and Schmidt, C. E. (2006). Optimizing neurotrophic factor combinations for neurite outgrowth, *J. Neural Eng.,* **3**, pp. 172–179.

89. Takagi, T., Kimura, Y., Shibata, S., Saito, H., Ishii, K., Okano, H. J., Toyama, Y., Okano, H., Tabata, Y., and Nakamura, M. (2012). Sustained bFGF-release tubes for peripheral nerve regeneration: Comparison with autograft, *Plast. Reconstr. Surg.,* **130**, pp. 866–876.

90. Hobson, M. I. (2002). Increased vascularisation enhances axonal regeneration within an acellular nerve conduit, *Ann. R. Coll. Surg. Eng.,* **84**, pp. 47–53.

91. Lee, A. C., Yu, V. M., Lowe, J. B., 3rd, Brenner, M. J., Hunter, D. A., Mackinnon, S. E., and Sakiyama-Elbert, S. E. (2003). Controlled release of nerve growth factor enhances sciatic nerve regeneration, *Exp. Neurol.,* **184**, pp. 295–303.

92. Goraltchouk, A., Scanga, V., Morshead, C. M., and Shoichet, M. S. (2006). Incorporation of protein-eluting microspheres into biodegradable nerve guidance channels for controlled release, *J. Control. Release,* **110**, pp. 400–407.

93. Piotrowicz, A., and Shoichet, M. S. (2006). Nerve guidance channels as drug delivery vehicles, *Biomaterials,* **27**, pp. 2018–2027.

94. Rosner, B. I., Siegel, R. A., Grosberg, A., and Tranquillo, R. T. (2003). Rational design of contact guiding, neurotrophic matrices for peripheral nerve regeneration, *Ann. Biomed. Eng.,* **31**, pp. 1383–1401.

95. Xu, X., Yee, W. C., Hwang, P. Y., Yu, H., Wan, A. C., Gao, S., Boon, K. L., Mao, H. Q., Leong, K. W., and Wang, S. (2003). Peripheral nerve regeneration with sustained release of poly(phosphoester) microencapsulated nerve growth factor within nerve guide conduits, *Biomaterials,* **24**, pp. 2405–2412.

96. Wood, M. D., MacEwan, M. R., French, A. R., Moore, A. M., Hunter, D. A., Mackinnon, S. E., Moran, D. W., Borschel, G. H., and Sakiyama-Elbert, S. E. (2010). Fibrin matrices with affinity-based delivery systems and neurotrophic factors promote functional nerve regeneration, *Biotechnol. Bioeng.*, **106**, pp. 970–979.

97. de Boer, R., Knight, A. M., Borntraeger, A., Hebert-Blouin, M. N., Spinner, R. J., Malessy, M. J., Yaszemski, M. J., and Windebank, A. J. (2011). Rat sciatic nerve repair with a poly-lactic-co-glycolic acid scaffold and nerve growth factor releasing microspheres, *Microsurgery*, **31**, pp. 293–302.

98. Bagnard, D., Thomasset, N., Lohrum, M., Puschel, A. W., and Bolz, J. (2000). Spatial distributions of guidance molecules regulate chemorepulsion and chemoattraction of growth cones, *J. Neurosci.*, **20**, pp. 1030–1035.

99. Li, G. N., Liu, J., and Hoffman-Kim, D. (2008). Multi-molecular gradients of permissive and inhibitory cues direct neurite outgrowth, *Ann. Biomed. Eng.*, **36**, pp. 889–904.

100. von Philipsborn, A. C., Lang, S., Loeschinger, J., Bernard, A., David, C., Lehnert, D., Bonhoeffer, F., and Bastmeyer, M. (2006). Growth cone navigation in substrate-bound ephrin gradients, *Development*, **133**, pp. 2487–2495.

101. Dodla, M. C., and Bellamkonda, R. V. (2008). Differences between the effect of anisotropic and isotropic laminin and nerve growth factor presenting scaffolds on nerve regeneration across long peripheral nerve gaps, *Biomaterials*, **29**, pp. 33–46.

102. Xu, H., Yan, Y., and Li, S. (2011). PDLLA/chondroitin sulfate/chitosan/ NGF conduits for peripheral nerve regeneration, *Biomaterials*, **32**, pp. 4506–4516.

103. Mohanna, P. N., Terenghi, G., and Wiberg, M. (2005). Composite PHB-GGF conduit for long nerve gap repair: A long-term evaluation, *Scand. J. Plast. Reconstr. Surg. Hand Surg.*, **39**, pp. 129–137.

104. Dowsing, B. J., Hayes, A., Bennett, T. M., Morrison, W. A., and Messina, A. (2000). Effects of LIF dose and laminin plus fibronectin on axotomized sciatic nerves, *Muscle Nerve*, **23**, pp. 1356–1364.

105. Lee, K., Silva, E. A., and Mooney, D. J. (2011). : General approaches and a review of recent developments, *J. R. Soc. Interface*, **8**, pp. 153–170.

106. Rosenstein, J. M., and Krum, J. M. (2004). New roles for VEGF in nervous tissue--beyond blood vessels, *Exp. Neurol.*, **187**, pp. 246–253.

107. Kokai, L. E., Ghaznavi, A. M., and Marra, K. G. (2010). Incorporation of double-walled microspheres into polymer nerve guides for the sustained delivery of glial cell line-derived neurotrophic factor, *Biomaterials,* **31**, pp. 2313–2322.

108. Yang, Y., De Laporte, L., Rives, C. B., Jang, J. H., Lin, W. C., Shull, K. R., and Shea, L. D. (2005). Neurotrophin releasing single and multiple lumen nerve conduits, *J. Control. Release,* **104**, pp. 433–446.

109. Yu, H., Peng, J., Guo, Q., Zhang, L., Li, Z., Zhao, B., Sui, X., Wang, Y., Xu, W., and Lu, S. (2009). Improvement of peripheral nerve regeneration in acellular nerve grafts with local release of nerve growth factor, *Microsurgery,* **29**, pp. 330–336.

110. Kuihua, Z., Chunyang, W., Cunyi, F., and Xiumei, M. (2013). Aligned SF/P(LLA-CL)-blended nanofibers encapsulating nerve growth factor for peripheral nerve regeneration, *J. Biomed. Mater. Res. A.*

111. Xu, H., Holzwarth, J. M., Yan, Y., Xu, P., Zheng, H., Yin, Y., Li, S., and Ma, P. X. (2014). Conductive PPY/PDLLA conduit for peripheral nerve regeneration, *Biomaterials,* **35**, pp. 225–235.

112. Arslantunali, D., Budak, G., and Hasirci, V. (2013). Multiwalled CNT-pHEMA composite conduit for peripheral nerve repair, *J. Biomed. Mater. Res. A,* **102**, pp. 828–841.

113. Shen, C. C., Yang, Y. C., Huang, T. B., Chan, S. C., and Liu, B. S. (2013). Neural regeneration in a novel nerve conduit across a large gap of the transected sciatic nerve in rats with low-level laser phototherapy, *J. Biomed. Mater. Res. A,* **101**, pp. 2763–2777.

# Chapter 9

# Biomimetic Scaffolds Integrated with Patterns of Exogenous Growth Factors

Silvia Minardi, Francesca Taraballi, Bayan Aghdasi, and Ennio Tasciotti

*The Methodist Hospital Research Institute, Houston, Texas, USA*

sminardi@houstonmethodist.org

## 9.1 Scaffolds and Bioactive Molecules in Orthopedic Surgery: Potential and Pitfalls

Protein- and peptide-based therapeutics represent 13% of the total sales in the biomedical field [1]. Growth factor (GF) signaling in tissue regrowth and homeostasis involves precise regulation of the concentration, temporal gradient, and spatial gradient of the factors, and these key parameters control the final outcome of regenerative therapies [2]. In fact, many efforts combined surgical and biological approaches in order to increase the success of regeneration. The augmentation of tissue healing in musculoskeletal surgery has benefitted from the surgical implantation of growth factors (GFs) [3], chemo/cytokines [4], and bioconductive scaffolds [5]. However, GFs' use in clinical procedures resulted in controversial

---

*Bio-Inspired Regenerative Medicine: Materials, Processes, and Clinical Applications*
Edited by Simone Sprio and Anna Tampieri
Copyright © 2016 Pan Stanford Publishing Pte. Ltd.
ISBN 978-981-4669-14-6 (Hardcover), 978-981-4669-15-3 (eBook)
www.panstanford.com

outcomes. Recombinant human bone morphogenetic protein two (rhBMP-2) has been successfully used with FDA approval to treat Grade III open tibia fractures [6]. On the other hand, recently, anterior cervical discectomy and fusion procedures (ACDF) suffered criticism with use of Medtronic's Infuse (BMP-2) product [7] because of the uncontrollable GF dosage and release kinetics. The dose-response effects was established to be crucial [8], and since an uncontrollable pharmacokinetics showed adverse side effects, such as respiratory compression and dysphagia, FDA revoked the BMP-2 approval [9]. This evidence brings attention to the fact that adverse outcomes could have been avoided managing a controlled or localized formulation of BMP-2. Burst and widespread tissue exposure to the GF together with an early dissipation from the fusion site (with irrigation, bleeding, edema, etc.) is not an ideal pharmacokinetic profile for tissue-regenerative indications [10]. During arthroscopic surgery, continuous saline infusion into the operative joint and over the repair site is commonly done, and this irrigation procedure and fluid delivery dilutes or washes away the growth factor [11] as already demonstrated using a platelet rich plasma (PRP) in rotator cuff repair [12]. One valuable approach to reducing and avoiding this problem is to use a functionalized scaffold able to localize over space and time GFs [13, 14].

The gold standard for osteochondral defect (OCD) repair remains microfracture—to which FDA-approved alternatives must submit a non-inferiority counterclaim [15]. A notable shortcoming of this intervention remains the bleeding-induced formation of fibrocartilage within the defect [16], not hyaline cartilage, with inferior tissue strength and functional characteristics [17]. As materials science advances, questions about fine-tuned surgical applications will find their answer in a multi-layered, multi-scale scaffold for delivery of two or more drugs with unique release kinetics and spatio-temporal integration [13, 18]. Extraordinary progress has been made over the past decade toward the design of scaffolds with a suitable multiscale hierarchical structure [19], and toward the design of delivery systems able to release active proteins according to any complex delivery pattern [2, 20, 21].

Bioactive factors can be incorporated within the scaffolds by layer deposition, or integrated into their fibrous mesh by either electrospinning or self-assembly techniques [22, 23]. Herein, we review the currently available techniques and approaches of fabrication of 3D scaffolds integrated with patterns of bioactive molecules.

## 9.2 Conventional Fabrication Methods of Scaffold Functionalized with Bioactive Molecules

### 9.2.1 Layer-by-Layer Assembly of Growth Factor-Coated Implants

Drug-eluting coatings can ameliorate the host's response to implants and favor tissue regeneration [24]. Materials' functionalization for biomedical applications with bioactive molecules is the strategy to reduce both the medical and financial burden of complications from implantation, which made this field highly attractive [25].

Layer-by-layer (LbL) polyelectrolyte multilayer films have attracted great interest as ultrathin reservoirs of biomelecules, as they allow for the coating of surfaces with complex geometries and for their tunability of incorporation and release profiles [26]. Macdonalds et al. described the first LbL films capable of microgram-scale release of Bone Morphogenetic Protein 2 (BMP-2), directing tissue response, by stimulating the differentiation of host's progenitor cells. With this technique they successfully decreased the BMP-2 burst release from 60% (commercial standard) to less than 1% in the first 3 h [27]. Ma et al. modified the LbL technique using a red-ox method to improve the coating [28]. In this way, they introduced a stable collagen layer incorporated with basic fibroblast growth factor (bFGF) on 3-D porous PLLA scaffold surface for applications of cartilage repair. They demonstrated that this functionalized device is able to improve chondrocyte spreading and growth. This convenient and effective method can be used to prepare bioactive scaffolds with extra cellular matrix (ECM)-mimic composition for tissue engineering [28]. Shah and coworkers described a complex polyelectrolyte multilayer (PEM) films that sequestered physiological amounts of osteogenic BMP-2 and angiogenic rhVEGF165 (recombinant human vascular endothelial growth factor) in different ratios. All was loaded onto a degradable [poly($\beta$-amino ester)/polyanion/

growth factor/polyanion] tetralayer repeated architecture where the biologic components scaled linearly with the number of tetralayers. Despite the complex architecture of the materials, they achieved the reduction of the GFs burst release and moreover they demonstrated that both growth factors retained their efficacy over time [29]. These promising results suggested the possibility to deliver precise doses of different GFs from many implant applications with an overall spatial and temporal control of the release profile and the final efficacy. Leipzig et al. developed a protein-biomaterial system combining pro-neural rat interferon-$\gamma$ (rIFN-$\gamma$) and the photo-crosslinkable biopolymer, methacrylamide chitosan. They demonstrated the ability of this material to trigger the differentiation of neural stem/progenitor cells into mature neurons and they put the basis of a new biomaterial able to regenerate lost or damaged central nervous tissue [30]. Suarez-Gonzales and colleagues developed mineral coatings on polycaprolactone scaffolds to serve as templates for GFs binding and release. Peptide versions of VEGF and BMP2 were bound with efficiencies up to 90% to mineral mineral-coated PCL scaffolds. They also demonstrated sustained release of all GFs with release kinetics that were strongly dependent in the solubility of the mineral coating [31]. In conclusion, LbL versatility to coat implanted devices to direct the molecular environment of this host cell/surface interface becomes crucially important. LbL has been developed and ad hoc modified as a convenient method to produce composite films with precise control over space and time. Localized release of GFs from implantable medical devices could represent a powerful tool able to increase tissue healing avoiding adverse side effects.

## 9.2.2 Electrospun Scaffolds Functionalized with Bioactive Molecules

Another way to functionalized scaffold with GFs is via electrospinning [32]. This consolidated technique allows the incorporation of GFs inside the bulk of the materials characterized by nanosized fibers. In fact, using coaxial electrospinning is possible to fabricate nanofibers with core–shell structures internally loaded with GFs [22]. Moreover, further adjustments in the thickness and porosity of the polymer shell may enhance the release kinetics GFs [33]. Due to the large surface area and high porosity of an electrospun material, the drug release can be easily controlled [34–36], and the drug-loaded electrospun mat could also be easily fabricated into various shapes (e.g., membrane, tube) for different applications, such as wound dressing and nerve conduits [37, 38]. However, to date, most studies of electrospun fibers for drug delivery have focused on the sustained release of a single drug, either by the method of coaxial electrospinning or by emulsion electrospinning [22, 39–41]. Zhang et al. [42] compared the blending and the coaxial method incorporating fluorescein isothiocyanate-conjugated BSA in poly($\varepsilon$-caprolactone) nanofibers. They demonstrated that the coaxial method resulted in a more sustained release behavior due to the presence of the polymer shell. Also, Han et al. proposed a novel dual drug delivery system using triaxial structured nanofibers, which provides different release profiles for model drugs separately loaded in either the sheath or the core of the fibers [43]. Sahoo et al. further confirmed these findings, by comparing two types of PLGA nanofibers functionalized with bFGF using the blending (Group I) or the coaxial electrospinning (Group II). They demonstrated that both scaffolds showed similar GF encapsulation efficiency and release over 1–2 weeks. This study also showed that the Group I scaffold upregulated gene expression of ECM proteins demonstrating that the materials was able to prolong GF release and that in combination with a nanofibrous structure could positively influence stem cell behavior and fate [44].

As already discussed, in order to accelerate wound healing and decrease the adverse effects of the therapeutics, the release of two or more different molecules at the proper time and in appropriate doses may be required during treatment [45]. Okuda et al. fabricated a multilayered electrospun polymer mat with two model drugs (spatially distributed in the first and third layers). The second and fourth electrospun layers, which were without drugs, were used to wrap the third layer, which was loaded with one of two drugs. They showed two different release profiles for the different drugs in the electrospun mat. However, the prepared multilayered electrospun mat was a macroscale release system in which two drugs had significantly different spatial distributions (one was on the top, and the other on the bottom). Thus, when the drugs were released from the system, it resulted in a non-uniform distribution of the two drugs in the surrounding environment that led to distinct concentration gradients, which might affect the efficiency of multi-drug combination therapy [46].

A significant step in the development of functional 3D engineered tissues is the proper vascularization of the constructs [47]. In an attempt to address this, Ekaputra and colleagues developed a hybrid mesh of poly($\varepsilon$-caprolactone)-collagen blend (PCL/Col) and hyaluronic acid (HA) hydrogel, synthesized by simultaneous deposition of HA and PCL/Col/. This allowed the dual loading and controlled release of two potent angiogenic GFs VEGF165 and PDGF-BB over a period of five weeks in vitro [47].

GFs functionalized electrospun scaffolds has been successfully employed also in the treatment of challenging fractures and large osseous defects [48]. One of outstanding approaches was conducted by Kolambkar et al., who proposed a hybrid system composed of electrospun polymeric tubes filled with an injectable peptide-modified alginate hydrogel [49]. They successfully tested the ability of this system to deliver recombinant bone morphogenetic protein-2 (rhBMP-2) for the repair of critically sized segmental bone defects in a rat model [49].

Thus, electrospinning is a method for preparing tissue-engineered scaffolds incorporated with therapeutics and GFs for controlled release in combination with the nanostructured features.

## 9.3 Mimicry of the Natural Biochemical Gradients

Cells are capable of responding to signaling molecules in a concentration-dependent way, can sense the concentration gradient, and respond to stimuli. In tissue regeneration and developmental biology, gradients of GFs have a crucial role, as they provide spatial and directional cues to cells [50]. In natural tissues, a GF is released from a localized source (e.g., a cell) and diffusing, it is bound to the matrix, typically resulting in local gradients [51]. The slope of the gradient depends on the affinity of the extracellular matrix, half-life, and the diffusion rate of the signaling molecule [50, 52]. Cellular mechanisms to sense spatial gradients are determined by their sensitivity to the relative steepness of the gradient, as well as their dependence on the absolute chemoattractant concentration [53]. Scaffolds mimicking the chemical [54], physical, and topographical [54] cues of the target tissue can be further engineered with nanostructured delivery systems to mimic the natural gradients of molecules of interest [55, 56]. This is of particular interest for applications of interface tissue engineering, which focus on the development of tissue engineered grafts capable of promoting integration between different types of tissue and between the implant and surrounding tissues [57]. Some of the most important targets for this discipline are ligament-to-bone [58], tendon-to-bone [59], and cartilage-to-bone [60] interfaces. Engineering tissue interfaces is very challenging, for the need to regenerate two different and adjacent tissues, thus requiring a combination of specialized biomaterials with spatially organized material composition, cell types, and signaling molecules [57]. Precise regulation of the concentration, temporal and spatial gradients of growth factors through the three-dimensional scaffolds is crucial to enhancing the signaling capability of the materials [53]. Several techniques have been employed to create growth factor gradients for various applications, including diffusion [61], gradient mixing [62], differential dipping [63], microstamping [64], and microfluidics [65].

## 9.3.1 Functionalization of Scaffolds with Nano- and Microstructured Delivery Systems

Engineering tridimensional scaffolds with nanostructured delivery systems represents a promising strategy to reach highly controlled release kinetics of molecules of therapeutic interest [66]. Recently, several efforts have been done to develop methods to spatially control the immobilization of different GFs in distinct volumes in 3D biomimetic scaffolds [67]. Although Kim et al. showed that two or more drugs could be easily incorporated into a PLGA-based electrospun mat through electrospinning, the release of two drugs with distinct behaviors could not be controlled due to the severe burst release of each drug [68]. The incorporation of drug-loaded silica particles into PLGA mats loaded with the other drug could solve the above-mentioned problem and deliver two drugs with different release rates to satisfy potential clinical application. In an effort to accomplish the combined release of multiple molecules from different compartments, Song et al. incorporated silica nanoparticles into electrospun fibers to realize a dual controlled release as well [69]. The composite could be loaded with two different model molecules: one included in the electrospun fibers, for a faster release, and the other in mesoporous silica nanoparticles integrated in the fibers, for a more sustained and slower release. Singh et al. introduced an interesting microparticle-based scaffold fabrication technique, as a method to create 3D scaffolds with spatial control over multiple model molecules using uniform PLGA microspheres [70]. The scaffold they proposed was assembled by flowing suspensions of microspheres (loaded with the molecules of interest) into a cylindrical glass mold, ultimately physically attaching the microspheres to form a continuous scaffold, using an ethanol treatment. In addition, bilayered, multilayered, and gradient scaffolds could be fabricated, exhibiting excellent spatial control and resolution [70]. Such novel fabrication technique could serve for the design of devices for the sustained release of heterogeneous signals in a continuous and seamless manner, particularly useful in interfacial tissue engineering applications. Recently the group of Oh [71] proposed a novel porous hydroxyapatite (HAp) scaffold with incorporated drug-releasing PLGA microspheres that enhanced bone regeneration releasing dexamethasone in vivo. With the same objective, Wenk et al. [72] developed a silk fibroin porous scaffold carrying microparticles (MP) that were loaded with insulin-like growth factor I (IGF-I). They demonstrated that embedding the PLGA MP into the scaffolds led to more sustained release of the payload. Recently, Minardi et al. presented a novel approach for the creation of multiscale biomimetic scaffold, capable of generating both spatial and temporal protein patterns [13].

This result was achieved by leveraging the natural ability of the collagen matrix to interact with PLGA-porous silicon microspheres (PLGA-pSi), effectively constructing a simple and tunable system for various tissue engineering applications. Optimizing the synthesis of monolithic multilayered collagen-based scaffolds, they stably integrated PLGA-pSi within the collagen matrix without altering collagen's nano- and microstructure.

The results demonstrated that this approach allowed for tissues mimicry at a multiscale level. At the nanoscale, the type

I collagen conserved its fibrillar structure and typical D-bands appearance, while the pSi nanostructure allowed the loading and release of reporter proteins. At the microscale, the PLGA coating of pSi created a composite delivery platform for the tunable release of the reporter proteins, while the collagen coating on PLGA-pSi enabled for their spatial confinement in the scaffold. Finally, at the macroscale, all these elements combined, without altering the feature of the material, such as pore size, porosity and swelling upon PLGA-pSi integration. pSi, PLGA, and collagen boundaries contributed to accomplishing the temporal patterning of the proteins in the multi-layered scaffold, through a triple controlled release, enabling for the zero-order release kinetics of reporter protein up to 50 days [13].

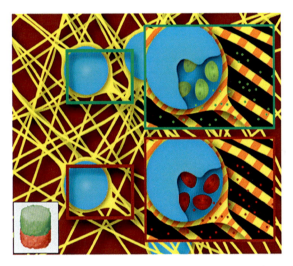

**Figure 9.1** Schematic showing the multiscale patterned scaffold for the spatially and temporally controlled release of multiple proteins within intrascaffold compartments, proposed by Minardi et al.

Hence, by grafting distinct sets of PLGA-pSi composites, one can envision the creation of multiple unique biochemical niches within a 3D scaffold, while protecting the payload and the delivery system itself. This might significantly impact the current clinical practice during surgical implantation of materials which comprise several steps of washing and fluid aspiration, during which the integrity of the material is challenged [66].

### 9.3.2 Spatial and Temporal Patterning of Biomimetic Scaffolds and Hydrogels with Multiple Proteins

Three-dimensional protein-patterned scaffolds provide a more biomimetic environment for cell culture than traditional two-dimensional surfaces, but concurrent 3D protein patterning has proved difficult [73]. Despite all of the efforts in applying nanotechnology to control the release of biological factors from scaffolds, the field is still developing compared with the great achievements of nanoparticle-based drug delivery [33].

Wylie and coworkers developed a method to spatially control the immobilization of different GF in distinct 3D compartments of hydrogels, and to specifically guide differentiation of progenitor cells [73]. In details, stem-cell differentiation factors sonic hedgehog (SHH) and ciliary neurotrophic factor (CNTF) were immobilized using physical binding pairs, barnase–barstar and streptavidin–biotin [74], respectively. Barnase and streptavidin were sequentially immobilized using two-photon chemistry to be ultimately complexed with fusion proteins barstar–SHH and biotin–CNTF, resulting in bioactive 3D patterned hydrogels. The technique was particularly attractive as it was applicable to a wide range of proteins [73].

T. A. Martin et al. developed a benzophenone (BP)-based direct photolithographic approach to spatially pattern solution phase biomolecules within collagen-GAG (CG) scaffolds [75]. It was proven the ability to immobilize biomolecules at surface densities of up to 1000 ligands per square micron on the scaffold surface andto depths limited by the penetration depth of the excitation source into the scaffold structure. Their findings established the use of direct BP photolithography as a methodology for covalently incorporating activity-improving biochemical cues within 3D collagen biomaterial scaffolds with spatial control over biomolecular deposition [75].

In an effort to add one level of complexity over the synthesis of biomimetic materials, Ker et al. [76] were able to orient sub-micron fibers, morphologically similar to musculoskeletal ECM, and to spatially pattern them with GFs using an inkjet-based bioprinter. This strategy allowed the creation of geometric patterns of biochemical cues to direct musculoskeletal cell alignment and differentiation in vitro according to fiber orientation and printed patterns, respectively. Functionalizing oriented submicron fibers with printed GFs provides instructive cues to spatially control cell fate and alignment to mimic native tissue organization [76].

Leslie-Barbick et al. developed poly(ethylene glycol) hydrogels presenting cell adhesion ligands and angiogenic signaling protein, which were demonstrated to induce spontaneous formation of endothelial tubules, restricted to the patterned micron-scale regions [77]. In details, arginine-glycine-aspartic acid-serine (RGDS) and vascular endothelial growth factor (VEGF) were covalently bound through photopolymerization via laser scanning lithography to the surface of poly(ethylene glycol) hydrogels in patterned micron-scale regions. Only the endothelial cells cultured in this restricted environment underwent accelerated tubulogenesis within 2 days. Additionally, tubules that formed on restricted areas of RGDS and VEGF expressed more VEGF receptor 1, VEGF receptor 2, and ephA7 surface markers, in addition to higher expression of laminin, than cells remaining spread on wide patterned lines [77].

## References

1. Sheridan, C., Fresh from the biologic pipeline[mdash] 2009. *Nat. Biotech.*, 2010. **28**(4), pp. 307–310.

2. Guldberg, R. E., Spatiotemporal delivery strategies for promoting musculoskeletal tissue regeneration. *J. Bone Mineral Res.*, 2009. **24**(9), pp. 1507–1511.

3. Anitua, E., M. H. Alkhraisat, and G. Orive, Perspectives and challenges in regenerative medicine using plasma rich in growth factors. *J. Control. Release*, 2012. **157**(1), pp. 29–38.

4. Garner, B. C., et al., Using animal models in osteoarthritis biomarker research. *J. Knee Surg.*, 2011. **24**(04), pp. 251–264.

5. Hsu, W. K., et al., Improving the clinical evidence of bone graft substitute technology in lumbar spine surgery. *Global Spine J.*, 2012. **2**(4), pp. 239–248.

6. Wei, S., et al., Recombinant human BMP-2 for the treatment of open tibial fractures. *Orthopedics*, 2012. **35**(6), pp. e847–e854.

7. Epstein, N. E., Complications due to the use of BMP/INFUSE in spine surgery: The evidence continues to mount. *Surg. Neurol. Int.*, 2013. **4**(Suppl 5), pp. S343–S352.

8. Shields, L. B. E., et al., Adverse effects associated with high-dose recombinant human bone morphogenetic protein-2 use in anterior cervical spine fusion. *Spine*, 2006. **31**(5), pp. 542–547.

9. McKie, J., et al., Trends in bone morphogenetic protein usage since the U.S. Food and Drug Administration Advisory in 2008: What Happens to Physician Practices When the Food and Drug Administration Issues an Advisory? *Global Spine J.*, 2014. **4**(2), pp. 71–76.

10. Lai, R.-F., et al., Effect of rhBMP-2 sustained-release nanocapsules on the ectopic osteogenesis process in Sprague-Dawley rats. *Asian Pac. J. Trop. Med.*, 2013. **6**(11), pp. 884–888.

11. Malavolta, E. A., et al., Platelet-rich plasma in rotator cuff repair: A prospective randomized study. *Am. J. Sports Med.*, 2014. **42**(10), pp. 2446–2454.

12. Angeline, M. E. and S. A. Rodeo, Biologics in the management of rotator cuff surgery. *Clin. Sports Med.*, 2012. **31**(4), pp. 645–663.

13. Minardi, S., et al., Multiscale patterning of a biomimetic scaffold integrated with composite microspheres. *Small*, 2014. **10**(19), pp. 3943–3953.

14. Kothapalli, C. R., et al., A high-throughput microfluidic assay to study neurite response to growth factor gradients. *Lab Chip*, 2011. **11**(3), pp. 497–507.

15. Nicolini, A. P., et al., Updates in biological therapies for knee injuries: Full thickness cartilage defect. *Curr. Rev. Musculoskelet. Med.*, 2014. **7**(3), pp. 256–262.

16. Thomopoulos, S., et al., Fibrocartilage tissue engineering: The role of the stress environment on cell morphology and matrix expression. *Tissue Eng. Part A*, 2011. **17**(7–8), pp. 1039–1053.

17. Carey, J. L., Fibrocartilage following microfracture is not as robust as native articular cartilage: Commentary on an article by Aaron J. Krych, MD, et al.: Activity levels are higher after osteochondral autograft transfer mosaicplasty than after microfracture for articular cartilage defects of the knee. A retrospective comparative study". *The Journal of Bone and Joint Surgery*. American Volume, 2012. **94**(11).

18. Chen, R. R., et al., Spatio–temporal VEGF and PDGF delivery patterns blood vessel formation and maturation. *Pharm. Res.*, 2007. **24**(2), pp. 258–264.

19. Tampieri, A., et al., From wood to bone: Multi-step process to convert wood hierarchical structures into biomimetic hydroxyapatite

scaffolds for bone tissue engineering. *J. Mater. Chem.*, 2009. **19**(28), pp. 4973–4980.

20. Biondi, M., et al., Controlled drug delivery in tissue engineering. *Adv. Drug Deliv. Rev.*, 2008. **60**(2), pp. 229–242.

21. Chen, F.-M., M. Zhang, and Z.-F. Wu, Toward delivery of multiple growth factors in tissue engineering. *Biomaterials*, 2010. **31**(24), pp. 6279–6308.

22. Sun, Z., et al., Compound core–shell polymer nanofibers by co-electrospinning. *Adv. Mater.*, 2003. **15**(22), pp. 1929–1932.

23. Hosseinkhani, H., et al., Enhanced angiogenesis through controlled release of basic fibroblast growth factor from peptide amphiphile for tissue regeneration. *Biomaterials*, 2006. **27**(34), pp. 5836–5844.

24. Peterson, A. M., et al., Growth factor release from polyelectrolyte-coated titanium for implant applications. *ACS Appl. Mater. Interfaces*, 2013. **6**(3), pp. 1866–1871.

25. Kretlow, J. D., L. Klouda, and A. G. Mikos, Injectable matrices and scaffolds for drug delivery in tissue engineering. *Adv. Drug Deliv. Rev.*, 2007. **59**(4), pp. 263–273.

26. Smith, R. C., et al., Layer-by-layer platform technology for small-molecule delivery. *Angew. Chem. Int. Ed.*, 2009. **48**(47), pp. 8974–8977.

27. Macdonald, M. L., et al., Tissue integration of growth factor-eluting layer-by-layer polyelectrolyte multilayer coated implants. *Biomaterials*, 2011. **32**(5), pp. 1446–1453.

28. Ma, Z., et al., Cartilage tissue engineering PLLA scaffold with surface immobilized collagen and basic fibroblast growth factor. *Biomaterials*, 2005. **26**(11), pp. 1253–1259.

29. Shah, N. J., et al., Tunable dual growth factor delivery from polyelectrolyte multilayer films. *Biomaterials*, 2011. **32**(26), pp. 6183–6193.

30. Leipzig, N. D., et al., Differentiation of neural stem cells in three-dimensional growth factor-immobilized chitosan hydrogel scaffolds. *Biomaterials*, 2011. **32**(1), pp. 57–64.

31. Suárez-González, D., et al., Controllable mineral coatings on PCL scaffolds as carriers for growth factor release. *Biomaterials*, 2012. **33**(2), pp. 713–721.

32. Li, C., et al., Electrospun silk-BMP-2 scaffolds for bone tissue engineering. *Biomaterials*, 2006. **27**(16), pp. 3115–3124.

33. Shi, J., et al., Nanotechnology in drug delivery and tissue engineering: From discovery to applications. *Nano Lett.*, 2010. **10**(9), pp. 3223–3230.

34. Chakraborty, S., et al., Electrohydrodynamics: A facile technique to fabricate drug delivery systems. *Adv. Drug Deliv. Rev.*, 2009. **61**(12), pp. 1043–1054.

35. Zhang, H., G. Wang, and H. Yang, Drug delivery systems for differential release in combination therapy. *Expert Opin. Drug Deliv.*, 2011. **8**(2), pp. 171–190.

36. Cui, W., et al., Investigation of drug release and matrix degradation of electrospun poly(DL-lactide) fibers with paracetanol inoculation. *Biomacromolecules*, 2006. **7**(5), pp. 1623–1629.

37. Liu, J. J., et al., Peripheral nerve regeneration using composite poly(lactic acid-caprolactone)/nerve growth factor conduits prepared by coaxial electrospinning. *J. Biomed. Mater. Res. Part A*, 2011. **96**(1), pp. 13–20.

38. Kenawy, E.-R., et al., Release of tetracycline hydrochloride from electrospun poly(ethylene-co-vinylacetate), poly(lactic acid), and a blend. *J. Control. Release*, 2002. **81**(1), pp. 57–64.

39. Yarin, A., Coaxial electrospinning and emulsion electrospinning of core–shell fibers. *Polym. Adv. Technol.*, 2011. **22**(3), pp. 310–317.

40. Ji, W., et al., Fibrous scaffolds loaded with protein prepared by blend or coaxial electrospinning. *Acta Biomater.*, 2010. **6**(11), pp. 4199–4207.

41. Han, F., et al., Diverse release behaviors of water-soluble bioactive substances from fibrous membranes prepared by emulsion and suspension electrospinning. *J. Biomater. Sci. Polym. Ed.*, 2013. **24**(10), pp. 1244–1259.

42. Zhang, Y. Z., et al., Coaxial electrospinning of (fluorescein isothiocyanate-conjugated bovine serum albumin)-encapsulated poly($\varepsilon$-caprolactone) nanofibers for sustained release. *Biomacromolecules*, 2006. **7**(4), pp. 1049–1057.

43. Han, D., and A. J. Steckl, Triaxial electrospun nanofiber membranes for controlled dual release of functional molecules. *ACS Appl. Mater. Interfaces*, 2013. **5**(16), pp. 8241–8245.

44. Sahoo, S., et al., Growth factor delivery through electrospun nanofibers in scaffolds for tissue engineering applications. *J. Biomed. Mater. Res. Part A*, 2010. **93A**(4), pp. 1539–1550.

45. Song, B., C. Wu, and J. Chang, Dual drug release from electrospun poly(lactic-co-glycolic acid)/mesoporous silica nanoparticles composite mats with distinct release profiles. *Acta Biomater.*, 2012. **8**(5), pp. 1901–1907.

46. Okuda, T., K. Tominaga, and S. Kidoaki, Time-programmed dual release formulation by multilayered drug-loaded nanofiber meshes. *J. Control. Release*, 2010. **143**(2), pp. 258–264.

47. Ekaputra, A. K., et al., The three-dimensional vascularization of growth factor-releasing hybrid scaffold of poly($\varepsilon$-caprolactone)/ collagen fibers and hyaluronic acid hydrogel. *Biomaterials*, 2011. **32**(32), pp. 8108–8117.

48. Schofer, M. D., et al., Electrospun PLLA nanofiber scaffolds and their use in combination with BMP-2 for reconstruction of bone defects. *PLoS One*, 2011. **6**(9), p. e25462.

49. Kolambkar, Y. M., et al., An alginate-based hybrid system for growth factor delivery in the functional repair of large bone defects. *Biomaterials*, 2011. **32**(1), pp. 65–74.

50. Tayalia, P., and D. J. Mooney, Controlled growth factor delivery for tissue engineering. *Adv. Mater.*, 2009. **21**(32–33), pp. 3269–3285.

51. Guo, X., et al., Creating 3D angiogenic growth factor gradients in fibrous constructs to guide fast angiogenesis. *Biomacromolecules*, 2012. **13**(10), pp. 3262–3271.

52. Mosadegh, B., et al., Generation of stable complex gradients across two-dimensional surfaces and three-dimensional gels. *Langmuir*, 2007. **23**(22), pp. 10910–10912.

53. Santo, V. E., et al., Controlled release strategies for bone, cartilage, and osteochondral engineering—part I: Recapitulation of native tissue healing and variables for the design of delivery systems. *Tissue Eng. Part B: Rev.*, 2013. **19**(4), pp. 308–326.

54. Xia, Z., et al., Fabrication and characterization of biomimetic collagen–apatite scaffolds with tunable structures for bone tissue engineering. *Acta Biomater.*, 2013. **9**(7), pp. 7308–7319.

55. Discher, D. E., D. J. Mooney, and P. W. Zandstra, Growth factors, matrices, and forces combine and control stem cells. *Science*, 2009. **324**(5935), pp. 1673–1677.

56. Lutolf, M. P., and J. A. Hubbell, Synthetic biomaterials as instructive extracellular microenvironments for morphogenesis in tissue engineering. *Nat. Biotech.*, 2005. **23**(1), pp. 47–55.

57. Seidi, A., et al., Gradient biomaterials for soft-to-hard interface tissue engineering. *Acta Biomater.*, 2011. **7**(4), pp. 1441–1451.

58. Spalazzi, J. P., et al., In vivo evaluation of a multiphased scaffold designed for orthopaedic interface tissue engineering and soft

tissue-to-bone integration. *J. Biomed. Mater. Res. Part A*, 2008. **86**(1), pp. 1–12.

59. Manning, C. N., et al., Sustained delivery of transforming growth factor beta three enhances tendon-to-bone healing in a rat model. *J. Orthop. Res.*, 2011. **29**(7), pp. 1099–1105.

60. Tampieri, A., et al., Design of graded biomimetic osteochondral composite scaffolds. *Biomaterials*, 2008. **29**(26), pp. 3539–3546.

61. Cao, X. and M. Shoichet, Defining the concentration gradient of nerve growth factor for guided neurite outgrowth. *Neuroscience*, 2001. **103**(3), pp. 831–840.

62. Wang, X., et al., Growth factor gradients via microsphere delivery in biopolymer scaffolds for osteochondral tissue engineering. *J. Control. Release*, 2009. **134**(2), pp. 81–90.

63. Mei, Y., et al., Tuning cell adhesion on gradient poly(2-hydroxyethyl methacrylate)-grafted surfaces. *Langmuir*, 2005. **21**(26), pp. 12309–12314.

64. Campbell, P. G., et al., Engineered spatial patterns of FGF-2 immobilized on fibrin direct cell organization. *Biomaterials*, 2005. **26**(33), pp. 6762–6770.

65. He, J., et al., Rapid generation of biologically relevant hydrogels containing long-range chemical gradients. *Adv. Funct. Mater.*, 2010. **20**(1), pp. 131–137.

66. Minardi, S., et al., Multiscale patterning of a biomimetic scaffold integrated with composite microspheres. *Small* (Weinheim an der Bergstrasse, Germany), 2014. **10**(19), pp. 3943–3953.

67. Lee, S.-H., J. J. Moon, and J. L. West, Three-dimensional micropatterning of bioactive hydrogels via two-photon laser scanning photolithography for guided 3D cell migration. *Biomaterials*, 2008. **29**(20), pp. 2962–2968.

68. Kim, K., et al., Incorporation and controlled release of a hydrophilic antibiotic using poly(lactide-co-glycolide)-based electrospun nanofibrous scaffolds. *J. Control. Release*, 2004. **98**(1), pp. 47–56.

69. Song, B., C. Wu, and J. Chang, Dual drug release from electrospun poly(lactic-co-glycolic acid)/mesoporous silica nanoparticles composite mats with distinct release profiles. *Acta Biomater.*, 2012. **8**(5), pp. 1901–1907.

70. Singh, M., et al., Microsphere-based seamless scaffolds containing macroscopic gradients of encapsulated factors for tissue engineering. *Tissue Eng. Part C Methods*, 2008. **14**(4), pp. 299–309.

71. Son, J. S., et al., Porous hydroxyapatite scaffold with three-dimensional localized drug delivery system using biodegradable microspheres. *J. Control. Release*, 2011. **153**(2), pp. 133–140.

72. Wenk, E., et al., Microporous silk fibroin scaffolds embedding PLGA microparticles for controlled growth factor delivery in tissue engineering. *Biomaterials*, 2009. **30**(13), pp. 2571–2581.

73. Wylie, R. G., et al., Spatially controlled simultaneous patterning of multiple growth factors in three-dimensional hydrogels. *Nat. Mater.*, 2011. **10**(10), pp. 799–806.

74. West, J. L., Protein-patterned hydrogels: Customized cell microenvironments. *Nat. Mater.*, 2011. **10**(10), pp. 727–729.

75. Martin, T. A., et al., The generation of biomolecular patterns in highly porous collagen-GAG scaffolds using direct photolithography. *Biomaterials*, 2011. **32**(16), pp. 3949–3957.

76. Ker, E. D., et al., Bioprinting of growth factors onto aligned sub-micron fibrous scaffolds for simultaneous control of cell differentiation and alignment. *Biomaterials*, 2011. **32**(32), pp. 8097–8107.

77. Leslie-Barbick, J. E., et al., Micron-scale spatially patterned, covalently immobilized vascular endothelial growth factor on hydrogels accelerates endothelial tubulogenesis and increases cellular angiogenic responses. *Tissue Eng. Part A*, 2010. **17**(1–2), pp. 221–229.

# Chapter 10

# Heart Failure and MicroRNA-Based Therapy: A Perspective on the Use of Nanocarriers

**Michele Miragoli, Michael V. G Latronico, Gianluigi Condorelli, and Daniele Catalucci**

*Humanitas Clinical and Research Center,*
*via Manzoni 113, Rozzano (MI) 20089, Italy*

michele.miragoli@humanitasresearch.it, daniele.catalucci@humanitasresearch.it

The incidence of heart failure has increased over the last decades, primarily because of the expansion of the "modern" lifestyle to developing countries and the lengthening of life expectancy in the West. Despite advancements in the management of heart failure, it still remains a leading cause of death worldwide. Excluding lifestyle changes, this situation can only be reversed through the development of novel therapeutic strategies. For this to occur, we need to improve our understanding of the mechanisms leading to heart failure and find new drugs. The unearthing of the microRNA-mediated gene expression network, its involvement in pathogenesis, and the ability to target/use microRNAs for therapeutic ends has produced much excitement in the scientific community

---

*Bio-Inspired Regenerative Medicine: Materials, Processes, and Clinical Applications*
Edited by Simone Sprio and Anna Tampieri
Copyright © 2016 Pan Stanford Publishing Pte. Ltd.
ISBN 978-981-4669-14-6 (Hardcover), 978-981-4669-15-3 (eBook)
www.panstanford.com

in this regard. However, before miRNA-based therapeutics can become a reality, we need a suitable cardiac-specific drug delivery system. In this chapter, we give brief overviews of heart failure and microRNAs, and discuss the development of an innovative therapeutic strategy based on novel biocompatible and bioresorbable nanoparticles for carrying miRNA-based therapeutics to the heart.

## 10.1 Introduction

Cardiovascular diseases (CVDs) are a heterogeneous collection of pathologies affecting the heart and circulatory system. Over the last 30 years, significant improvements have been made in the way CVDs are diagnosed and treated surgically [1]. Despite this—and a better awareness of the impact of diet and life-style—mortality and morbidity from CVD remains unacceptably high: In fact, CVD remains a leading reason for hospitalization and the largest cause of mortality, claiming more lives than cancer in the Western world.

For many types of CVD, therapy is palliative, slowing the progression of disease: The only real cure remains heart transplantation because there are no regenerative therapies available to overcome the cardiomyocyte loss that is part of the common final stage of many CVDs, known as *heart failure* [2]. Therefore, novel strategies are needed if we are to make any new advancement in the treatment of CVD. To this end, a better understanding of cardiovascular pathophysiology is paramount, as are parallel advances in the development of new classes of pharmaceuticals and innovative and organ-specific modes of drug delivery. The relatively recent discovery of non-protein coding RNAs (ncRNAs) as modulators of gene expression has opened up these areas of research. In fact, as we will see in this chapter, an abundant class of ncRNAs intimately linked to cardiac development and physiology may be central to the pathological modifications underlying CVDs, and, thus, may be taken advantage of therapeutically. In addition, cutting-edge nanoparticle-mediated drug delivery approaches may be instrumental for this innovative therapeutic strategy to come about.

## 10.2 The Pathophysiology of Cardiac Hypertrophy and Failure

The heart has an extraordinary adaptive potential for maintaining contractile function in the face of a wide range of intrinsic and extrinsic factors [3]. During development, proliferation of the cells constituting the myocardium—a process termed *hyperplasia*—allows the heart to increase in size along with the increasing metabolic demands of the growing organism. Postnatally, the heart compensates subacute intensification of cardiac workload—such as that produced by running—by increasing cardiac output through augmenting the beating frequency (tachycardia) and the volume of blood expelled per beat (the stroke volume) [4]. However, when workload is increased chronically—such as with training or a due to a CVD—the heart adapts by undergoing more permanent changes in its morphology and physiology. This is done primarily by increasing the thickness of the heart wall in order to offset the increased tension produced within the ventricles. Because cardiomyocytes—the contractile elements of the heart—are terminally differentiated and, thus, unable to replicate, the heart does this by increasing the size of individual myocardial fibers, a process termed *hypertrophy* [5]. When the stimulus for this chronic increase in mass is physiological—such as postnatal growth, exercise, training, or pregnancy—the changes occurring within the myocardium—termed its *remodeling*—are harmonious [6]. In other words, the coronary blood supply and the cardiac extracellular matrix grow appropriately with the increased thickness of the myocardium. In contrast, when the heart is subjected to an increase in workload due to a CVD—such as hypertension, aortic stenosis, or cardiac infarction—cardiac remodeling is deemed detrimental, even if it may initially seem to be compensatory. In this case, there is poor myocardial vascularization, inappropriate collagen deposition (*fibrosis*), and increased cardiomyocyte death. At the organ level, pathological remodeling ultimately causes a reduction of contractility, impairing the ability of the heart to eject blood (i.e., systolic dysfunction), and hinders the filling of the ventricles by increasing the stiffness of the myocardium (i.e., diastolic dysfunction). Eventually, cardiac function cannot meet the body's metabolic needs any longer—and in extreme cases even at rest—and the heart is said to be "failing." Heart failure is therefore a syndrome that is often encountered as the endpoint of many CVDs, when not caused directly by genetic mutations.

Pathological remodeling of the heart occurs at various levels: Morphological remodeling refers to changes in heart size and shape brought about by alterations at the cellular (cardiomyocyte hypertrophy) and extracellular matrix (fibrosis) levels [7]; metabolic remodeling involves a transition from fatty acids to carbohydrates as the substrate of choice [8]; and ion channel, electrical, and calcium-handling remodeling [9] lead to arrhythmias and contraction defects. Transcriptional remodeling is at the basis of most of these phenomena: For example, a hallmark of pathological hypertrophy is the re-activation of a *fetal cardiac gene program* [10], such as increased expression of a fetal isoform of myosin heavy chain, an event that may improve energy expenditure on the one hand, but that has unfavorable effects on contraction on the other [11].

## 10.2.1 Cardiac Ion Channel Remodeling and Arrhythmogenesis

The generation of arrhythmias is a major aspect of pathological hypertrophy and contributes significantly to the clinical picture [12]. In fact, degeneration of ventricular tachycardia into ventricular fibrillation is a primary cause of sudden death in heart-failure patients. Fibrosis and altered electronic coupling in the hypertrophic myocardium create an arrhythmogenic substrate by inducing non-homogeneity in the progression of conduction. This is mainly related to an uncontrolled production of collagen by the re-activation and proliferation of myofibroblasts, which affect the orderly three-dimensional organization of the myocardium. The presence of collagenous septa between cardiomyocyte bundles affects impulse propagation indirectly by causing impulse propagation to "zig-zag" and, hence, causes unidirectional conduction block by creating a substrate for reentrant arrhythmias [13]. We have described how myofibroblasts can exert a direct pathological effect on cardiomyocytes through heterocellular coupling, generating membrane potential depolarization, a decrement in conduction velocity, and ectopic activity [14–16]. Thus, attention has now veered toward the myofibroblast as a target for "non-cardiomyocyte-centered" anti-arrhythmic therapy. The interest in this area encompasses not only the development of conventional myofibroblast-centered pharmaceutical drugs [17, 18], but also the new avenues opened up by the discovery of microRNAs (see Section 10.3) [19].

This scenario is further aggravated by the electrical and structural remodeling of hypertrophic cardiomyocytes, which apart from altering passive cellular properties (membrane resistance, membrane capacitance), mainly modulates action potential characteristics. Indeed, the re-expression of fetal genes, mentioned above, includes the re-expression of T-type calcium channels ($ICa_{T-type}$), the overproduction of several voltage-dependent channels—i.e., potassium transient outward channels ($I_{to}$), L-type calcium channels ($ICa_{L-type}$), potassium repolarizing channels ($IKr$)—and redistribution of connexins (Cx). These all result in an increment in action potential duration (APD), induction of delayed after depolarization (DAD), and calcium alternans, a well-known substrate for ventricular fibrillation [20].

## 10.3 MicroRNA: A Class of Abundant Non-Protein Regulators

Only ~2% of the human genome encodes for protein. This fact was perplexing up until recently, principally because—apart from the special case of infrastructural RNAs, namely transfer RNA and ribosomal RNA—proteins were thought to be the inescapable final outcome of transcription, their being the wherewithal not only for cellular structure and function but also for all the accompanying regulatory processes. Under this perspective, the rest of the genome was thought to represent "junk," a vestige of evolution, DNA duplication, viral infection, etc. The last couple of decades have seen great advances in our understanding of this genomic "dark matter": In fact, it is now known that a vast proportion of the transcriptional output (~98%) of the cell is represented by non-protein coding—but, nevertheless, functional—RNA, and that this non-coding RNA (ncRNA) is a fundamental part of the control architecture of the cell. An increasing complexity of ncRNA-mediated regulatory networks is also thought to be at the basis of increasing phenotypic diversity and developmental complexity in eukaryotes, vastly reducing the need for expansion of the proteome in these processes [21].

To date, two main ncRNA families have been categorized: long non-coding RNA (lcnRNA), with a length of between 0.2 and 2Kb [22], and small RNA, which are <200 nucleotides long [23]. One of the largest classes, found in all eukaryotes, is microRNA (miRNA)—evolutionarily conserved, single-stranded ~21-nucleotide-long transcripts.

## 10.3.1 MicroRNA Biogenesis

The suggestion that gene expression could be regulated by an RNA–RNA interaction was put forward in the early 1990s when the short transcript *lin-4*—found earlier to be involved in the inhibition of the heterochronic genes *lin-14* and *lin-2* in the nematode *Caenorabditis elegans*—was found not to encode for a protein [24, 25]. Since then, miRNA discovery has been exponential, with thousands of miRNAs having been annotated and cataloged to date in an ad hoc online repository [26].

miRNA genes are transcribed by RNA polymerase II to generate primary (pri-) miRNAs [27]. Pri-miRNAs, which can be thousands of bases long and fold into characteristic loop–stem structures, are capped at their 5′ end and adenylated at the 3′ end [28]. While still within the nucleus, the ends of the pri-miRNAs are cleaved by the RNAse III drosha to form ~70-nucleotide-long hairpin structures called precursor (pre-) miRNAs [29]. The helical structure of the pre-miRNAs is recognized by the nuclear export factor exportin 5, and shuttled out [30, 31]. Within the cytoplasm, another RNAse III, called dicer [32], cleaves the pre-miRNAs at the looped end to generate an RNA duplex composed of the mature miRNA strand and a *passenger strand* (or *miRNA\**) [33]. The miRNA\* is then stripped away, leaving the mature miRNA associated with argonaute [34], the core protein component of the final effector complex, called the miRNA-induced silencing complex (miRISC) [35] (Fig. 10.1).

In addition to this "canonical" pathway of miRNA biogenesis, non-canonical pathways have been discovered, such as that of miR-451 [36], the splicing-derived miRNAs (mirtrons) [37], and the splicing-independent mirtron-like miRNAs (simtrons) [38].

The biogenesis of these types of miRNAs bypasses various initial steps of the canonical pathway but eventually converges on it at some later stage.

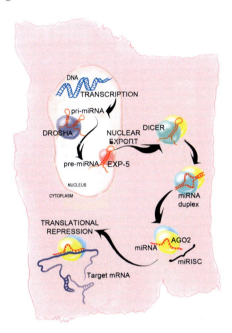

**Figure 10.1** Schematic representation of the canonical microRNA biogenesis pathway. miRNA genes are transcribed into characteristic stem–loop-structured preliminary (pri-miRNA) transcripts that are cleaved in the nucleus by the RNase drosha into shorter preliminary (pre-miRNA) transcripts. Pre-miRNA are shuttled out of the nucleus by exportin-5 (EXP-5) and then cleaved further by dicer to form double-stranded miRNAs. The mature miRNA stand is handed over to argonaute 2 (AGO2) to form the active miRNA-induced silencing complex (miRISC).

## 10.3.2 Function and Mechanism of Action of MicroRNA

miRNAs control gene expression by acting as "guides" for the miRISCs: In fact, the nucleotide sequences of miRNAs are (partially) complementary to binding site(s) present on the 3′ untranslated region (UTR) of mRNAs [39]. miRNAs have been described as "micromanagers" of gene expression, acting as "fine-tuners" of the abundance of mRNA in a particular cell type, and as "on–off switches" that repress proteins that should not be expressed at a particular time or in a particular tissue [40].

A major determiner of miRNA–mRNA hybridization is the *seed* sequence, a perfectly complementary tract of six/seven bases at the 5' end of the miRNA. It is here where interaction with the target is thought to be initiated [41]. When miRNAs bind to their target mRNAs, the latter are degraded and/or their translation repressed [42–44]. A single miRNA can regulate hundreds of targets, and multiple miRNAs can cooperate in the regulation of a single mRNA. Thus, miRNAs are posttranscriptional gene silencers, although it seems that they may also stimulate gene expression under rare circumstances [45]. In mammals, more than 60% of all protein-coding genes are thought to be regulated by miRNAs; these mRNAs encode proteins of all major cellular functions, such as differentiation, proliferation, and apoptosis [46]. Bioinformatics tools aid in the identification of these targets; however, they must be validated experimentally [47].

### 10.3.3  MicroRNA and Cardiac Pathophysiology

The study of miRNA expression patterns has revealed the presence of highly conserved miRNAs across phyla, but also of species-, developmental-, tissue-, and cell-specific miRNAs. The particular miRNA transcriptome profile—or *miRNome*—is thought to be fundamental for tissue specification and cell lineage commitment [48]. Regarding the heart, a recent deep-sequencing effort has demonstrated that >800 miRNAs are expressed in healthy human myocardial tissue, most of which have not been annotated yet and some of which are unique to primates [49]. Deep sequencing of the transcriptome has the advantage of being able to pick up miRNAs in a genome-wide manner, irrespective of whether they are known or not. Up until recently, miRNome assessment was carried out mainly with microarrays, in which chips containing thousands of predetermined probes are used to capture the transcripts of interest. With this technology, a number of miRNAs have been found to be particularly enriched in striated muscle, such as miR-1, miR-133, and miR-208 [50]. miR-208 is the only cardiac–specific miRNA known [51]. The 18 most abundant heart miRNAs account for >90% of the known cardiac miRNome [52].

Of potential clinical importance is the fact that the miRNome has been found to be altered in pathological settings. For instance, one deep-sequencing study found <250 miRNAs differentially expressed in forms of cardiomyopathy [49]. In humans, miR-1, miR-30, miR-133, and miR-150 have been found downregulated, and miR-21, miR-23a, miR-125, miR-195, miR-199, and miR-214 have been found upregulated in diseased heart. In addition, cardiac expression of DICER was found to be very low in patients with dilated cardiomyopathy [53]. Above all, it has been suggested that the dysregulation of some of miRNAs has a role in the progression and/or pathogenesis of CVD, i.e., an alteration in miRNA expression is the cause, rather than an effect, of disease. For example, miR-23a, miR-23b, miR-24, miR-195, and miR-214 produced hypertrophy when overexpressed in cardiomyocytes in vitro; transgenic overexpression of miR-195 has also been shown to generate increased heart size in mice [54]. In contrast, inhibition of miR-133a with an *antagomiR*—an oligonucleotide that is chemically engineered to be complementary to a given miRNA and, thus, that binds to the targeted miRNA, effectively silencing it [55]— was found to induce cardiac hypertrophy in wild-type mice [56], whereas overexpression of miR-1 was found to blunt hypertrophic growth [57].

### 10.3.3.1 Cardiac miRNAs: A close-up on miR-1 and miR-133

miR-1—one of the most highly conserved miRNAs—is an abundant miRNA in cardiomyocytes. It is transcribed from two loci— located respectively on chromosomes 20 and 18 in humans—the products of which are designated miR-1-1 and miR-1-2. As for many miRNAs, the miR-1 family of miRNAs—which includes the skeletal-muscle-specific miRNA miR-206—are transcribed from polycistronic genes. In fact, the miR-1 family members are found in bicistronic units with miR-133: In particular, miR-1-1 is clustered with miR133a-1, miR-1-2 with miR-133a-1, and miR-206 with miR-133b (the suffixes *a* and *b* indicate that the miRNAs differ in a small number of nucleotides but have the same seed sequence) [58].

In the embryo, the miR-1/miR-133 cluster is regulated by the transcription factor SRF [59], and promotes mesoderm specification while inhibiting differentiation of endoderm and ectoderm [60]. Later on in heart development, these two miRNAs often have opposing roles. Importantly, miR-133a was found to be important for repressing a slew of smooth-muscle-restricted proteins in the heart [61], an example of the fundamental role of miRNAs in the repression of unwanted transcripts [40]. More recently, an innovative method for the detection of miRNA targets in vivo identified 209 targets for miR-133a in mouse heart [62]. Table 10.1 gives a list of some validated targets of miR-1 and miR-133.

**Table 10.1**    Validated cardiac targets of miR-1 and miR-133

| miRNA | Species/model or disease | Dysregulation | Targets | Ref |
|---|---|---|---|---|
| miR-1 | m/miR1-Tg | ↑ | *Hand2* | [59] |
| | m/miR1-KO | ↓ | *Irx2* | [66] |
| | m/TAC, h/iCMP | ↓ | *Cdk9, Fn1, Rheb, RasGAP* | [57] |
| | m/TAC, h/AM | ↓ | *Igf1* | [68] |
| | m/fasted, m/Akt-Tg, h/GHD | ↑ | *Fabp3* | [69] |
| | m/TAC, h/AS, h/AM | ↓ | *Fabp3* | [69] |
| miR-133 | m/miR133a-KO | ↓ | *Ccnd2, Srf,* | [61] |
| | m/TAC, m/training, m/Akt-Tg, h/iCMP | ↓ | *Cdc42, Rhoa, Whsc2* | [56] |

- ↑, upregulation/overxpression of the miRNA; m, mouse; miR1-Tg, miR-1 transgenic model; miR1-KO, miR-1-2 knockout model; TAC, transverse aortic constriction; h, human; iCMP, idiopathic cardiomyopathy; ↓, downregulation/knockdown of the miRNA; AM, acromegaly; Akt-Tg, transgenic Akt model; GHD, growth hormone deficiency AS, aortic valve stenosis; miR133a-KO, miR-133a knockout model.

miRNAs have been implicated in the regulation of cardiac ion channels and in ion channel remodeling [63, 64]. For example, cardiac-specific deletion of *Dicer* in mice heart was associated with upregulation of the gap junction protein connexin 45—through the loss of inhibition on its mRNA, *Gjc1*—leading to conduction defects [53]. Overexpression of miR-1 in rat heart reduced conduction through inhibition of the potassium channel subunit

*Kcnj2* and *Gja1*, the mRNA of connexin 43 [65]. miR-1 has also been reported to target *Irx5*, a repressor of the potassium channel Kcnd2 [66]. Moreover, miR-133a overexpression reduced potassium channel accessory subunit KChIP2, probably through an indirect mechanism [67]. Therefore, dysregulation of miRNAs targeting cardiac ion-channel mRNAs could very well be involved in heart failure-associated arrhythmogenesis.

### 10.3.4 MicroRNA-Based Therapies

End-stage heart failure was thought to be an irreversible state. However, placement of a left ventricle assist device (LVAD)—a mechanical pump that reduces the cardiac workload by aiding with blood circulation [70]—can induce *reverse remodeling*. This is a phenomenon characterized by reduced hypertrophy and apoptosis, and improved $\beta$-adrenergic responsiveness and contractility, which lead to better heart function and, hence, patient survival [71]. Moreover, cardiac expression of DICER has been shown to be significantly improved in cardiomyopathy patients receiving an LVAD [53].

Because misexpression of specific miRNAs may have a causative role for disease, methods to counteract these miRNAs are being pursued as novel therapeutic avenues [72]. In essence, antagomiRs can be administrated to silence and sequester disease-causing upregulated miRNAs, whereas synthetic miRNA mimics can be used in replacement therapies for pathology-related miRNAs that are downregulated (Fig. 10.2). The mimics are RNA duplexes that contain a strand identical to the miRNA in question, which are processed and loaded onto the RISCs by the endogenous machinery present in the target cells. The pharmacological manipulation of miRNAs for therapeutic ends is still in its infancy, however, and many obstacles must be overcome. A main hurdle is developing organ-specific delivery of miRNA-based pharmaceuticals. This is especially important if untoward effects of miRNA manipulation are to be avoided in non-target organs. As we shall see in the following sections, nanoparticle-based delivery systems may provide an answer to at least some of these problems.

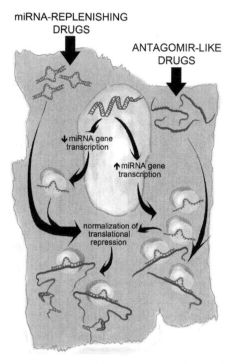

**Figure 10.2** Schematic representation of miRNA-based therapy. Disease can be associated with either increased or decreased transcription of miRNA genes. In the former condition, the delivery of a drug that binds to and sequesters excess miRNAs, such as antagomiRs, can be used to normalize increased translational repression. In the latter condition, inappropriately reduced translational repression can be reversed by the administration of synthetic oligonucleotides that co-opt the miRNA biosynthetic machinery to form "functional" miRISCs.

## 10.4 Nanoparticles and the Heart

Despite the almost epidemic spreading of CVDs in the West and developing countries, improvements in clinical management have not been delivered at the needed pace. This may be explained by the reluctance of the industrial sector to invest massively in the cardiovascular field—because of the prohibitive costs of mortality trials and the difficulty in establishing the clinical benefit of any new medication beyond current conventional pharmacological therapies—but also by a lack of new, ground-breaking targets for novel medications and preventive therapies.

This may change with the recent attention given to nanoparticles as a drug delivery system for the pathological heart [73]. In this capacity, nanoparticles need to be engineered so that they can bind to the drug, carry the drug to the heart, and release it directly in the myocardium. While this may sound straightforward, unfortunately it is not. In fact, two main concerns need to be addressed: Nanoparticles are potentially cardiotoxic, so naturally non-toxic ones that are rapidly biodegradable need to be found (discussed in Section 10.4.1, Side A of the Coin); in addition, the physicochemical nature of the nanoparticles, the administration route, and the interactions with organs/cells/proteins need to be understood (discussed in Section 10.4.2, Side B of the Coin).

### 10.4.1 Side A of the Coin: Nanoparticle Cardiotoxicity

In light of recent studies on particulate matter, a pressing need to better understand the interactions of nanoparticles within the body, and in particular with the cardiovascular system, has arisen. In fact, electrically charged nanoparticles with a hydrodynamic diameter of 6–34 nm can readily cross the pulmonary alveolar–epithelial barrier and enter into the systemic circulation [74]. This has as a potentially adverse effect on the cardiovascular system on account of anti-arrhythmic effects [75], but, incidentally, can be taken advantage of as the delivery route of nanoparticulate drugs. Indeed, a release of prothrombotic and inflammatory cytokines by the lung when exposed to nanoparticles may set up a cascade of vascular reactivity. Such events could result in electrical desynchronization of cardiac activity and autonomic function [76]. It has also been proposed that nanoparticles play a role in the inflammatory process by enhancing oxidative stress [77]. Of note, neither of these explanations considers the physicochemical nature of the nanoparticles.

### 10.4.2 Side B of the Coin: The Physicochemical Nature of Nanoparticles

The nanoparticles found in urban air are highly heterogeneous. However, the majority, which are emitted from diesel exhaust and are electrically charged, have a primary aerodynamic diameter of ~20 nm [78]. Whether and how the surface charge of such nanoparticles affects an electrically excitable tissue, such as the myocardium, is still only incompletely investigated.

To address this issue, we recently evaluated the effect of positively and negatively charged nanoparticles on neonatal rat ventricular cardiomyocytes [79]. We assessed not only classical markers of cardiotoxicity (such as apoptosis and necrosis), but also whether direct interaction of the charged nanoparticles with the excitable cardiac membrane led to changes in electrophysiology. We found that there is an interaction between the surface charge of a nanoparticle and the cardiomyocyte, and that this possibly affects the excitable nature of the heart. The most important observation was that the negatively charged (carboxyl-modified) nanoparticles studied—even if not as cytotoxic as the positively charged (amino-modified) ones—induced arrhythmias. Moreover, the use of positively charged nanoparticles as nanocarriers was excluded a priori because they created a "woodworm"-like disruption of the sarcolemma, increasing necrosis and apoptosis of cardiomyocytes after a 2 h exposure (Fig. 10.3). This scenario was accompanied by a significant dose–response increment in the percentage of cardiomyocyte clusters with intracellular $Ca^{2+}$ alternans. The negatively charged nanoparticles were highly pro-arrhythmogenic—inducing DADs, $APD_{90}$ prolongation, and $Ca_i^{2+}$ overload—and reduced the beating rate and conduction velocity, but only at the highest doses. More interestingly, the negatively charged polystyrene latex nanoparticles studied induced the formation of life-compatible nanopores (i.e., that were the same diameter as the nanoparticles) in the cardiomyocytes. Although the nanopores acted as potentially pathogenic "doors" for ion fluxes—for example, causing rapid accumulation of $Ca^{2+}$ within the cell—the intriguing perspective emerges that the presence of such nanopores might be clinically relevant for drug delivery and cardiac rhythm management. A key future study would be aimed at defining the interaction between infarcted tissue and charged nanoparticles. Because fibrotic areas are themselves pro-arrhythmogenic, the delivery of therapeutic miRNAs on these nanoparticles may be used to control the hypertrophic phenotype in a direct fashion by reducing the electrical interaction between cardiomyocytes and myofibroblasts.

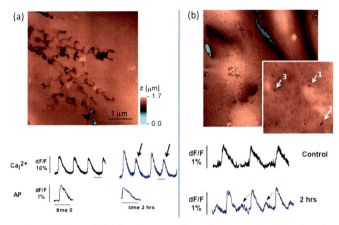

**Figure 10.3** Effect of high doses of positive- and negative-charged nanoparticles on cardiac tissue. (a) 50 µg/ml amino-modified positively charged nanoparticles disrupting the membrane of a neonatal ventricular cardiomyocyte (top panel), inducing calcium alternans (arrows in lower panel). (b) 50 µg/ml carboxyl-modified negatively charged nanoparticles inducing 50 nm nanopores (three have been highlighted by arrows in the inset of the top panel), which were compatible with life. This high dose induced delayed after depolarizaiton (arrows in the lower panel). Modified with permission from ref. [79].

## 10.5 Nanoparticle-Mediated Delivery of MicroRNA to the Heart: Future Perspectives

The development of miRNA-based therapy would open new avenues in the treatment of cardiac hypertrophy. However, the "handling" of such a small molecule is still challenging because of their nature, the lack of appropriate delivery technologies, obstacles in overcoming organ barriers, and their potential off-target effects. The requirement for an efficient, biocompatible miRNA carrier is imperative for minimizing side-effects.

Nanocarriers can be produced from materials ranging from inorganic compounds to organic or biological materials, once the above-mentioned concerns are satisfied. One pursuable candidate is hydroxylapatite (HA), which possesses ideal properties of biocompatibility, bioresorbability, and biodegradability on account of its structural and chemical similarity with the mineral component of bones and teeth. Moreover, HA is known for its capability to bind to a wide variety of molecules and therapeutic agents, because of the presence of available ($Ca^{2+}$ and $PO_4^{3-}$) surface sites, and for its easy dissolution, which would avoid undesirable accumulation of nanoparticles in cells and tissues—a drawback often encountered with other inorganic and metallic nanoparticles [80]. To improve the guiding of HA to the target site, novel bioresorbable iron-substituted HA nanoparticles, which have super-paramagnetic properties, have been developed. This new material also avoids the presence of poorly tolerated magnetic phases, like iron oxide, whose long-term effects on the human body are not yet completely assessed [81, 82].

Another class of interesting nanocarriers is represented by polymeric nanocapsules made of, for example, polyurethanes or cyanoacrylates [83; 84]. These are biocompatible and biodegradable with a rate of degradation depending on the choice of building blocks. More important, all of these nanoparticles are flexible regarding the modification of their surface properties, since we do believe that a negative surface charge is a *sine qua non conditio* for the development of a cardiac-specific nanocarrier.

A separate perspective needs to be described for the new avenues opened up by graphene, and its oxides, as a possible nanocarrier. A number of groups have been devoted to exploring the effects of graphene oxide, but one critical issue still remaining is that it induces toxicity when applied at 50 mg/ml in vitro and 10 mg/kg BW in vivo (our unpublished data and [85]). On the other hand, this is only the beginning of the graphene story—Sony Corporation has recently applied for a patent using graphene for drug delivery (US 20120289613). Although graphene research has progressed very rapidly because of cheap and fast laboratory procedures, we do not know at the moment if this "miracle" material could become the next *disruptive* technology. However, functionalization with DNA and RNA is possible, and graphene is lipophilic, so penetrates membrane barriers [86].

There is a cautious optimism in the selection, characterization, and functionalization of nanoparticles for drug delivery. At the moment, we can ascertain that the "nanoworld" will, in the near future, impose new interdisciplinary collaborations involving physicists, biologists, MDs, engineers, mathematicians, and chemists, with a reinvigorated outlook.

# References

1. Roger, V. L., Go, A. S., Lloyd-Jones, D. M., Benjamin, E. J., Berry, J. D., Borden, W. B., Bravata, D. M., Dai, S., Ford, E. S., Fox, C. S., Fullerton, H. J., Gillespie, C., Hailpern, S. M., Heit, J. A., Howard, V. J., Kissela, B. M., Kittner, S. J., Lackland, D. T., Lichtman, J. H., Lisabeth, L. D., Makuc, D. M., Marcus, G. M., Marelli, A., Matchar, D. B., Moy, C. S., Mozaffarian, D., Mussolino, M. E., Nichol, G., Paynter, N. P., Soliman, E. Z., Sorlie, P. D., Sotoodehnia, N., Turan, T. N., Virani, S. S., Wong, N. D., Woo, D., and Turner, M. B. (2012). Heart disease and stroke statistics–2012 update: A report from the American Heart Association, *Circulation*, **125**, pp. e2–e220.

2. McMurray, J. J., Adamopoulos, S., Anker, S. D., Auricchio, A., Bohm, M., Dickstein, K., Falk, V., Filippatos, G., Fonseca, C., Gomez-Sanchez, M. A., Jaarsma, T., Kober, L., Lip, G. Y., Maggioni, A. P., Parkhomenko, A., Pieske, B. M., Popescu, B. A., Ronnevik, P. K., Rutten, F. H., Schwitter, J., Seferovic, P., Stepinska, J., Trindade, P. T., Voors, A. A., Zannad, F., Zeiher, A., Bax, J. J., Baumgartner, H., Ceconi, C., Dean, V., Deaton, C., Fagard, R., Funck-Brentano, C., Hasdai, D., Hoes, A., Kirchhof, P., Knuuti, J., Kolh, P., McDonagh, T., Moulin, C., Reiner, Z., Sechtem, U., Sirnes, P. A., Tendera, M., Torbicki, A., Vahanian, A., Windecker, S., Bonet, L. A., Avraamides, P., Ben Lamin, H. A., Brignole, M., Coca, A., Cowburn, P., Dargie, H., Elliott, P., Flachskampf, F. A., Guida, G. F., Hardman, S., Iung, B., Merkely, B., Mueller, C., Nanas, J. N., Nielsen, O. W., Orn, S., Parissis, J. T., and Ponikowski, P. (2012). ESC guidelines for the diagnosis and treatment of acute and chronic heart failure 2012: The Task Force for the Diagnosis and Treatment of Acute and Chronic Heart Failure 2012 of the European Society of Cardiology. Developed in collaboration with the Heart Failure Association (HFA) of the ESC, *Eur. J. Heart Fail.*, **14**, pp. 803–869.

3. Hill, J. A., and Olson, E. N. (2008). Cardiac plasticity, *N. Engl. J. Med.*, **358**, pp. 1370–1380.

4. Rivera-Brown, A. M., and Frontera, W. R. (2012). Principles of exercise physiology: Responses to acute exercise and long-term adaptations to training, *PM R*, **4**, pp. 797–804.

5. Soonpaa, M. H., Kim, K. K., Pajak, L., Franklin, M., and Field, L. J. (1996). Cardiomyocyte DNA synthesis and binucleation during murine development, *Am. J. Physiol.*, **271**, pp. H2183–H2189.

6. Maillet, M., van Berlo, J. H., and Molkentin, J. D. (2013). Molecular basis of physiological heart growth: Fundamental concepts and new players, *Nat. Rev. Mol. Cell Biol.*, **14**, pp. 38–48.

7. Khan, R., and Sheppard, R. (2006). Fibrosis in heart disease: Understanding the role of transforming growth factor-beta in cardiomyopathy, valvular disease and arrhythmia, *Immunology*, **118**, pp. 10–24.

8. Stanley, W. C., Recchia, F. A., and Lopaschuk, G. D. (2005). Myocardial substrate metabolism in the normal and failing heart, *Physiol. Rev.*, **85**, pp. 1093–1129.

9. Nass, R. D., Aiba, T., Tomaselli, G. F., and Akar, F. G. (2008). Mechanisms of disease: Ion channel remodeling in the failing ventricle, *Nat. Clin. Pract. Cardiovasc. Med.*, **5**, pp. 196–207.

10. Clerk, A., Cullingford, T. E., Fuller, S. J., Giraldo, A., Markou, T., Pikkarainen, S., and Sugden, P. H. (2007). Signaling pathways mediating cardiac myocyte gene expression in physiological and stress responses, *J. Cell Physiol.*, **212**, pp. 311–322.

11. Gupta, M. P. (2007). Factors controlling cardiac myosin-isoform shift during hypertrophy and heart failure, *J. Mol. Cell Cardiol.*, **43**, pp. 388–403.

12. Michael, G., Xiao, L., Qi, X. Y., Dobrev, D., and Nattel, S. (2009). Remodelling of cardiac repolarization: How homeostatic responses can lead to arrhythmogenesis, *Cardiovasc. Res.*, **81**, pp. 491–499.

13. Rohr, S. (2012). Arrhythmogenic implications of fibroblast-myocyte interactions, *Circ. Arrhythm Electrophysiol.*, **5**, pp. 442–452.

14. Gaudesius, G., Miragoli, M., Thomas, S. P., and Rohr, S. (2003). Coupling of cardiac electrical activity over extended distances by fibroblasts of cardiac origin, *Circ. Res.*, **93**, pp. 421–428.

15. Miragoli, M., Gaudesius, G., and Rohr, S. (2006). Electrotonic modulation of cardiac impulse conduction by myofibroblasts, *Circ. Res.*, **98**, pp. 801–810.

16. Miragoli, M., Salvarani, N., and Rohr, S. (2007). Myofibroblasts induce ectopic activity in cardiac tissue, *Circ. Res.*, **101**, pp. 755–758.

17. Miragoli, M., Kadir, S. H., Sheppard, M. N., Salvarani, N., Virta, M., Wells, S., Lab, M. J., Nikolaev, V. O., Moshkov, A., Hague, W. M., Rohr, S., Williamson, C., and Gorelik, J. (2011). A protective antiarrhythmic role of ursodeoxycholic acid in an in vitro rat model of the cholestatic fetal heart, *Hepatology*, **54**, pp. 1282–1292.

18. Rosker, C., Salvarani, N., Schmutz, S., Grand, T., and Rohr, S. (2011). Abolishing myofibroblast arrhythmogeneicity by pharmacological ablation of alpha-smooth muscle actin containing stress fibers, *Circ. Res.*, **109**, pp. 1120–1131.

19. Turner, N. A., and Porter, K. E. (2013). Function and fate of myofibroblasts after myocardial infarction, *Fibrogenesis Tissue Repair*, **6**, p. 5.

20. Wilson, L. D., and Rosenbaum, D. S. (2007). Mechanisms of arrythmogenic cardiac alternans, *Europace*, **9 Suppl 6**, pp. vi77–82.

21. Mattick, J. S. (2001). Non-coding RNAs: The architects of eukaryotic complexity, *EMBO Rep.*, **2**, pp. 986–991.

22. Wang, K. C., and Chang, H. Y. (2011). Molecular mechanisms of long noncoding RNAs, *Mol. Cell*, **43**, pp. 904–914.

23. Farazi, T. A., Juranek, S. A., and Tuschl, T. (2008). The growing catalog of small RNAs and their association with distinct Argonaute/Piwi family members, *Development*, **135**, pp. 1201–1214.

24. Lee, R. C., Feinbaum, R. L., and Ambros, V. (1993). The C. elegans heterochronic gene lin-4 encodes small RNAs with antisense complementarity to lin-14, *Cell*, **75**, pp. 843–854.

25. Wightman, B., Ha, I., and Ruvkun, G. (1993). Posttranscriptional regulation of the heterochronic gene lin-14 by lin-4 mediates temporal pattern formation in C. elegans, *Cell*, **75**, pp. 855–862.

26. Kozomara, A., and Griffiths-Jones, S. (2011). miRBase: Integrating microRNA annotation and deep-sequencing data, *Nucleic Acids Res.*, **39**, pp. D152–D157.

27. Lee, Y., Kim, M., Han, J., Yeom, K. H., Lee, S., Baek, S. H., and Kim, V. N. (2004). MicroRNA genes are transcribed by RNA polymerase II, *EMBO J.*, **23**, pp. 4051–4060.

28. Cai, X., Hagedorn, C. H., and Cullen, B. R. (2004). Human microRNAs are processed from capped, polyadenylated transcripts that can also function as mRNAs, *RNA*, **10**, pp. 1957–1966.

29. Lee, Y., Ahn, C., Han, J., Choi, H., Kim, J., Yim, J., Lee, J., Provost, P., Radmark, O., Kim, S., and Kim, V. N. (2003). The nuclear RNase III Drosha initiates microRNA processing, *Nature*, **425**, pp. 415–419.

30. Bohnsack, M. T., Czaplinski, K., and Gorlich, D. (2004). Exportin 5 is a RanGTP-dependent dsRNA-binding protein that mediates nuclear export of pre-miRNAs, *RNA*, **10**, pp. 185–191.

31. Yi, R., Qin, Y., Macara, I. G., and Cullen, B. R. (2003). Exportin-5 mediates the nuclear export of pre-microRNAs and short hairpin RNAs, *Genes Dev.*, **17**, pp. 3011–3016.

32. Bernstein, E., Caudy, A. A., Hammond, S. M., and Hannon, G. J. (2001). Role for a bidentate ribonuclease in the initiation step of RNA interference, *Nature*, **409**, pp. 363–366.

33. Lau, N. C., Lim, L. P., Weinstein, E. G., and Bartel, D. P. (2001). An abundant class of tiny RNAs with probable regulatory roles in Caenorhabditis elegans, *Science*, **294**, pp. 858–862.

34. Schwarz, D. S., Hutvagner, G., Du, T., Xu, Z., Aronin, N., and Zamore, P. D. (2003). Asymmetry in the assembly of the RNAi enzyme complex, *Cell*, **115**, pp. 199–208.

35. Mourelatos, Z., Dostie, J., Paushkin, S., Sharma, A., Charroux, B., Abel, L., Rappsilber, J., Mann, M., and Dreyfuss, G. (2002). miRNPs: A novel class of ribonucleoproteins containing numerous microRNAs, *Genes Dev.*, **16**, pp. 720–728.

36. Cheloufi, S., Dos Santos, C. O., Chong, M. M., and Hannon, G. J. (2010). A dicer-independent miRNA biogenesis pathway that requires Ago catalysis, *Nature*, **465**, pp. 584–589.

37. Berezikov, E., Chung, W. J., Willis, J., Cuppen, E., and Lai, E. C. (2007). Mammalian mirtron genes, *Mol. Cell*, **28**, pp. 328–336.

38. Havens, M. A., Reich, A. A., Duelli, D. M., and Hastings, M. L. (2012). Biogenesis of mammalian microRNAs by a non-canonical processing pathway, *Nucleic Acids Res.*, **40**, pp. 4626–4640.

39. Bartel, D. P. (2009). MicroRNAs: Target recognition and regulatory functions, *Cell*, **136**, pp. 215–233.

40. Bartel, D. P., and Chen, C. Z. (2004). Micromanagers of gene expression: The potentially widespread influence of metazoan microRNAs, *Nat. Rev. Genet*, **5**, pp. 396–400.

41. Brodersen, P., and Voinnet, O. (2009). Revisiting the principles of microRNA target recognition and mode of action, *Nat. Rev. Mol. Cell Biol.*, **10**, pp. 141–148.

42. Fabian, M. R., and Sonenberg, N. (2012). The mechanics of miRNA-mediated gene silencing: A look under the hood of miRISC, *Nat. Struct. Mol. Biol.*, **19**, pp. 586–593.

43. Huntzinger, E., and Izaurralde, E. (2011). Gene silencing by microRNAs: Contributions of translational repression and mRNA decay, *Nat. Rev. Genet*, **12**, pp. 99–110.

44. Wu, L., and Belasco, J. G. (2008). Let me count the ways: Mechanisms of gene regulation by miRNAs and siRNAs, *Mol. Cell*, **29**, pp. 1–7.

45. Vasudevan, S., Tong, Y., and Steitz, J. A. (2007). Switching from repression to activation: MicroRNAs can up-regulate translation, *Science*, **318**, pp. 1931–1934.

46. Bushati, N., and Cohen, S. M. (2007). microRNA functions, *Annu. Rev. Cell Dev. Biol.*, **23**, pp. 175–205.

47. Schmitz, U., and Wolkenhauer, O. (2013). Web resources for microRNA research, *Adv. Exp. Med. Biol.*, **774**, pp. 225–250.

48. Lagos-Quintana, M., Rauhut, R., Yalcin, A., Meyer, J., Lendeckel, W., and Tuschl, T. (2002). Identification of tissue-specific microRNAs from mouse, *Curr. Biol.*, **12**, pp. 735–739.

49. Leptidis, S., El Azzouzi, H., Lok, S. I., de Weger, R., Olieslagers, S., Kisters, N., Silva, G. J., Heymans, S., Cuppen, E., Berezikov, E., De Windt, L. J., and da Costa Martins, P. (2013). A deep sequencing approach to uncover the miRNOME in the human heart, *PLoS One*, **8**, p. e57800.

50. Lee, E. J., Baek, M., Gusev, Y., Brackett, D. J., Nuovo, G. J., and Schmittgen, T. D. (2008). Systematic evaluation of microRNA processing patterns in tissues, cell lines, and tumors, *RNA*, **14**, pp. 35–42.

51. van Rooij, E., Sutherland, L. B., Qi, X., Richardson, J. A., Hill, J., and Olson, E. N. (2007). Control of stress-dependent cardiac growth and gene expression by a microRNA, *Science*, **316**, pp. 575–579.

52. Rao, P. K., Toyama, Y., Chiang, H. R., Gupta, S., Bauer, M., Medvid, R., Reinhardt, F., Liao, R., Krieger, M., Jaenisch, R., Lodish, H. F., and Blelloch, R. (2009). Loss of cardiac microRNA-mediated regulation leads to dilated cardiomyopathy and heart failure, *Circ. Res.*, **105**, pp. 585–594.

53. Chen, J. F., Murchison, E. P., Tang, R., Callis, T. E., Tatsuguchi, M., Deng, Z., Rojas, M., Hammond, S. M., Schneider, M. D., Selzman, C. H., Meissner, G., Patterson, C., Hannon, G. J., and Wang, D. Z. (2008). Targeted deletion of Dicer in the heart leads to dilated cardiomyopathy and heart failure, *Proc. Natl. Acad. Sci. U. S. A.*, **105**, pp. 2111–2116.

54. van Rooij, E., Sutherland, L. B., Thatcher, J. E., DiMaio, J. M., Naseem, R. H., Marshall, W. S., Hill, J. A., and Olson, E. N. (2008). Dysregulation of microRNAs after myocardial infarction reveals a role of miR-29 in cardiac fibrosis, *Proc. Natl. Acad. Sci. U. S. A.*, **105**, pp. 13027–13032.

55. Krutzfeldt, J., Rajewsky, N., Braich, R., Rajeev, K. G., Tuschl, T., Manoharan, M., and Stoffel, M. (2005). Silencing of microRNAs in vivo with "antagomirs", *Nature*, **438**, pp. 685–689.

56. Care, A., Catalucci, D., Felicetti, F., Bonci, D., Addario, A., Gallo, P., Bang, M. L., Segnalini, P., Gu, Y., Dalton, N. D., Elia, L., Latronico, M. V., Hoydal, M., Autore, C., Russo, M. A., Dorn, G. W., 2nd, Ellingsen, O., Ruiz-Lozano, P., Peterson, K. L., Croce, C. M., Peschle, C., and Condorelli, G. (2007). MicroRNA-133 controls cardiac hypertrophy, *Nat. Med.*, **13**, pp. 613–618.

57. Sayed, D., Hong, C., Chen, I. Y., Lypowy, J., and Abdellatif, M. (2007). MicroRNAs play an essential role in the development of cardiac hypertrophy, *Circ. Res.*, **100**, pp. 416–424.

58. van Rooij, E., Liu, N., and Olson, E. N. (2008). MicroRNAs flex their muscles, *Trends Genet*, **24**, pp. 159–166.

59. Zhao, Y., Samal, E., and Srivastava, D. (2005). Serum response factor regulates a muscle-specific microRNA that targets Hand2 during cardiogenesis, *Nature*, **436**, pp. 214–220.

60. Ivey, K. N., Muth, A., Arnold, J., King, F. W., Yeh, R. F., Fish, J. E., Hsiao, E. C., Schwartz, R. J., Conklin, B. R., Bernstein, H. S., and Srivastava, D. (2008). MicroRNA regulation of cell lineages in mouse and human embryonic stem cells, *Cell Stem Cell*, **2**, pp. 219–229.

61. Liu, N., Bezprozvannaya, S., Williams, A. H., Qi, X., Richardson, J. A., Bassel-Duby, R., and Olson, E. N. (2008). microRNA-133a regulates cardiomyocyte proliferation and suppresses smooth muscle gene expression in the heart, *Genes Dev.*, **22**, pp. 3242–3254.

62. Matkovich, S. J., Van Booven, D. J., Eschenbacher, W. H., and Dorn, G. W., 2nd (2011). RISC RNA sequencing for context-specific identification of in vivo microRNA targets, *Circ. Res.*, **108**, pp. 18–26.

63. Kim, G. H. (2013). MicroRNA regulation of cardiac conduction and arrhythmias, *Transl. Res.*, **161**, pp. 381–392.

64. Latronico, M. V., and Condorelli, G. (2009). RNA silencing: Small RNA-mediated posttranscriptional regulation of mRNA and the implications for heart electropathophysiology, *J. Cardiovasc. Electrophysiol.*, **20**, pp. 230–237.

65. Yang, B., Lin, H., Xiao, J., Lu, Y., Luo, X., Li, B., Zhang, Y., Xu, C., Bai, Y., Wang, H., Chen, G., and Wang, Z. (2007). The muscle-specific microRNA miR-1 regulates cardiac arrhythmogenic potential by targeting GJA1 and KCNJ2, *Nat. Med.*, **13**, pp. 486–491.

66. Zhao, Y., Ransom, J. F., Li, A., Vedantham, V., von Drehle, M., Muth, A. N., Tsuchihashi, T., McManus, M. T., Schwartz, R. J., and Srivastava, D. (2007). Dysregulation of cardiogenesis, cardiac conduction, and cell cycle in mice lacking miRNA-1-2, *Cell*, **129**, pp. 303–317.

67. Matkovich, S. J., Wang, W., Tu, Y., Eschenbacher, W. H., Dorn, L. E., Condorelli, G., Diwan, A., Nerbonne, J. M., and Dorn, G. W., 2nd (2010). MicroRNA-133a protects against myocardial fibrosis and modulates electrical repolarization without affecting hypertrophy in pressure-overloaded adult hearts, *Circ. Res.*, **106**, pp. 166–175.

68. Elia, L., Contu, R., Quintavalle, M., Varrone, F., Chimenti, C., Russo, M. A., Cimino, V., De Marinis, L., Frustaci, A., Catalucci, D., and Condorelli, G. (2009). Reciprocal regulation of microRNA-1 and insulin-like growth factor-1 signal transduction cascade in cardiac and skeletal muscle in physiological and pathological conditions, *Circulation*, **120**, pp. 2377–2385.

69. Varrone, F., Gargano, B., Carullo, P., Di Silvestre, D., De Palma, A., Grasso, L., Di Somma, C., Mauri, P., Benazzi, L., Franzone, A., Jotti, G. S., Bang, M. L., Esposito, G., Colao, A., Condorelli, G., and Catalucci, D. (2013). The circulating level of FABP3 is an indirect biomarker of microRNA-1, *J. Am. Coll Cardiol.*, **61**, pp. 88–95.

70. Rose, E. A., Gelijns, A. C., Moskowitz, A. J., Heitjan, D. F., Stevenson, L. W., Dembitsky, W., Long, J. W., Ascheim, D. D., Tierney, A. R., Levitan, R. G., Watson, J. T., Meier, P., Ronan, N. S., Shapiro, P. A., Lazar, R. M., Miller, L. W., Gupta, L., Frazier, O. H., Desvigne-Nickens, P., Oz, M. C., and Poirier, V. L. (2001). Long-term use of a left ventricular assist device for end-stage heart failure, *N. Engl. J. Med.*, **345**, pp. 1435–1443.

71. Koitabashi, N., and Kass, D. A. (2012). Reverse remodeling in heart failure–mechanisms and therapeutic opportunities, *Nat. Rev. Cardiol.*, **9**, pp. 147–157.

72. van Rooij, E., and Olson, E. N. (2012). MicroRNA therapeutics for cardiovascular disease: Opportunities and obstacles, *Nat. Rev. Drug Discov.*, **11**, pp. 860–872.

73. Dvir, T., Bauer, M., Schroeder, A., Tsui, J. H., Anderson, D. G., Langer, R., Liao, R., and Kohane, D. S. (2011). Nanoparticles targeting the infarcted heart, *Nano Lett.*, **11**, pp. 4411–4414.

74. Choi, H. S., Ashitate, Y., Lee, J. H., Kim, S. H., Matsui, A., Insin, N., Bawendi, M. G., Semmler-Behnke, M., Frangioni, J. V., and Tsuda, A. (2010). Rapid translocation of nanoparticles from the lung airspaces to the body, *Nat. Biotechnol.*, **28**, pp. 1300–1303.

75. Mills, N. L., Donaldson, K., Hadoke, P. W., Boon, N. A., MacNee, W., Cassee, F. R., Sandstrom, T., Blomberg, A., and Newby, D. E. (2009). Adverse cardiovascular effects of air pollution, *Nat. Clin. Pract. Cardiovasc. Med.*, **6**, pp. 36–44.

76. Brook, R. D., Rajagopalan, S., Pope, C. A., 3rd, Brook, J. R., Bhatnagar, A., Diez-Roux, A. V., Holguin, F., Hong, Y., Luepker, R. V., Mittleman, M. A., Peters, A., Siscovick, D., Smith, S. C., Jr., Whitsel, L., and Kaufman, J. D. (2010). Particulate matter air pollution and cardiovascular disease: An update to the scientific statement from the American Heart Association, *Circulation*, **121**, pp. 2331–2378.

77. Yokota, S., Seki, T., Furuya, M., and Ohara, N. (2005). Acute functional enhancement of circulatory neutrophils after intratracheal instillation with diesel exhaust particles in rats, *Inhal. Toxicol.*, **17**, pp. 671–679.

78. Gidney, J. T., Twigg, M. V., and Kittelson, D. B. (2010). Effect of organometallic fuel additives on nanoparticle emissions from a gasoline passenger car, *Environ. Sci. Technol.*, **44**, pp. 2562–2569.

79. Miragoli, M., Novak, P., Ruenraroengsak, P., Shevchuk, A. I., Korchev, Y. E., Lab, M. J., Tetley, T. D., and Gorelik, J. (2013). Functional interaction between charged nanoparticles and cardiac tissue: A new paradigm for cardiac arrhythmia?, *Nanomedicine (Lond)*, **8**, pp. 725–737.

80. Lacerda, L., Bianco, A., Prato, M., and Kostarelos, K. (2006). Carbon nanotubes as nanomedicines: From toxicology to pharmacology, *Adv. Drug Deliv. Rev.*, **58**, pp. 1460–1470.

81. Mahmoudi, M., Hofmann, H., Rothen-Rutishauser, B., and Petri-Fink, A. (2012). Assessing the in vitro and in vivo toxicity of superparamagnetic iron oxide nanoparticles, *Chem. Rev.*, **112**, pp. 2323–2338.

82. Panseri, S., Cunha, C., D'Alessandro, T., Sandri, M., Giavaresi, G., Marcacci, M., Hung, C. T., and Tampieri, A. (2012). Intrinsically superparamagnetic Fe-hydroxyapatite nanoparticles positively influence osteoblast-like cell behaviour, *J. Nanobiotechnol.*, **10**, p. 32.

83. Chiou, G. Y., Cherng, J. Y., Hsu, H. S., Wang, M. L., Tsai, C. M., Lu, K. H., Chien, Y., Hung, S. C., Chen, Y. W., Wong, C. I., Tseng, L. M., Huang, P. I., Yu, C. C., Hsu, W. H., and Chiou, S. H. (2012). Cationic polyurethanes-short branch PEI-mediated delivery of Mir145 inhibited epithelial-mesenchymal transdifferentiation and cancer stem-like properties and in lung adenocarcinoma, *J. Control. Release*, **159**, pp. 240–250.

84. Yang, Y. P., Chien, Y., Chiou, G. Y., Cherng, J. Y., Wang, M. L., Lo, W. L., Chang, Y. L., Huang, P. I., Chen, Y. W., Shih, Y. H., Chen, M. T., and Chiou, S. H. (2012). Inhibition of cancer stem cell-like properties and reduced chemoradioresistance of glioblastoma using microRNA145 with cationic polyurethane-short branch PEI, *Biomaterials*, **33**, pp. 1462–1476.

85. Wang, K., Ruan, J., Song, H., Zhang, J., Wo, Y., Guo, S., and Cui, D. (2011). Biocompatibility of graphene oxide, *Nanoscale Res Lett.*, **6**, p. 8.

86. Novoselov, K. S., Fal'ko, V. I., Colombo, L., Gellert, P. R., Schwab, M. G., and Kim, K. (2012). A roadmap for graphene, *Nature*, **490**, pp. 192–200.

# Chapter 11

# Triggering Cell–Biomaterial Interaction: Recent Approaches for Osteochondral Regeneration

**Monica Montesi and Silvia Panseri**

*Institute of Science and Technology for Ceramics—National Research Council of Italy—ISTEC—CNR, Via Granarolo 64, 48018 Faenza, Italy*

monica.montesi@istec.cnr.it

## 11.1 Introduction

Osteoarthritis (OA) is the most common form of degenerative joint disease and a leading cause of pain primarily associated with aging [1, 2]. OA is a leading cause of chronic disability in the USA and EU. Numbers are impressive, accounting for over 25 million diseased people in the USA and over 50 million in EU, registering as much as 25% of the total visits to primary care physicians, and half of all non-steroidal anti-inflammatory drugs (NSAID) prescriptions. The number of people with OA-related disability is expected to double by the year 2020, thereby increasing the already significant economic burden resulting from the condition [3]. OA is characterized by typical structural alterations of the joint, including focal degradation of articular cartilage and remodeling

---

*Bio-Inspired Regenerative Medicine: Materials, Processes, and Clinical Applications*
Edited by Simone Sprio and Anna Tampieri
Copyright © 2016 Pan Stanford Publishing Pte. Ltd.
ISBN 978-981-4669-14-6 (Hardcover), 978-981-4669-15-3 (eBook)
www.panstanford.com

of subchondral bone [4]; the situation is complicated by the fact that injuries to articular cartilage are one of the most challenging issues of musculoskeletal medicine due to the poor intrinsic ability of this tissue for repair. Despite centuries of progress in medicine and science, there is currently no successful and universally accepted approach for the treatment of damaged articular cartilage [5]. Pharmacological treatments available to date are modestly efficacious, and are frequently associated with substantial side effects or costs [6]; in addition, surgical intervention is frequently required to repair bone and cartilage damage. This evidence highlights the need for new and efficacious treatments and therapeutics. In this respect, tissue engineering (TE) offers an integrative strategy to reconstitute a tissue both structurally and functionally. TE usually involves the use of biomaterials, cells and bioactive factors (signaling cues/regulators) [7] in various combinations to facilitate the regeneration of lost or injured tissue in order to modulate cellular processes including proliferation, differentiation and tissue morphogenesis [8]. The emerging trends in cartilage tissue engineering and regenerative medicine [9] rely on biomaterial-based therapies, still in the developmental stages, with the use of biomaterials as a central delivery system for microenvironmental cues and regulators to manipulate transplanted or ingrowth cells and to orchestrate host cell response in vivo [10]. Initially, biomaterials for cartilage tissue engineering applications have been evaluated for their physical (e.g., porosity and mechanical compressive strength) and chemical (e.g., degradation) properties [11]. Only in recent years, design of these biomaterials includes signaling cues incorporated within the synthetic microenvironment [12, 13]. The situation becomes more complex when OA damage includes deep lesions penetrating to the subchondral bone [14]. TE requires a tissue-conductive system in order to mimic the 3-D environment of the extracellular matrix (ECM), provide structural support to the regenerate and surrounding tissues, and provide an increased surface area to volume ratio for cellular migration, adhesion, differentiation [15, 16]. Note that the cellular growth and subsequent tissue regeneration depend in part on the characteristics and porosity of the scaffold. It must be biodegradable and biocompatible and it must present a suitable fixation to the defect site, facilitate cell attachment, regulate cell expression, and promote the supply of nutrients and growth factors. This chapter addresses the most promising TE approaches in improving cell–material interactions for articular cartilage and subchondral bone regeneration.

## 11.2   Biomaterial Chemical Features

A wide range of materials are currently being used for both three-dimensional (3D) cell culture and for cartilage and bone defects repair [15, 16]. They include synthetic and natural ones, in turn further distinguished as protein-based [17] and polysaccharide-based [18] biomaterials. Some of these materials, such as collagen [19], hyaluronan [20] and fibrin [21, 22], are already clinically used for cartilage repair. Among the protein-based biomaterials, membranes formed of type I and III collagens are clinically used [23] for autologous chondrocyte implantation (i.e., MACI®, Verigen, Leverkusen, Germany; Maix® Matricel, Hezoenrath, Germany; Chondro-gide® Geistlich Biomaterials, Wolhusen, Switzerland; Atelocollagen® Koken Co. Ltd, Tokyo, Japan). In this scenario, it is envisaged that improvements in osteochondral defect repair and regeneration would be achieved through development of innovative biomaterial systems (possibly associated to ease of clinical application).

In order to control and direct cell behavior, a well-defined biomimetic environment, which surrounds the cells and promotes specific cell interactions, is necessary. Scaffold properties depend primarily on the nature of the biomaterial and the fabrication process. The nature of the biomaterial has been the subject of extensive studies including different materials such as natural, synthetic materials, ceramics, or composite of these compounds.

Natural materials provide a more physiological environment for cell adhesion and proliferation and may be further divided into protein-based matrices such as collagen and fibrin, and carbohydrate-based matrices such as alginate, agarose, chitosan, and hyaluronan [24–26]. Natural materials are biocompatible, biodegradable and they have the ability to mimic certain aspects of native ECM, thus facilitating cell adhesion, migration, differentiation, and ECM deposition. However, natural materials have several disadvantages such as immunogenecity, difficulty in processing, and a potential risk of transmitting animal-originated pathogens. Moreover, despite the biocompatibility, these materials are mechanically weak and undergo rapid degradation upon implantation if not cross-linked with appropriate chemical reagents [27].

## 11.3 View within Article

Synthetic materials have been used extensively both in vitro and in vivo due to their easy molding characteristics, relatively easy production, and the ability to control dissolution and degradation they are fully employed in tissue engineering [28]. The most popular biodegradable synthetic polymers include poly($\alpha$-hydroxy acids), especially poly(lactic acid) (PLA), poly(glycolic acid) (PGA) and their co-polymers (PLGA), poly($\varepsilon$-caprolactone), poly(propylene fumarate), poly(dioxanone) [29].

Although synthetic materials are biocompatible, they do not have natural sites for cell adhesion, and these often need to be added. Further, their in vivo degradation by a hydrolytic reaction causes a local reduction in pH and possible inflammation response [30].

Ceramics, such as hydroxyapatite (HA) or other calcium phosphate (Ca-P) ceramics (including tricalcium phosphate, TCP) or bioactive glasses are known to promote, when implanted, the formation of a bone-like apatite layer on their surfaces [31, 32]. They have been investigated extensively during the last decades and are widely used for bone replacement, due to their osteoconductivity and high biocompatibility, also associated with stem cells therapy [19].

The main purpose for osteochondral TE is to recreate a more biomimetic scaffold combining synthetic materials with cell-recognition sites of naturally derived materials [31, 33, 34]. In addition, looking to the architectures of native tissues, novel graded scaffolds represent the challenge for osteochondral defect treatment. In fact bone and cartilage have complete different properties. For bone, mechanically stiff biomaterials with options for medium perfusion and vascularization are required to support cell expansion, as well as the production of bone matrix rich in type I collagen and hydroxyapatite. By contrast, native cartilage matrix consists of an avascular highly hydrated proteoglycan hydrogel embedded into a type II collagen network.

Although several studies focus on the design and optimization of a stratified osteochondral graft with biomimetic multi-tissue regions, only few show good results in experiments in vivo. Here, some encouraging examples are mentioned.

A multi-phased scaffold of agarose hydrogel and sintered microspheres of PLGA-bioactive glass composite has shown in vitro a controlled chondrocyte and osteoblast culture on each scaffold region, resulting in the formation of three distinct yet continuous regions of cartilage, calcified cartilage and bone-like matrices [35]. Very recently, a poly vinyl alcohol/gelatin-nano-hydroxyapatite/polyamide6 (PVA-n-HA/PA6) bilayered scaffold seeded with induced bone marrow stem cells (BMSCs) showed ectopic neocartilage formation in the PVA layer and reconstitution of the subchondral bone, confined within the n-HA/PA6 layer, when implanted into the rabbit muscle pouch for up to 12 weeks [36]. A biphasic scaffold combining hyaluronic acid and atelocollagen for the chondral phase and combining HA and β-TCP for the osseous phase has proved to be effective for repairing osteochondral defects, when implanted in the knee joint of a porcine model [37]. Another biphasic scaffold based on collagen-glycosaminoglycan and nano calcium phosphate has been developed to mimic the composition and structure of articular cartilage on one side, subchondral bone on the other side and the continuous, gradual soft interface between these tissues. The different properties of the osseous and cartilaginous compartments seem to be promising, but, as far as we know, this scaffold has not yet been tested in a biological system.

Very recently, a 3D biomimetic scaffold (MaioRegen, Fin-Ceramica Faenza S.p.A., Italy) was obtained by nucleating type I collagen fibrils with HA nanoparticles, in two configurations, bi- and tri-layered, to reproduce, respectively, chondral and osteochondral anatomy [38]. In vivo results showed that the growth of trabecular bone in the osteochondral lesion was evident and newly formed fibrocartilaginous tissue was present [39]. The same scaffold has been used already in an early stability clinical trial with 15 degenerative chondral lesions. The mean size of the defects was 2.8 $cm^2$ and MRI evaluation at short-term follow-up has demonstrated good stability of the scaffold without any other fixation device and the histological analysis showed the formation of subchondral bone without the presence of biomaterial and the cartilage repair tissue appeared to be engaged in an ongoing maturation process [38]. Presently, an extensive clinical trial is ongoing involving 11 European centers and 150 patients (http://clinicaltrialsfeeds.org/clinical-trials/show/NCT01282034).

## 11.4 Scaffold Architecture: From Macro- to Molecular Level

To understand the mechanism of cell–material interaction, the structure of biological tissue is one of the most important characteristics that has to be taken in consideration during the biomaterials designing process [40]. Therefore, one of the most stimulating challenge of the tissue engineering is to obtain materials able to mimic a specific biological microenvironment and able to trigger the natural process of cell-driven tissues regeneration.

Not only the chemical compositions is crucial to improve the efficiency of biomaterials, but also the overall structure and architecture of the scaffold should be appropriate, especially focusing on the biomimesis of bone substitutes [41].

It has been shown in several studies that surface topography (random/ordered reliefs, patterns, etc.) could drive cell adhesion, proliferation, migration, and differentiation [42, 43]. The single molecules of the ECM exhibit a nanometer scale topographies, by which they exert the signaling for the cell-matrix interaction; the intrinsic capacity of the ECM proteins to form a tertiary conformation (i.e., collagen type I fibrils, one of the most abundant protein of the bone ECM), contribute to the microscale topographies of the tissue [44].

Focusing on bone tissue engineering, the trigger of the cell–material interaction depends on the scaffold design; in fact, the combination of macro-, micro-, and nanostructures could provide a platform influencing bone cell adhesion, spreading, proliferation, and differentiation [45, 46] (Fig. 11.1). The cellular interaction with a nanoscale topography occurs through integrin-mediated adhesions focal clustering. The binding of integrin heterodimers (i.e., $\alpha 5\ \beta 3$) to specific amino acid sequences, such as arginine-glycine-aspartic acid (Arg-Gly-Asp or RGD) largely present in many ECM proteins, results in a focal contact formation, and that process can be influenced when the surface topography is within the nanometer range [40, 47]. However, cell–nanotopography interactions can induce different effects within a single cell type but affects basic cell function in almost all types of mammalian cells. Langer and collaborators in 2009 described the important role of the biomaterial nanotopography as an alternative signaling mechanism to precisely control cell morphology, migration, function and differentiation [44]. It has been shown that the scale and order topography could modulate the gene expression during the mesenchymal stem cells (MSCs) osteogenetic differentiation. In a Dalby M. J. and collaborators study, both human osteoprogenitors and MSCs cells, grown in disordered square array with dots displaced randomly by up to 50 nm on both axes from their position, showed an increasing in osteoblast phenotype and in osteospecific markers expression, as osteopontin, osteocalcin, alkaline phosphatase, collagens, matrix metallopeptidase 8; as well as high expression level of important osteoblast adhesion molecules among which ICAM1 and different kinds of integrin [48].

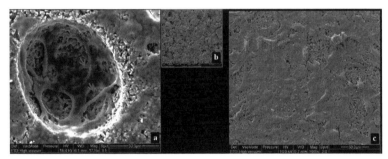

**Figure 11.1** Scanning electron microscopy images of cellular interactions with Hydroxyapatite-forming calcium phosphate cements (H-CPC). MG63 cells, grown on the H-CPC surface, showed tight interactions with the materials. Red arrows indicate cellular body processes in contact with the cements (a, magnification 1775×) and (c, magnification 1000×). In (b) a detail of H-CPC microstructures (magnification 4000×).

It has been also shown that the osteogenetic commitment of MSCs was also mediated by changing in substrate stiffness, by directly modulating integrin-adhesion ligand bond formation [49]. Through integrin-mediated focal adhesions, cells are able to anchor onto the underlying substrate, sense the surrounding microenvironment, and react to the specific signaling pathway such us bone morphogenetic protein (BMP) signaling pathway that plays a vital role for bone development and regeneration [50, 51].

Structurally, the bone is hierarchically organized from macro-, micro-, to nanoscale, where the basic building blocks are the plate-like HA nanocrystals incorporated collagen nanofibers [52]. Thus, in the bone tissue engineering researches a rational strategy to develop composites scaffolds with nanofiber ultrastructure to recapitalize the ECM of bone exist.

In recent years, this tendency has been well documented in literature and demonstrated great promise of the nanofiber-based bone substitutes and/or replacements for bone regeneration [53, 54]. Nanostructured scaffolds, made of biomimetic apatite with a high level of porosity that simulate the morphology of spongy bone (porosity varying from micro-porosity of >1 μm to a macroporosity in the range 300–2000 μm), and chitosan-based hydroxyapatite (HAp/CTS) biocomposites, have been widely used in bone tissue engineering [55, 56]. Besides, the development of new specific hybrids to be applied as multifunctional and bioinspired systems is an important progress in field of bone regenerative medicine [57]. Recent advanced techniques permitted the manufacturing of 3D porous scaffolds, by using bioactive materials ranging over inorganic phases (i.e., nanostructured calcium phosphates, biomimetic HA, and high-strength ceramics) and organic phases (i.e., natural and bio-erodible polymers) [58–60]. High level of the bone tissue biomimesis has been obtained with the develop of the hybrid composites formed by the bone-like hydroxyapatite nanocrystals nucleated on self-assembling collagen fibers (collagen/HA) [21]. The reproduction of the complex bone structure, made of elements characterized by a defined chemistry and with a morphology hierarchically organized down to the molecular scale, can be obtained by using techniques in which hybrid organic–inorganic composites are spontaneously built, driven by biological mechanisms [58].

These bone-like composites showed an high level of biological compatibility (biodegradability and absence of any cytotoxic effects); because of the bioavailability of these elements and their topographic structure from macro- to nanoscale, they play a crucial role in the adhesion and integration of cells on the scaffold and the subsequent activity of bone formation and remodeling [46, 61–63].

Based on all the above described, the hybrid organic-inorganic scaffold has shown a promising prospects for clinical applications in a wide range of bone replacement needs, on this basis several patents and commercial products have been developed and commercialized (e.g., RegenOss® and MaioRegen®).

## 11.5 Biosignals to Enhance the Cellular Interactions with Biomaterials

The main goal of tissue engineering and regenerative medicine strategies is to restore the function of damaged tissues combining cells and biomaterials, on which cells must adhere, organize and develop similarly to native tissue, and also a controlled delivery of biological. The cell fates, in vivo, are determined by a complex interaction between cell receptors and nanoscale biological, physical and chemical signals; for these reasons a pivotal approach in tissue engineering consist of the mimicking of the submicron-scale spatial orientation of extracellular signaling molecules for enhancing cell–biomaterial communication and inducing cell behaviors [64]. In recent decades, a range of new strategies to increase the interaction between cells and materials have been developed; many surface modification techniques such as $\gamma$-ray irradiation, plasma treatment, engrafting, ozone oxidization, or in situ polymerization have already been considered to modify the materials surface properties with the aim to improve the cytocompatibility of the polymeric materials without altering their bulk properties [65, 66]. Moreover, the self-assembly approach, in which smaller molecules spontaneously formed an ordered structures, is an important nanotechnology tool which may be utilized for spatially orienting peptides with nanoscale precision [67].

The scaffolds for tissue engineering often incorporate biosignals to create a controlled, bioinspired extracellular environment to direct tissue specific cell responses. Some functionalization strategies use the nanoscale ECM-derived peptides, such as collagens, elastin, and laminin, glycoproteins such as fibronectin and vitronectin, as well as glycosaminoglycans such as chondroitin sulfate [68]; in other cases, the strategy consists of the use of *cell recognition motifs* functionalization. The RGD motif is the most often employed peptide sequence that not only triggers cell adhesion but also can be used to address selectively certain cell lines and elicit specific cell responses [69, 70].

The RGD motives, but also other peptides motives such as integrin-binding modules of fibronectin, are recognized by integrin receptors. It is well known that integrins are a family of cell-surface transmembrane receptors, each of which consists of $\alpha$ and $\beta$ subunits associate to form 24 distinct $\alpha\beta$ domains and each of these domains have unique binding characteristics. The interaction between an integrin domain and its specific RDG motifs acts as a upstream regulator of several molecular pathways, involved in the definition of cell fate in terms of survival, adhesion, proliferation and differentiation [71]. Thanks to its characteristics, in the last years the effects of RGD micro- and nano distribution have been extensively explored by using molecular scaffolds or new materials that allow controlled RGD spatial arrangement [72–75].

Other bioinspired approaches have focused on incorporating soluble signals into tissue engineering scaffolds, with the aim of promoting stem cell proliferation and differentiation. Soluble signals include growth factors such as epidermal growth factor (EGF), vascular endothelial growth factor (VEGF) and fibroblast growth factor (FGF), as well as cytokines and chemokines, have been also used in combination with adhesive peptides to direct cell functions for tissue engineering, or in many applications of biomaterial delivery systems for growth factors or drug delivery in tissue engineering [76, 77].

Recently, the study of interaction between biomolecules, with anabolic effects in bone, and different kinds of bone biomimetic materials is a growing topic in bioengineering field, not only as a strategy to improve the cellular–biomaterial interaction, but also with the aim to develop new delivery systems for therapy based on local release of the therapeutic factors [78, 79].

Moreover other techniques have been studied in the field of tissue engineering to improve the strategies of biomimesis of the material, some examples include the self-assembled monolayers (SAMs), polymer-assisted patterning, the use of DNA templating, nanoimprint lithography, electron beam lithography, and 3D peptide patterning.

## 11.6 Magnetic Remote Control: Innovative Solution for Tissue Regeneration

The increasing need of reducing invasivity and increasing efficacy of regenerative therapies is pushing the recent advances in tissue engineering, stem cell research, nanotechnology as well as in understanding of organogenesis, toward the development of new biomedical solutions based on smart devices [80, 81]. In this respect, recent research evidences that tissue regeneration assisted by external magnetic fields is an issue of increasing interest.

In the last decades, it has been demonstrated that weak magnetic or pulse electromagnetic fields are effective stimuli that promoted bone fracture healing, spinal fusion and bone ingrowth in animal models [82–85]. Strong static magnetic field (SMF) of 5–10 T was reported to have the ability to regulate in vitro and in vivo the orientation of protein matrices and cells along the field lines [86, 87]. Therefore, the association of magnetic stimulationand suitable biochemical agents could lead to more efficient treatments for the regeneration of extended bone and osteochondral regions.

Recently, the use of magnetic nanoparticles (MNPs) for biological and medical purposes has been increasing and their biocompatibility is validated by several studies [88–90]. MNPs are unique in their reaction applications (e.g., hyperthermia, contrast agent for magnetic resonance imaging (MRI), magnetic drug delivery and cell mechanosensitive receptor manipulation to induce cell differentiation), whereas few authors have proposed approaches for their use in tissue engineering [91–93]. There are several limitations to the clinical application of a magnetic field for targeted therapy of a magnetic drug or for cell delivery. In fact, since the magnetic gradient decreases with the distance to the target, the main limitation of magnetic delivery relates to the strength of the external field that can be applied to obtain the necessary magnetic gradient to control the residence time of MNPs in the desired area or which triggers the drug desorption [94, 95]. The limitations inherent to the use of external magnetic fields can be circumvented by introduction of internal magnets located in the proximity of the target by minimally invasive surgery or by using a superparamagnetic scaffold under the influence of an externally applied magnetic field. In the latter, the magnetic moment of these scaffolds affords the potential for their continuous control and reloading with several tissue growth factors [96, 97].

For the reasons just mentioned, the preparation of magnetic scaffolds, mimicking the complexity of bone/cartilage structure from the macro to the molecular scale and enabling to activate cell adhesion and proliferation under the stimulus of magnetic field can be an appealing solution in tissue engineering. Recently, several works have demonstrated that MNPs embedded in polymeric or inorganic scaffolds have effect on the osteoinduction with and without external magnetic force. In particular, it was reported that the introduction of MNPs to CaP bioceramics promoted bone formation and growth in vitro and in vivo [98, 99] and the addition of MNPs in fibrous polymeric scaffolds induced higher cell proliferation and faster differentiation in osteoblasts in vitro, and enhanced osteogenesis and new bone tissue formation in animal model; moreover their magnetic behavior can allow to label the scaffold to be visualized in vivo by MRI [100–103].

In this view, magnetic scaffolds may offer great potential in bone regenerative medicine and magnetic forces could influence the orientation of scaffold architecture and subsequently the tissue regeneration. Our recent results demonstrated as a proof of principle how magnetic scaffolds implanted in vivo can induce controlled bone tissue regeneration in a well-defined 3D pattern according to an applied SMF. The collagen-based scaffolds tested, due to their MNPs component, under the effect of the magnetic field are "activated" and determine the orientation of the scaffold according with the magnetic lines. This effect, modulated by the SMF, could be used to obtain an aligned scaffold that will work as a template for new oriented ECM deposition mimicking the site-specific collagen/apatite orientation [104, 105]. In addition, the magnetic fixation was investigated as a promising approach to prevent micromotion at the scaffold/tissue interface. Nowadays suturing of cartilage grafts, pin fixation and transosseous fixation of the scaffolds show several limits [106–108]. The configuration studied by finite element modeling, shows how four small permanent magnet pins implanted into the subchondral bone under the scaffold can fix the magnetic scaffold avoiding micromotion and enhancing tissue regeneration [107].

One of the most important criteria in using MNPs is the absence of any toxicity. Nowadays all the MNPs presented on the market are made by iron oxides phases (i.e., magnetite, maghemite) whose long-term cytotoxic effects in the human body are not yet completely assessed and their use is becoming a critical issue due to their accumulation in soft tissues and organs such as liver and kidney [109, 110]. Over the last decade, the surface of MNPs has been modified through the creation of biocompatible layers made of organic polymers, inorganic phases or metals deposited on the existing surface [111]. Due to the importance of having non-toxic MNPs for the above-mentioned applications, recently our group developed a new biocompatible and bioresorbable superparamagnetic-like phase by doping hydroxyapatite (HA) with $Fe^{2+}/Fe^{3+}$ ions (FeHA) avoiding the presence of poorly tolerated magnetic secondary phases. This new magnetic apatite could represent, by virtue of its bioactivity, a conceptually new type of scaffold for hard tissue regeneration. In vitro study revealed that FeHA nanoparticles not only did not reduce cell viability, but they enhanced cell proliferation compared to HA particles. This effect was even significantly increased when a magnetic field was applied [106]. Moreover a pilot animal study of bone repair (a rabbit critical bone defect model) demonstrated the in vivo biocompatibility and biodegradability of FeHA [98, 106]. FeHA nanoparticles have been also recently used to prepare magnetic hybrid inorganic-polymeric composites in the form of films and hollow micro-nanospheres [112].

Recently FeHA was directly nucleated on self-assembling collagen (type I) fibers using a biologically inspired mineralization process [34, 63]. Magnetic hybrid FeHA/Coll composites were prepared at different temperatures and the effect of synthesis parameters have been correlated to the reaction yield in terms of mineralization degree and magnetization. The influence of scaffold properties on cellular response was investigated: MG63 human osteoblast-like cells were seeded on magnetic scaffolds and differences in terms of cell viability, adhesion, proliferation were studied with respect to the non-magnetic HA/Coll scaffold (paper in preparation). Under an external magnetic field, this scaffold can be activated and function like a magnet, attracting functionalized magnetic nanoparticles injected close to the scaffold. Using this approach, strategies for drug delivery using nanoparticles could be made more effective by reducing nanoparticle loss [94, 95]. Thus, there is potential to enhance tissue regeneration via delivery of several growth factors that can be accurately released close to or into the scaffold.

## References

1. Helmick, C. G., et al., Estimates of the prevalence of arthritis and other rheumatic conditions in the United States. Part I. *Arthritis Rheum.*, 2008. **58**(1): pp. 15–25.

2. Lohmander, S., Osteoarthritis year 2012 in review. *Osteoarthritis Cartilage/OARS*, Osteoarthritis Research Society, 2012. **20**(12): p. 1439.

3. Zhang, Y., and J. M. Jordan, Epidemiology of osteoarthritis. *Clin. Geriatr. Med.*, 2010. **26**(3): pp. 355–369.

4. van der Kraan, P. M., Osteoarthritis year 2012 in review: Biology. Osteoarthritis and cartilage/OARS, *Osteoarthritis Res. Soc.*, 2012. **20**(12): pp. 1447–1450.

5. Kalson, N. S., P. D. Gikas, and T. W. R. Briggs, Current strategies for knee cartlage repair. *Int. J. Clin. Pract.*, 2010. **64**: pp. 1444–1442.

6. Lohmander, L. S., and E. M. Roos, Clinical update: Treating osteoarthritis. *Lancet*, 2007. **370**(9605): pp. 2082–2084.

7. Koepsel, J. T., and W. L. Murphy, Patterned self-assembled monolayers: Efficient, chemically defined tools for cell biology. *Chembiochem: Eur. J. Chem. Biol.*, 2012. **13**(12): pp. 1717–1724.

8. Pashuck, E. T., and M. M. Stevens, Designing regenerative biomaterial therapies for the clinic. *Sci. Translational Med.*, 2012. **4**(160): p. 160sr4.

9. Toh, W. S., et al., Biomaterial-mediated delivery of microenvironmental cues for repair and regeneration of articular cartilage. *Mol. Pharm.*, 2011. **8**(4): pp. 994–1001.

10. Elisseeff, J., Injectable cartilage tissue engineering. *Expert Opin. Biol. Therapy*, 2004. **4**(12): pp. 1849–1859.

11. Hutmacher, D. W., Scaffolds in tissue engineering bone and cartilage. *Biomaterials*, 2000. **21**(24): pp. 2529–2543.

12. Kim, T. G., H. Shin, and D. Wo, Biomimetic scaffolds for tissue engineering. *Adv. Funct. Mater.*, 2012. **22**: pp. 2446–2468.

13. Lutolf, M. P., and J. A. Hubbell, Synthetic biomaterials as instructive extracellular microenvironments for morphogenesis in tissue engineering. *Nat. Biotechnol.*, 2005. **23**: pp. 47–55.

14. Liu, Y., X. Z. Shu, and G. D. Prestwich, Osteochondral defect repair with autologous bone marrow-derived mesenchymal stem cells in an

injectable, in situ, cross-linked synthetic extracellular matrix. *Tissue Eng.*, 2006. **12**(12): pp. 3405–3416.

15. Vinatier, C., et al., Cartilage engineering: A crucial combination of cells, biomaterials and biofactors. *Trends Biotechnol.*, 2009. **27**(5): pp. 307–314.

16. Chung, C., and J. A. Burdick, Engineering cartilage tissue. *Adv. Drug Deliv. Rev.*, 2008. **60**(2): pp. 243–262.

17. Ma, P. X., Biomimetic materials for tissue engineering. *Adv. Drug Deliv. Rev.*, 2008. **60**(2): pp. 184–198.

18. Selmi, T. A., et al., Autologous chondrocyte implantation in a novel alginate-agarose hydrogel: Outcome at two years. *J. Bone Joint Surg Br*, 2008. **90**: pp. 597–604.

19. Marcacci, M., et al., Stem cells associated with macroporous bioceramics for long bone repair: 6- to 7-year outcome of a pilot clinical study. *Tissue Eng.*, 2007. **13**(5): pp. 947–955.

20. Nehrer, S., et al., Results of chondrocyte implantation with a fibrin-hyaluronan matrix: A preliminary study. *Clin. Orthop. Relat. Res.*, 2008. **466**(8): pp. 1849–1855.

21. Tampieri, A., et al., Biologically inspired synthesis of bone-like composite: Self-assembled collagen fibers/hydroxyapatite nanocrystals. *J. Biomed. Mater. Res. A*, 2003. **67**(2): pp. 618–625.

22. Tampieri, A., et al., Design of graded biomimetic osteochondral composite scaffolds. *Biomaterials*, 2008. **29**(26): pp. 3539–3546.

23. Abou Neel, E. A., et al., Collagen–emerging collagen based therapies hit the patient. *Adv. Drug Deliv. Rev.*, 2013. **65**(4): pp. 429–456.

24. Ng, K. W., et al., A layered agarose approach to fabricate depth-dependent inhomogeneity in chondrocyte-seeded constructs. *J. Orthop. Res.*, 2005. **23**(1): pp. 134–141.

25. Ochi, M., et al., Current concepts in tissue engineering technique for repair of cartilage defect. *Artif. Organs*, 2001. **25**(3): pp. 172–179.

26. Pabbruwe, M. B., et al., Induction of cartilage integration by a chondrocyte/collagen-scaffold implant. *Biomaterials*, 2009. **30**(26): pp. 4277–4286.

27. Lee, S. H., and H. Shin, Matrices and scaffolds for delivery of bioactive molecules in bone and cartilage tissue engineering. *Adv. Drug Deliv. Rev.*, 2007. **59**(4–5): pp. 339–359.

28. Capito, R. M., and M. Spector, Scaffold-based articular cartilage repair. *IEEE Eng. Med. Biol. Mag.*, 2003. **22**(5): pp. 42–50.

29. Mano, J. F., and R. L. Reis, Osteochondral defects: Present situation and tissue engineering approaches. *J. Tissue Eng. Regen. Med.*, 2007. **1**(4): pp. 261–273.

30. Getgood, A., et al., Articular cartilage tissue engineering: Today's research, tomorrow's practice? *J. Bone Joint Surg. Br.*, 2009. **91**(5): pp. 565–576.

31. Bernhardt, A., et al., Mineralised collagen–an artificial, extracellular bone matrix–improves osteogenic differentiation of bone marrow stromal cells. *J. Mater. Sci. Mater. Med.*, 2008. **19**(1): pp. 269–275.

32. Mastrogiacomo, M., et al., Tissue engineering of bone: Search for a better scaffold. *Orthod. Craniofac. Res.*, 2005. **8**(4): pp. 277–284.

33. Martin, I., et al., Osteochondral tissue engineering. *J. Biomech.*, 2007. **40**(4): pp. 750–765.

34. Tampieri, A., et al., Biologically inspired synthesis of bone-like composite: Self-assembled collagen fibers/hydroxyapatite nanocrystals. *J. Biomed. Mater. Res. Part A*, 2003. **67**(2): pp. 618–625.

35. Jiang, J., et al., Bioactive stratified polymer ceramic-hydrogel scaffold for integrative osteochondral repair. *Ann. Biomed. Eng.*, 2010. **38**(6): pp. 2183–2196.

36. Qu, D., et al., Ectopic osteochondral formation of biomimetic porous PVA-n-HA/PA6 bilayered scaffold and BMSCs construct in rabbit. *J. Biomed. Mater. Res. B Appl. Biomater.*, 2011. **96**(1): pp. 9–15.

37. Im, G. I., et al., A hyaluronate-atelocollagen/beta-tricalcium phosphate-hydroxyapatite biphasic scaffold for the repair of osteochondral defects: A porcine study. *Tissue Eng. Part A*, 2010. **16**(4): pp. 1189–1200.

38. Kon, E., et al., A novel nano-composite multi-layered biomaterial for treatment of osteochondral lesions: Technique note and an early stability pilot clinical trial. *Injury*, 2010. **41**(7): pp. 693–701.

39. Kon, E., et al., Novel nanostructured scaffold for osteochondral regeneration: Pilot study in horses. *J. Tissue Eng. Regen. Med.*, 2010. **4**(4): pp. 300–308.

40. Gloria, A., et al., Three-dimensional poly(epsilon-caprolactone) bioactive scaffolds with controlled structural and surface properties. *Biomacromolecules*, 2012. **13**(11): pp. 3510–3521.

41. Scaglione, S., et al., Order versus Disorder: In vivo bone formation within osteoconductive scaffolds. *Sci. Rep.*, 2012. **2**: p. 274.

42. Martino, S., et al., Stem cell-biomaterial interactions for regenerative medicine. *Biotechnol. Adv.*, 2012. **30**(1): pp. 338–351.

43. Flemming, R. G., et al., Effects of synthetic micro- and nano-structured surfaces on cell behavior. *Biomaterials*, 1999. **20**(6): pp. 573–588.

44. Bettinger, C. J., R. Langer, and J. T. Borenstein, Engineering substrate topography at the micro- and nanoscale to control cell function. *Angew. Chem. Int. Ed. Engl.*, 2009. **48**(30): pp. 5406–5415.

45. Saranya, N., et al., Enhanced osteoblast adhesion on polymeric nanoscaffolds for bone tissue engineering. *J. Biomed. Nanotechnol.*, 2011. **7**(2): pp. 238–244.

46. Cunha, C., et al., Bio-inspired artificial scaffolds and the quest to replicate biology. *Materrialstoday*, 2012. **15**(5): p. 223.

47. Biggs, M. J., et al., Interactions with nanoscale topography: Adhesion quantification and signal transduction in cells of osteogenic and multipotent lineage. *J. Biomed. Mater. Res. A*, 2009. **91**(1): pp. 195–208.

48. Dalby, M. J., et al., The control of human mesenchymal cell differentiation using nanoscale symmetry and disorder. *Nat. Mater.*, 2007. **6**(12): pp. 997–1003.

49. Huebsch, N., et al., Harnessing traction-mediated manipulation of the cell/matrix interface to control stem-cell fate. *Nat. Mater.*, 2010. **9**(6): pp. 518–526.

50. Nava, M. M., M. T. Raimondi, and R. Pietrabissa, Controlling self-renewal and differentiation of stem cells via mechanical cues. *J. Biomed. Biotechnol.*, 2012. **2012**: p. 797410.

51. Liu, H., et al., The promotion of bone regeneration by nanofibrous hydroxyapatite/chitosan scaffolds by effects on integrin-BMP/Smad signaling pathway in BMSCs. *Biomaterials*, 2013. **34**(18): pp. 4404–4417.

52. Rho, J. Y., L. Kuhn-Spearing, and P. Zioupos, Mechanical properties and the hierarchical structure of bone. *Med. Eng. Phys.*, 1998. **20**(2): pp. 92–102.

53. Wei, G., et al., The enhancement of osteogenesis by nano-fibrous scaffolds incorporating rhBMP-7 nanospheres. *Biomaterials*, 2007. **28**(12): pp. 2087–2096.

54. Holzwarth, J. M., and P. X. Ma, Biomimetic nanofibrous scaffolds for bone tissue engineering. *Biomaterials*, 2011. **32**(36): pp. 9622–9629.

55. Oliveira, J. M., et al., Novel hydroxyapatite/chitosan bilayered scaffold for osteochondral tissue-engineering applications: Scaffold design and its performance when seeded with goat bone marrow stromal cells. *Biomaterials*, 2006. **27**(36): pp. 6123–6137.

56. Costa-Pinto, A. R., R. L. Reis, and N. M. Neves, Scaffolds based bone tissue engineering: The role of chitosan. *Tissue Eng. Part B Rev.*, 2011. **17**(5): pp. 331–347.

57. Tampieri, A., G. Celotti, and E. Landi, From biomimetic apatites to biologically inspired composites. *Anal. Bioanal. Chem.*, 2005. **381**(3): pp. 568–576.

58. Tampieri, A., et al., Mimicking natural bio-mineralization processes: A new tool for osteochondral scaffold development. *Trends Biotechnol.*, 2011. **29**(10): pp. 526–535.

59. Sprio, S., et al., Biomimesis and biomorphic transformations: New concepts applied to bone regeneration. *J. Biotechnol.*, 2010. **156**(4): pp. 347–355.

60. Landi, E., F. Valentini, and A. Tampieri, Porous hydroxyapatite/gelatine scaffolds with ice-designed channel-like porosity for biomedical applications. *Acta Biomater.*, 2008. **4**(6): pp. 1620–1626.

61. Ning, L., H. Malmstrom, and Y. F. Ren, Porous collagen-hydroxyapatite scaffolds with mesenchymal stem cells for bone regeneration. *J. Oral Implantol.*, 2013. **41**(1): pp. 45–49.

62. Fu, S., et al., Injectable and thermo-sensitive PEG-PCL-PEG copolymer/collagen/n-HA hydrogel composite for guided bone regeneration. *Biomaterials*, 2012. **33**(19): pp. 4801–4809.

63. Sprio, S., et al., Hybrid scaffolds for tissue regeneration: Chemotaxis and physical confinement as sources of biomimesis. *J. Nanomater.*, 2012. **2012**: pp. 418281-1–10.

64. Romano, N. H., et al., Protein-engineered biomaterials: Nanoscale mimics of the extracellular matrix. *Biochim. Biophys. Acta*, 2011. **1810**(3): pp. 339–349.

65. Ko, Y. G., et al., Immobilization of poly(ethylene glycol) or its sulfonate onto polymer surfaces by ozone oxidation. *Biomaterials*, 2001. **22**(15): pp. 2115–2123.

66. Causa, F., et al., Surface investigation on biomimetic materials to control cell adhesion: The case of RGD conjugation on PCL. *Langmuir*, 2010. **26**(12): pp. 9875–9884.

67. Hersel, U., C. Dahmen, and H. Kessler, RGD modified polymers: Biomaterials for stimulated cell adhesion and beyond. *Biomaterials*, 2003. **24**(24): pp. 4385–4415.

68. Shekaran, A., and A. J. Garcia, Nanoscale engineering of extracellular matrix-mimetic bioadhesive surfaces and implants for tissue engineering. *Biochim. Biophys. Acta*, 2011. **1810**(3): pp. 350–360.

69. Ruoslahti, E., and M. D. Pierschbacher, New perspectives in cell adhesion: RGD and integrins. *Science*, 1987. **238**(4826): pp. 491–497.

70. Travis, J., Biotech gets a grip on cell adhesion. *Science*, 1993. **260**(5110): pp. 906–908.

71. Hynes, R. O., Integrins: Bidirectional, allosteric signaling machines. *Cell*, 2002. **110**(6): pp. 673–687.

72. Kantlehner, M., et al., Surface coating with cyclic RGD peptides stimulates osteoblast adhesion and proliferation as well as bone formation. *Chembiochem*, 2000. **1**(2): pp. 107–114.

73. Lin, Y. S., et al., Growth of endothelial cells on different concentrations of Gly-Arg-Gly-Asp photochemically grafted in polyethylene glycol modified polyurethane. *Artif. Organs*, 2001. **25**(8): pp. 617–621.

74. Sugawara, T., and T. Matsuda, Photochemical surface derivatization of a peptide containing Arg-Gly-Asp (RGD). *J. Biomed. Mater. Res.*, 1995. **29**(9): pp. 1047–1052.

75. Lin, H. B., et al., Endothelial cell adhesion on polyurethanes containing covalently attached RGD-peptides. *Biomaterials*, 1992. **13**(13): pp. 905–914.

76. Chen, R. R., and D. J. Mooney, Polymeric growth factor delivery strategies for tissue engineering. *Pharm. Res.*, 2003. **20**(8): pp. 1103–1112.

77. Anitua, E., et al., Delivering growth factors for therapeutics. *Trends Pharmacol. Sci.*, 2008. **29**(1): pp. 37–41.

78. Latour, R. A., Molecular simulation of protein-surface interactions: benefits, problems, solutions, and future directions. *Biointerphases*, 2008. **3**(3): pp. FC2–FC12.

79. Iafisco, M., et al., Adsorption and spectroscopic characterization of lactoferrin on hydroxyapatite nanocrystals. *Dalton Trans.*, 2011. **40**(4): pp. 820–827.

80. Korbling, M., and Z. Estrov, Adult stem cells for tissue repair—a new therapeutic concept? *N. Engl. J. Med.*, 2003. **349**(6): pp. 570–582.

81. Rossi, C. A., M. Pozzobon, and P. De Coppi, Advances in musculoskeletal tissue engineering: Moving towards therapy. *Organogenesis*, 2010. **6**(3): pp. 167–172.

82. Assiotis, A., N. P. Sachinis, and B. E. Chalidis, Pulsed electromagnetic fields for the treatment of tibial delayed unions and nonunions. A prospective clinical study and review of the literature. *J. Orthop. Surg. Res.*, 2012. **7**: p. 24.

83. Barnaba, S. A., et al., Clinical significance of different effects of static and pulsed electromagnetic fields on human osteoclast cultures. *Rheumatol. Int.*, 2012. **32**(4): pp. 1025–1031.

84. Inoue, N., et al., Effect of pulsed electromagnetic fields (PEMF) on late-phase osteotomy gap healing in a canine tibial model. *J. Orthop. Res.*, 2002. **20**(5): pp. 1106–1114.

85. Markov, M. S., Magnetic field therapy: A review. *Electromagn. Biol. Med.*, 2007. **26**(1): pp. 1–23.

86. Ba, X., et al., The role of moderate static magnetic fields on biomineralization of osteoblasts on sulfonated polystyrene films. *Biomaterials*, 2011. **32**(31): pp. 7831–7838.

87. Kotani, H., et al., Strong static magnetic field stimulates bone formation to a definite orientation in vitro and in vivo. *J. Bone Miner Res.*, 2002. **17**(10): pp. 1814–1821.

88. Jain, T. K., et al., Biodistribution, clearance, and biocompatibility of iron oxide magnetic nanoparticles in rats. *Mol. Pharm.*, 2008. **5**(2): pp. 316–327.

89. Prijic, S., et al., Increased cellular uptake of biocompatible superparamagnetic iron oxide nanoparticles into malignant cells by an external magnetic field. *J. Membr. Biol.*, 2010. **236**(1): pp. 167–179.

90. Sun, C., et al., PEG-mediated synthesis of highly dispersive multifunctional superparamagnetic nanoparticles: Their physicochemical properties and function in vivo. *ACS Nano*, 2010. **4**(4): pp. 2402–2410.

91. Amirfazli, A., Nanomedicine: Magnetic nanoparticles hit the target. *Nat. Nanotechnol.*, 2007. **2**(8): pp. 467–468.

92. Arruebo, M., et al., Magnetic nanoparticles for drug delivery. *Nano Today*, 2007. **2**: pp. 22–32.

93. Gould, P., Nanomagnetism shows in vivo potential. *Nano Today*, 2006. **1**: pp. 34–39.

94. Foy, S. P., et al., Optical imaging and magnetic field targeting of magnetic nanoparticles in tumors. *ACS Nano*, 2010. **4**(9): pp. 5217–5224.

95. Hua, M. Y., et al., Magnetic-nanoparticle-modified paclitaxel for targeted therapy for prostate cancer. *Biomaterials*, 2010. **31**(28): pp. 7355–7363.

96. Phillips, M. A., M. L. Gran, and N. A. Peppas, Targeted nanodelivery of drugs and diagnostics. *Nano Today*, 2010. **5**: pp. 143–159.

97. Polyak, B., et al., High field gradient targeting of magnetic nanoparticle-loaded endothelial cells to the surfaces of steel stents. *Proc. Natl. Acad. Sci. U. S. A.*, 2008. **105**: pp. 698–703.

98. Panseri, S., et al., Magnetic hydroxyapatite bone substitutes to enhance tissue regeneration: evaluation in vitro using osteoblast-like cells and in vivo in a bone defect. *PLoS One*, 2012. **7**(6): p. e38710.

99. Wu, Y., et al., A novel calcium phosphate ceramic-magnetic nanoparticle composite as a potential bone substitute. *Biomed. Mater.*, 2010. **5**(1): p. 15001.

100. Meng, J., et al., Super-paramagnetic responsive nanofibrous scaffolds under static magnetic field enhance osteogenesis for bone repair in vivo. *Sci. Rep.*, 2013. **3**: p. 2655.

101. Meng, J., et al., Paramagnetic nanofibrous composite films enhance the osteogenic responses of pre-osteoblast cells. *Nanoscale*, 2010. **2**(12): pp. 2565–2569.

102. Panseri, S., et al., Modifying bone scaffold architecture in vivo with permanent magnets to facilitate fixation of magnetic scaffolds. *Bone*, 2013. **56**(2): pp. 432–439.

103. Shan, D., et al., Electrospun magnetic poly(L-lactide) (PLLA) nanofibers by incorporating PLLA-stabilized $Fe_3O_4$ nanoparticles. *Mater. Sci. Eng. C Mater. Biol. Appl.*, 2013. **33**(6): pp. 3498–3505.

104. Ascenzi, A., The micromechanics versus the macromechanics of cortical bone–a comprehensive presentation. *J. Biomech. Eng.*, 1988. **110**(4): pp. 357–363.

105. Bakbak, S., R. Kayacan, and O. Akkus, Effect of collagen fiber orientation on mechanical properties of cortical bone. *J. Biomech.*, 2011. **44**: p. 11.

106. Panseri, S., et al., Intrinsically superparamagnetic Fe-hydroxyapatite nanoparticles positively influence osteoblast-like cell behaviour. *J. Nanobiotechnol.*, 2012. **10**: p. 32.

107. Russo, A., et al., A new approach to scaffold fixation by magnetic forces: Application to large osteochondral defects. *Med. Eng. Phys.*, 2012. **34**(9): pp. 1287–1293.

108. Zelle, S., et al., Arthroscopic techniques for the fixation of a three-dimensional scaffold for autologous chondrocyte transplantation: Structural properties in an in vitro model. *Arthroscopy*, 2007. **23**(10): pp. 1073–1078.

109. Lewinski, N., V. Colvin, and R. Drezek, Cytotoxicity of nanoparticles. *Small*, 2008. **4**(1): pp. 26–49.

110. Singh, N., et al., Potential toxicity of superparamagnetic iron oxide nanoparticles (SPION). *Nano Rev.*, 2010. **1**: pp. 53–58.

111. Berry, C. C., and A. S. G. Curtis, Functionalisation of magnetic nanoparticles for applications in biomedicine. *J. Phys. D. Appl. Phys.*, 2003. **36**: pp. 198–206.

112. Iafisco, M., et al., Magnetic bioactive and biodegradable hollow Fe-doped hydroxyapatite coated poly(L-lactic) acid micro-nanospheres. *Chem. Mater.*, 2013. **25**(13): pp. 2610–2617.

# Chapter 12

# Biomimetic Materials in Regenerative Medicine: A Clinical Perspective

**Maurilio Marcacci, Giuseppe Filardo, Giulia Venieri, Lorenzo Milani, and Elizaveta Kon**

*II Clinic—Biomechanics Laboratory, Rizzoli Orthopaedic Institute, Bologna, Italy*

m.marcacci@biomec.ior.it

The high prevalence of degenerative or traumatic musculoskeletal diseases is a challenge for the orthopedic surgeon, who has to restore limb or joint functionality. Unfortunately, because of the poor intrinsic regenerative capacity of musculoskeletal tissues, the treatments available in this field consist primarily of surgical replacements of the damaged tissue, namely tissue transplantation and joint prosthesis, with several drawbacks, such as donor site scarcity, harvesting costs and post-operative morbidity; moreover, cadaveric transplantation may be responsible for disease transmission, risk of infections, and immunological rejections of the host to the cadaveric graft. To address these shortcomings, tissue engineering research has emerged as an alternative potential solution to tissue transplantation and grafting. In the past 50 years, the evolution of biomaterials in the orthopedic field has led to the introduction of a new class of intelligent engineering

---

*Bio-Inspired Regenerative Medicine: Materials, Processes, and Clinical Applications*
Edited by Simone Sprio and Anna Tampieri
Copyright © 2016 Pan Stanford Publishing Pte. Ltd.
ISBN 978-981-4669-14-6 (Hardcover), 978-981-4669-15-3 (eBook)
www.panstanford.com

products, which, besides being necessarily biocompatible, are also smart, biomimetic, and biodegradable. This chapter has been written with the purpose of briefly illustrating the clinical use of these smart biomimetic biomaterials, thus giving the reader an overview of the main areas of their application in the orthopedic field.

## 12.1 Introduction

Orthopedic diseases often imply a degenerative or traumatic loss of musculoskeletal tissue with poor intrinsic regenerative capacity. Nowadays these disorders afflict millions of people worldwide and the orthopedic surgeon has to satisfy the increased need for treatments that allow the restoration of limb or joint functionality. Unfortunately, the treatments available in this field consist primarily of surgical replacements of the damaged tissue, including tissue transplantations or joint prosthesis, with several limitations. Tissue transplantations include allografts, xenografts, and autografts, whose use presents several drawbacks, above all donor site scarcity, harvesting costs and post-operative morbidity [1–3]. Moreover, cadaveric transplantation may be responsible for viral disease transmission, such as HIV or Hepatitis C; although the sterilization process may protect the host from the risk of infection, a weakening of the allograft may be caused. Not least, immunological rejections of the host to the cadaveric graft have been recorded [4, 5]. Therefore, to overcome these limitations, tissue engineering research has emerged as an alternative potential solution to tissue transplantation and grafting. Several biomaterials have been developed as constituents of devices that are designed to perform certain biological functions by substituting or repairing different tissues, such as bone, cartilage, ligaments, or tendons [6]. Over time, biomaterials have evolved through three generations that differ in the evoked tissue response of the host to the graft [7]. The first generation of constructs includes metallic, ceramic, and polymeric solid prostheses, which are first characterized by their inertness: They are made of biocompatible materials, mainly aimed at ensuring a structural support for the replaced tissue with no induction of foreign body response by the host [8]. The second generation of products, besides biocompatibility, is characterized by their bioactivity, namely the ability to interact with the internal and external environment and to enhance biological response and tissue-surface bonding. Finally, the third generation consists of materials designed to stimulate specific cellular responses at the molecular level [6]. Recent development in tissue engineering research has led to a regenerative medicine aimed at repairing and regenerating tissues by using the natural signaling pathways induced by the implantation of scaffolds [6, 9]. The purpose of this chapter is to briefly illustrate the state-of-the-art in the clinical application of this new class of engineering technology, so called "smart biomaterials" or "biomimetic materials," thus giving the reader an overview of the main areas of their application in the orthopedic field.

## 12.2 Smart Biomimetic Materials

After more than 50 years of research, the evolution of biomaterials in the orthopedic field has seen the recent introduction of a new class of intelligent engineering products, in which the principles of biology meet bioengineering in order to obtain functional substitutes for damaged tissues [10]. These materials, besides the obvious requirement of being biocompatible, are also smart, biomimetic, and biodegradable. There is still no common definition of these materials. From a clinical point of view, the word "smart" means a biomaterial with an intrinsic ability to promote actively the inherent ability of tissue to heal and self-repair by responding to internal and external environment stimuli, thus taking part in the regeneration of the damaged tissue [10, 11]. To achieve this interaction, a smart biomaterial may also have biomimetic abilities, meaning the ability to mimic the function of extracellular matrix to stimulate cellular invasion, attachment, and proliferation [12]. Biomimetic properties have been obtained by technological adaptation of the macro, micro, and nanostructure, by trying to rearrange the natural hierarchical organization of tissues. The modification of the scaffold surface, such as roughness, topography, and chemistry lead to a better interaction for cell responsiveness; the three-dimensional morphological properties, including porosity and pore size are optimized in order to enhance vascularization and nutrient supply, thus improving tissue in-growth [13, 14]. Finally, to obtain an ideal mimicry, the implanted

# 308 | *Biomimetic Materials in Regenerative Medicine*

material should reabsorb gradually and ensure the preservation of local healthy tissue while new host tissue is regenerated [10].

## 12.3 Tendons

The management of acute and chronic tendon disorders is difficult primarily because of the limited healing capacity of this tissue and the peculiarity of the structural organization responsible for its functional properties. The clinical presentation can vary from a severe full-thickness rupture to an inflammatory peritendonitis, which is not of surgical management [15]. The state-of-the-art in tendon reconstruction techniques is the use of autografts, allografts, or biomaterials. Although the autograft is the gold standard thanks to its compatibility and its tendency to restore original mechanical strength, there is marked donor site morbidity [16]. Concerning allograft implantation, limitations are related to an inflammatory responses evoked in the host and the risk of disease transmission. These shortcomings have prompted continuous research in tissue engineering to investigate alternative solutions, and nowadays several biological and synthetic scaffolds are available for tendon reconstruction [17].

Biological scaffolds are made from mammalian (bovine, porcine, equine, and human) collagenous tissues, including fascia lata, small intestine submucosa (SIS), dermis, and pericardium, specifically treated to retain its native collagen structure with its chemical and mechanical properties, by removing cellular and non-collagenous components [18]. Despite their popular application, some problems have been reported, namely non-specific inflammatory reactions and foreign body-like reactions after the implantation of certain xenografts, which may cause failure of the implant due to its rapid biodegradation [17]. Even though the implantation of biological scaffolds is becoming popular, the literature lacks well-conducted clinical trials and data on their efficacy and adverse effects are still insufficient.

With regard to synthetic scaffolds, there is notable interest in developing synthetic extracellular matrix (ECM) temporary grafts. Preclinical studies have investigated the benefit of augmenting rotator cuff repair using synthetic ECMs and showed promising results for cellular and fibrotic growth: Histological analysis revealed an increased fibroblast rate and collagen formation, with a smaller risk of provoking an inflammatory response compared with allograft ECMs. However, results about mechanical strength are still controversial [19–21] and further studies are required to verify its effectiveness.

## 12.4 Ligaments

Among ligament ruptures, anterior cruciate ligament (ACL) reconstruction is a common subject in orthopedic surgery since ACL Injuries frequently occur as a result of sports injuries. There are several options available for the surgical management of ACL and the choice can vary between the implantation of autografts, allografts, or synthetic grafts. Among autologous grafts, those most commonly used are the patellar tendon and the semitendinosus-gracilis tendons, which show good clinical results, despite some complications: Patellar tendon autograft may lead to patellar fractures, patellar tendon ruptures, tendinopathy, localized tenderness, and numbness [22]. Allograft inserts have shown good clinical results, but not free from shortcomings [4, 5]. Since the 1980s, various synthetic materials have been proposed as permanent ACL replacement devices, such as carbon fibers, polytetrafluoroethylene, polyethylene terephthalate, and braided polypropylene, but subsequent adverse effects led to a marked decline in their use [23]. Dandy et al. first implanted a carbon fiber reinforced substitute for ACL via arthroscopy and obtained encouraging results in the early stage of the study. However, long-term results showed an early rupture of the neoligament due to its poor biomechanical strength [24]. Later a second generation of synthetic ligaments was clinically tested, but also in this case many complications were reported. The foreign-body reaction induced by the synthetic material led to immunoreaction mediated by an aggregation of giant cells that caused a synovial hypertrophy close to the wear debris. All types of grafts caused an increased expression of inflammatory cytokines such as inteleukin-1 and MMPs, producing a cartilage matrix degradation process that is responsible for the development of osteoarthritis. Moreover, the inflammatory reaction caused by wear particles of the foreign synthetic material leads to a peculiar modification in the composition of the synovial fluid, thus determining a clinical outcome with persistent pain and swelling [4, 5]. Finally, a new class of synthetic ligament was designed to overcome the issues of graft failure and synovitis. A polyethylene terephthalate (PET) graft was processed to obtain a material with high resistance to fatigue and high biocompatibility [23]. The Ligament Augmentation and Reconstruction System (LARS) was approved by the Food and Drug Administration (FDA) to treat complex cases, even if experimental and clinical applications of this product are not free from complications. The most commonly reported adverse events are effusion and reactive synovitis in the mid-long term of follow-up, which might damage the device, thus causing an early graft rupture and failure of the ligament.

Although numerous synthetic grafts have been tested in ACL reconstruction, every material has been found to present serious drawbacks: cross-infections, immunological responses, breakage, debris dispersion leading to synovitis, chronic effusion, recurrent instability, and knee osteoarthritis. Currently, research is still far from identifying the ideal artificial ligament, which should combine a high biocompatibility with as similar mechanical characteristics as possible to those of the natural ligament. Therefore, despite the significant rate of morbidities of the donor site, currently the most commonly used technique for ACL reconstruction is a tissue graft of autologous origin, more often the mid-third of the patella tendon or the semi-tendinous and gracilis tendons.

## 12.5 Menisci

Meniscus damage, as a consequence of injuries or degenerative processes, is one of the most common problems in the knee joint that leads to pain and knee dysfunction; unfortunately the intrinsic repair capacity of this kind of tissue is poor, and an arthroscopic meniscectomy is often necessary as the only way to improve knee symptoms. However, menisci are well known to play an important role in the maintenance of the joint homeostasis: In fact, both partial and total meniscectomy elicit a biomechanical alteration in load transmission, which is correlated with a high rate of secondary osteoarthritic changes [25]. Therefore, to minimize the deleterious effects of meniscus loss, different solutions for meniscal replacement are now clinically available: cadaveric donor transplantation, collagen meniscus implant (CMI, Ivy Sports

Medicine, Montvale, New Jersey) and the more recent polyurethane scaffold (Actifit®, Orteq Sports Medicine, London, UK). Allograft transplantation is indicated, with encouraging long-term results, for the treatment of patients who have undergone total meniscectomy and the entire menisci need to be restored [26]. Conversely, in the case of partial meniscectomy, a biomaterial substitution is suitable, since it can restore the injured menisci by attachment to the meniscal rim [27]. Concerning CMI, Zaffagnini et al. reported a comparative study of 33 patients affected by medial meniscal tears treated with arthroscopic CMI or partial medial meniscectomy. The evaluation was performed from basal level up to 10 years of follow-up, using clinical scores IKDC, VAS, and SF-36, and radiological images. The results showed a significant improvement in all scores and fewer signs of degeneration at the radiological evaluation in the CMI group [28, 29]. Kon et al. published a study of 18 patients who required partial meniscectomy, affected by partial meniscal tears or patients with a chronic loss of meniscal tissue, treated by arthroscopic polyurethane meniscal scaffold implantation (Actifit®, Orteq Sports Medicine, London, UK). The scaffold facilitates vascular ingrowth and meniscal tissue regeneration to replace the surgically removed tissue, thus preventing chondral degenerative changes. The clinical follow-up performed for up to 2 years by the IKDC and Tegner scores showed a significant improvement in all parameters and no major adverse effects [30]. These studies show the safety and potential effectiveness of these procedures to treat partial meniscal loss, but long-term studies are needed to confirm their role in preventing or slowing down the joint degenerative process.

## 12.6 Osteochondral Defects

Chondral and osteochondral lesions are a challenging problem for the orthopedic surgeon, and different regenerative techniques have been proposed in recent years to recreate a hyaline-like tissue to restore as similar an articular surface as possible to the physiological one. The first regenerative technique was introduced in 1994 by Brittberg et al. with autologous chondrocyte implantation (ACI), which gave satisfactory results in the treatment of isolated femoral condyle cartilage lesions [31]. Although its clinical efficacy has been shown by several studies, the ACI technique has numerous biological and surgical drawbacks, above all transplant hypertrophy, delamination, and graft failure. For these reasons many studies have turned to the research of new biomaterials and surgical approaches to address these shortcomings: Thanks to progress in tissue bioengineering research, second-generation ACI procedures have been developed, characterized by a three-dimensional biodegradable scaffold employed as a cell carrier, implanted ether by mini-arthrotomy or arthroscopically. However, cell-based strategies are costly and time consuming for the ex vivo cell processing; thus, particular interest has been aroused by applying acellular implants for osteochondral regeneration. Currently, there are two osteochondral scaffolds on the market for clinical application: a bilayer porous PLGA-calcium-sulfate biopolymer (TruFit®, Smith&Nephew, Andover, MA) and a nanostructured biomimetic scaffold with a porous 3-D three-layer composite structure (Maioregen®, Fin-Ceramica S.p.A., Faenza, Italy) [32]. Whereas the former has shown doubtful results and its use is rapidly decreasing, the latter is gaining increasing interest. This scaffold mimics the whole osteochondral anatomy and is composed of three layers: a cartilaginous type I collagen layer characterized by a smooth surface, an intermediate tide-mark-like layer consisting of a combination of type I collagen (60%) and hydroxyapatite (HA) (40%), and a lower layer, which consists of a mineralized blend of type I collagen (30%) and HA (70%), thus reproducing the subchondral bone [33]. Preclinical evaluations [34, 35] have showed encouraging results: When implanting scaffolds loaded with autologous chondrocytes or a scaffold alone similar macroscopic, histological, and radiographic results have been found, probably by inducing an in situ regeneration through stem cells coming from the surrounding bone marrow. In a clinical application of the scaffold, thirteen patients (15 lesions) affected by osteochondral lesions were treated with the implantation of the novel three-layer composite graft. Analyses were performed at an early post-operative time, 4 to 8 weeks by clinical and MRI evaluation, and, at the same time, the mechanical stability of the implanted graft was assessed [36]. Thirteen of the implantation sites had complete attachment and adherence, whereas in two patients partial attachment was found: The weak mechanical fixation was probably due to an inadequate surgical technique with insufficient shoulder coverage of the prepared implantation site. Further analysis performed at 6 months revealed partial reabsorption of the graft in one case with an incomplete cartilage layer and a complete subchondral structure, and in the other case an inhomogeneous tissue filled in the entire treated area. However, further studies have subsequently reported good clinical results at longer follow-ups, thus showing the potential of this osteochondral one-step procedure even for the treatment of complex salvage lesions, and a recent study documented medium-term 5-year results [37–42]. Even though MRI findings improve over time, some abnormalities persisted, but no correlation was found between imaging and clinical results. A statistically significant improvement in all clinical scores was obtained from the basal evaluation to the 2- and 5-year follow-ups, and the results were stable over time. Thus, the study results highlighted the safety and potential of this procedure, which offered a good clinical outcome with stable results up to a midterm follow-up [33].

## 12.7 Bone

Unlike cartilage, tendons, and menisci, bone has a spontaneous healing ability and achieves a complete restoration of its function after fractures. However, even for bone tissue there are several defects where this ability is compromised, usually caused by traumatic injury, osteomyelitis, or bone tumor resection. The critical-sized bone defect is defined as the smallest size of intraosseous wound that will not spontaneously heal completely with bone tissue [43], and its treatment represents a current challenge for orthopedic surgeons. Available approaches for large bone defects are mainly restricted to the Ilizarov technique without grafts and autograft or allograft implantation. The first procedure consists of an osteotomy followed by bone distraction, which avoids problems related to the graft transplantation at the expense of marked inconvenience for the patients; the latter are surgical techniques that have a high success rate, but risk of infection, limited availability, and donor site morbidity are hitches related to the graft. Even in this field, to address these drawbacks, in recent decades several solutions have been proposed thanks to the development of smart biomaterials; a variety of scaffolds are now marketed as biomimetic bone grafts, but clinical evidence for their efficacy is still in its infancy [44]. Among these, HA and other calcium phosphate ceramics have shown to be the most promising materials in terms of clinical results, due to their osteoinductive properties, unlimited availability, inertness, and no risk of disease transmission [45, 46]. Bone is naturally composed of 70% mineral (HA), 22% organic matrix (collagen and cells), and 8% water. HA, the main mineral component of natural bone has been combined with osteoinductive materials, such as magnesium and type I collagen, thus attempting to mimic the natural hierarchical structure of the bone. Marcacci et al. first published a pilot clinical study of 4 patients affected by large bone defects treated with a culture-expanded osteoprogenitor cells isolated form bone marrow and expanded on a porous bioceramic scaffold made of HA (ENGIpore®, FinCeramica, Faenza, Italy). Patients were followed up for 6 years, evaluated clinically, radiographically, and by CT (computed tomography) scans. For all patients, limb function was recovered and radiological investigations revealed abundant callus formation along the implants and good integration at the interfaces two months after surgery [47, 48]. Recently it has emerged how the inclusion of magnesium ions in HA improves its interaction with water and enables the HA crystal cell structure to become more biologically active, further stimulating cell-mediated material resorption, new bone formation, and remodeling. SINTlife® (JRI Orthopaedics, London, United Kingdom) is a synthetic fully resorbable graft made of magnesium-substituted HA nano-crystals, that once implanted are resorbed in a mean of 18 months, thus allowing time for the formation and maturation of new bone. Clinical indications are limited to use as a bone-void filler in trauma and knee and spinal surgery. A recent small randomized controlled trial showed promising results using SINTlife® in the treatment of medial compartment osteoarthritis of the knee treated with a high tibial osteotomy supplemented with internal fixation, when it was compared with the use of lyophilized bone chips [49].

Despite the aforementioned promising results, only a few clinical trials are available about biomimetic bone graft application and further studies are necessary to better clarify the effectiveness and the long duration of these benefits.

## 12.8 Conclusions

In the last 50 years, research into biomaterials has led to the development of smart biomimetic materials. A lot of products are still under preclinical study, and the clinical application of this new class of constructs shows encouraging but controversial results as presented in this chapter.

With regard to tendon-ligament reconstruction, the perfect graft continues to be just an abstract idea. Preliminary studies on the use of such implants in tendon injury repair are encouraging in terms of enhancement and acceleration of the biology of tissue repair, but results on mechanical strength are still controversial and further preclinical and clinical studies are required to assess its effectiveness. Concerning the ACL synthetic graft, its biocompatibility is still insufficient considering the complications and the immunological reaction related to its implantation in humans, which is the reason for its declining use in the clinical setting. In this field further studies are needed to find a material that better mimics the natural hierarchical structure of tendons and ligaments and achieves an appropriate inertness for the host with mechanical resistance to load and stress.

In meniscus transplantation, promising clinical results have been published on the application of two biomaterials in patients who underwent partial meniscectomy or with partial degeneration of the menisci. Collagen and polyurethane scaffolds differ in their biomaterial composition and microstructure, but both give good clinical outcomes and seem to facilitate vascular ingrowth and meniscal tissue regeneration to replace the surgically removed tissue, thus possibly preventing arthritic degenerative changes of cartilage and subchondral bone.

Also for the treatment of chondral and osteochondral lesions the implantation of a biomimetic nanostructured scaffold shows promising results as a regenerative procedure. However, further randomized controlled trials are necessary to evaluate this new regenerative approach and show disadvantages and advantages with respect to the more traditional procedures.

Finally, biomimetic materials obtained by the combination of HA with osteoinductive materials, such as magnesium and type

I collagen, have been successfully clinically tested. Numerous biomimetic scaffolds are now marketed with clinical indications, despite the still scarce evidence for their use. In the state-of-the-art, HA mimetic scaffold are indicated as a bone-void filler in trauma, knee and spinal surgery, but further studies are required to define the real effectiveness of these treatments.

Despite the wide use of these products, the ideal biomimetic scaffold that fulfills all the requirements, namely biocompatibility, bioactivity, and biodegradability is still lacking. Research into biomimetic scaffolds or bioengineered tissues has allowed the elaboration of new materials that permit a rapid scaffold-tissue integration and an adequate biodegradability, but further studies are still needed to optimize the mechanical, chemical, physical, and biological properties of these materials for an optimal regeneration of damaged musculoskeletal tissues.

## References

1. Banwart, J. C., Asher, M. A., Hassanein, R. S. (1995) Iliac crest bone graft harvest donor site morbidity. A statistical evaluation. *Spine* (Phila Pa 1976), **20**, pp. 1055–1060.

2. Fernyhough, J. C., Schimandle, J. J., Weigel, M. C., Edwards, C. C., Levine, A. M. (1992) Chronic donor site pain complicating bone graft harvesting from the posterior iliac crest for spinal fusion. *Spine* (Phila Pa 1976), **17**, pp. 1474–1480.

3. Goulet, J. A., Senunas, L. E., DeSilva, G. L., Greenfield, M. L. (1997) Autogenous iliac crest bone graft. Complications and functional assessment. *Clin. Orthop. Relat. Res.*, Jun 339, pp. 76–81.

4. Dheerendra, S. K., Khan, W. S., Singhal, R., Shivarathre, D. G., Pydisetty, R., Johnstone, D. (2012) Anterior cruciate ligament graft choices: A review of current concepts. *Open Orthop. J.*, **6**, pp. 281–286.

5. Legnani, C., Ventura, A., Terzaghi, C., Borgo, E., Albisetti, W. (2010) Anterior cruciate ligament reconstruction with synthetic grafts. A review of literature. *Int. Orthop.*, **34**, pp. 465–471.

6. Navarro, M., Michiardi, A., Castaño, O., Planell, J. A. (2008) Biomaterials in orthopaedics. *J. R. Soc. Interface*, Oct 6, pp. 1137–1158.

7. Hench, L. L., Polak, J. M. (2002) Third-generation biomedical materials. *Science*, Feb 8, pp. 1014–1017.

8. Hench, L. L. (1980) Biomaterials. *Science*, May 23, pp. 826–831.

9. Hardouin, P., Anselme, K., Flautre, B., Bianchi, F., Bascoulenguet, G., Bouxin, B. (2000) Tissue engineering and skeletal diseases. *Jt. Bone Spine*, **67**, pp. 419–424.

10. Holzapfel, B. M., Reichert, J. C., Schantz, J. T., Gbureck, U., Rackwitz, L., Nöth, U., Jakob, F., Rudert, M., Groll, J., Hutmacher, D. W. (2013) How smart do biomaterials need to be? A translational science and clinical point of view. *Adv. Drug Deliv. Rev.*, **68**, pp. 581–603.

11. Furth, M. E., Atala, A., Van Dyke, M. E. (2007) Smart biomaterials design for tissue engineering and regenerative medicine. *Biomaterials*, **28**, pp. 5068–5073.

12. Rosso, F., Giordano, A., Barbarisi, M., Barbarisi A. (2004) From cell–ECM interactions to tissue engineering. *J. Cell. Physiol.*, **199**, pp. 174–180.

13. Das, A., Botchwey, E. (2011) Evaluation of angiogenesis and osteogenesis. *Tissue Eng. Part. B. Rev.*, **17**, pp. 403–414.

14. Karageorgiou, V., Kaplan, D. (2005) Porosity of 3D biomaterial scaffolds and osteogenesis, *Biomaterials*, **26**, pp. 5474–5549.

15. Filardo, G., Presti, M. L., Kon, E., Marcacci, M. (2010) Nonoperative biological treatment approach for partial achilles tendon lesion. *Orthopedics*, **33**, pp. 120–123.

16. Janssen, R. P. A., Van der Wijk, J., Fiedler, A., Schmidt, T., Sala, H. A. G. M., Scheffler, S. U. (2011) Remodelling of human hamstring autografts after anterior cruciate ligament reconstruction. *Knee Surg. Sports Traumatol. Arthrosc.*, **19**, pp. 1299–1306.

17. Longo, U. G., Lamberti, A., Maffulli, N., Denaro, V. (2010) Tendon augmentation grafts: A systematic review. *Br. Med. Bull.*, **94**, pp. 165–188.

18. Chen, J., Xu, J., Wang, A., Zheng, M. (2009) Scaffolds for tendon and ligament repair: Review of the efficacy of commercial products. *Expert Rev. Med. Devices*, **6**, pp. 61–73.

19. Funakoshi, T., Majima, T., Suenaga, N., Iwasaki, N., Yamane, S., Minami, A. (2006) Rotator cuff regeneration using chitin fabric as an acellular matrix. *J. Shoulder Elbow Surg.*, **15**, pp. 112118.

20. MacGillivray, J. D., Fealy, S., Terry, M. A., Koh, J. L., Nixon, A. J., Warren, R. F. (2006) Biomechanical evaluation of a rotator cuff defect model augmented with a bioresorbable scaffold in goats. *J. Shoulder Elbow Surg.*, **15**, pp. 639–644.

21. Yokoya, S., Mochizuki, Y., Nagata, Y., Deie, M., Ochi, M. (2008) Tendon-bone insertion repair and regeneration using polyglycolic acid sheet in the rabbit rotator cuff injury model. *Am. J. Sports Med.*, **36**, pp. 1298–1309.

22. West, R. V., Harner, C. D. (2005) Graft selection in anterior cruciate ligament reconstruction. *J. Am. Acad. Orthop. Surg.*, **13**, pp. 197–207.

23. Newman, S. D., Atkinson, H. D., Willis-Owen, C. A. (2013) Anterior cruciate ligament reconstruction with the ligament augmentation and reconstruction system: A systematic review. *Int. Orthop.*, **37** pp. 321–326.

24. Rushton, N., Dandy, D. J., Naylor, C. P. (1983) The clinical, arthroscopic and histological findings after replacement of the anterior cruciate ligament with carbon-fibre. *J. Bone Joint. Surg. Br.*, **65**, pp. 308–309.

25. Heijink, A., Gomoll, A. H., Madry, H., Drobnič, M., Filardo, G., Espregueira-Mendes, J., Van Dijk, C. N. (2012) Biomechanical considerations in the pathogenesis of osteoarthritis of the knee. *Knee Surg. Sports Traumatol. Arthrosc.*, **20**, pp. 423–435.

26. Wirth, C. J., Peters, G., Milachowski, K. A., Weismeier, K. G., Kohn, D. (2002) Long-term results of meniscal allograft transplantation. *Am. J. Sports Med.*, **30**, pp. 174–181.

27. Gomoll, A. H., Filardo, G., Almqvist, F. K., Bugbee, W. D., Jelic, M., Monllau, J. C., Puddu, G., Rodkey, W. G., Verdonk, P., Verdonk, R., Zaffagnini, S., Marcacci, M. (2012) Surgical treatment for early osteoarthritis. Part II: Allografts and concurrent procedures. *Knee Surg. Sports Traumatol. Arthrosc.*, **20**, pp. 468–486.

28. Zaffagnini, S., Marcheggiani Muccioli, G. M., Lopomo, N., Bruni, D., Giordano, G., Ravazzolo, G., Molinari, M., Marcacci, M. (2011) Prospective long-term outcomes of the medial collagen meniscus implant versus partial medial meniscectomy: A minimum 10-year follow-up study. *Am. J. Sports Med.*, **39**, pp. 977–985.

29. Zaffagnini, S., Marcheggiani Muccioli, G. M., Bulgheroni, P., Bulgheroni, E., Grassi, A., Bonanzinga, T., Kon, E., Filardo, G., Busacca, M., Marcacci, M. (2012) Arthroscopic collagen meniscus implantation for partial lateral meniscal defects: A 2-year minimum follow-up study. *Am. J. Sports Med.*, **40**, pp. 2281–2288.

30. Kon E, Filardo G, Zaffagnini S, Di Martino A, Di Matteo B, Marcheggiani Muccioli GM, Busacca M, Marcacci M. Biodegradable polyurethane meniscal scaffold for isolated partial lesions or as combined procedure for knees with multiple comorbidities: clinical results at 2 years. *Knee Surg Sports Traumatol Arthrosc*. 2014 Jan; **22**(1): 128–34.

31. Brittberg, M., Lindahl, A., Nilsson, A., Ohlsson, C., Isaksson, O., Peterson, L. (1994) Treatment of deep cartilage defects in the knee with autologous chondrocyte transplantation. *N. Engl. J. Med.*, **331**, pp. 889–895.

32. Filardo, G., Kon, E., Roffi, A., Di Martino, A., Marcacci, M. (2013) Scaffold-based repair for cartilage healing: A systematic review and technical note. *Arthroscopy*, **29**, pp. 174–186.

33. Kon E, Filardo G, Di Martino A, Busacca M, Moio A, Perdisa F, Marcacci M. (2014) Clinical results and MRI evolution of a nano-composite multilayered biomaterial for osteochondral regeneration at 5 years. *Am J Sports Med.*, **42**(1): 158–65.

34. Kon, E., Mutini, A., Arcangeli, E., Delcogliano, M., Filardo, G., Nicoli Aldini, N., Pressato, D., Quarto, R., Zaffagnini, S., Marcacci, M. (2010) Novel nanostructured scaffold for osteochondral regeneration: Pilot study in horses. *J. Tissue Eng. Regen. Med.*, **4**, pp. 300–308.

35. Kon, E., Delcogliano, M., Filardo, G., Fini, M., Giavaresi, G., Francioli, S., Martin, I., Pressato, D., Arcangeli, E., Quarto, R., Sandri, M., Marcacci, M. (2010) Orderly ostechondral regeneration in a sheep model using a novel nano-composite multilayered biomaterial. *J. Orthop. Res.*, **28**, pp. 116–124.

36. Kon, E., Delcogliano, M., Filardo, G., Pressato, D., Busacca, M., Grigolo, B., Desando, G., Marcacci, M. (2010) A novel nano-composite multi-layered biomaterial for treatment of osteochondral lesions: Technique note and an early stability pilot clinical trial. *Injury*, **4**, pp. 693–701.

37. Filardo, G., Di Martino, A., Kon, E., Delcogliano, M., Marcacci, M. (2012) Midterm results of a combined biological and mechanical approach for the treatment of a complex knee lesion. *Cartilage*, **3**, pp. 288–292.

38. Filardo, G., Kon, E., Di Martino, A., Busacca, M., Altadonna, G., Marcacci, M. (2013) Treatment of knee osteochondritis dissecans with a cell-free biomimetic osteochondral scaffold: Clinical and imaging evaluation at 2-year follow-up. *Am. J. Sports Med.*, **41**, pp. 1786–1793.

39. Filardo G, Kon E, Perdisa F, Di Matteo B, Di Martino A, Iacono F, Zaffagnini S, Balboni F, Vaccari V, Marcacci M. (2013) Osteochondral scaffold reconstruction for complex knee lesions: a comparative evaluation. *Knee.*, **20**(6): 570–6.

40. Kon, E., Delcogliano, M., Filardo, G., Altadonna, G., Marcacci, M. (2009) Novel nano-composite multi-layered biomaterial for the treatment of multifocal degenerative cartilage lesions. *Knee Surg. Sports Traumatol. Arthrosc.*, **17**, pp. 1312–1315.

41. Kon, E., Delcogliano, M., Filardo, G., Busacca, M., Di Martino, A., Marcacci, M. (2011) Novel nano-composite multilayered biomaterial for osteochondral regeneration: A pilot clinical trial. *Am. J. Sports Med.*, **39**, pp. 1180–1190.

42. Marcacci M, Zaffagnini S, Kon E, Marcheggiani Muccioli GM, Di Martino A, Di Matteo B, Bonanzinga T, Iacono F, Filardo G. (2013) Unicompartmental osteoarthritis: an integrated biomechanical and biological approach as alternative to metal resurfacing. *Knee Surg Sports Traumatol Arthrosc.*, **21**(11): 2509–17.

43. Schmitz, J. P. and Hollinger, J. O. (1986) The critical size defect as an experimental model for craniomandibulofacial nonunions. *Clin. Orthop. Relat. Res.*, **205**, pp. 299–308.

44. Kurien, T., Pearson, R. G., Scammell, B. E. (2013) Bone graft substitutes currently available in orthopaedic practice: The evidence for their use. *Bone Joint J.*, **95**, pp. 583–597.

45. Heise, U., Osborn, J. F., Duwe, F. (1990) Hydroxyapatite ceramic as a bone substitute, *Int. Orthop.*, **14**, pp. 329–338.

46. Sartoris, D. J., Holmes, R. E., Resnick, D. (1992) Coralline hydroxyapatite bone graft substitutes: Radiographic evaluation. *J. Foot Surg.*, **31**, pp. 301–313.

47. Marcacci, M., Kon, E., Moukhachev, V., Lavroukov, A., Kutepov, S., Quarto, R., Mastrogiacomo, M., Cancedda, R. (2007) Stem cells associated with macroporous bioceramics for long bone repair: 6- to 7-year outcome of a pilot clinical study. *Tissue Eng.*, **13**, pp. 947–955.

48. Quarto, R., Mastrogiacomo, M., Cancedda, R., Kutepov, S. M., Mukhachev, V., Lavroukov, A., Kon, E., Marcacci, M. (2001) Repair of large bone defects with the use of autologous bone marrow stromal cells. *N. Engl. J. Med.*, **344**, pp. 385–386.

49. Dallari, D., Savarino, L., Albisinni, U., Fornasari, P., Ferruzzi, A., Baldini, N., Giannini, S. (2012) A prospective, randomised, controlled trial using a Mg-hydroxyapatite-demineralized bone matrix nanocomposite in tibial osteotomy. *Biomaterials*, **33**, pp. 72–79.

Chapter 13

# Clinical Aspects in Regeneration of Articular Regions: New Biologically Inspired Multifunctional Scaffolds

Elizaveta Kon, Giuseppe Filardo, Francesco Tentoni, Andrea Sessa, and Maurilio Marcacci

*II Clinic—Biomechanics Laboratory; Rizzoli Orthopaedic Institute, Bologna, Italy*

e.kon@biomec.ior.it

## 13.1 Introduction

The rationale for using scaffolds for regenerating the damaged articular surface is to have a temporary three-dimensional structure of biodegradable polymers for the growth of living cells and subsequent tissue formation. The ideal scaffold should mimic the biology, architecture, and structural properties of the native tissue in order to facilitate cell infiltration, attachment, proliferation, and differentiation. Other key properties include biocompatibility and biodegradability through safe biochemical pathways at suitable time intervals to support the first phases of tissue formation and gradually be replaced by the regenerating tissue [1]. From a clinical perspective, the ideal graft should be an off-the-shelf product, which is able to avoid the practical, economic, and regulatory limitations related to the use of cells.

---

*Bio-Inspired Regenerative Medicine: Materials, Processes, and Clinical Applications*
Edited by Simone Sprio and Anna Tampieri
Copyright © 2016 Pan Stanford Publishing Pte. Ltd.
ISBN 978-981-4669-14-6 (Hardcover), 978-981-4669-15-3 (eBook)
www.panstanford.com

This explains the most recent trend in cartilage regeneration. In fact, whereas the use of cell-based scaffolds has been documented with overall satisfactory clinical results up to a medium/long-term follow-up [2, 3], there is increasing effort in developing one-step, possibly cell-free products.

This new treatment strategy involves implanting various biomaterials for "in situ" cartilage repair by exploiting the bone marrow stem cell differentiation induced by the scaffold properties [1, 2]. The possibility to produce a cell-free implant that is "smart" enough to provide the joint with appropriate stimuli to induce orderly and durable tissue regeneration is really attractive, and new biomaterials are claiming to induce "in situ" cartilage regeneration after direct transplantation into the defect site. One of these cell-free procedures is Autologous Matrix-Induced Chondrogenesis—AMIC®, which combines microfractures with the implantation of a porcine collagen type-I/III bilayer matrix to stabilize the blood clot and has proved to be a valid one-step treatment for cartilage defects: Gille et al. reported highly satisfactory results in 87% of the 27 patients followed up for a mean of 37 months, with MRI showing moderate-to-complete filling and a normal-to-hyper intense signal in most cases [4]. After standard microfractures, Patrascu et al. [5] applied another scaffold, an absorbable non-woven polyglycolic acid textile treated with hyaluronic acid (BioTissue AG, Zurich, Switzerland), as a sponge to hold the blood clot and progenitor cells, fixed to the lesion site with resorbable threads, and reported the successful treatment of a 6 cm$^2$ post-traumatic medial femoral condyle defect after 2 years. Surgical variants to increase the healing potential involve hand-made perforations with a Kirschner wire, to gain the advantages of the Pridie technique with a greater number of MSCs to enrich the membrane, or augmentation with platelet-rich plasma to further enhance the healing response through the platelet-derived growth factors [6–9]. However, despite some promising preliminary results and increasing application of these techniques in the clinical practice, results are still controversial and treatment indications are mainly restricted to small focal defects, whereas the real benefit for other lesions has still to be determined.

## 13.2 The Osteochondral Strategy

Most previously developed surgical options have aimed at reconstructing a functional joint surface by focusing on the cartilage layer, but there is increasing awareness about the role of the subchondral bone for many of the articular surface pathologies [10]. In fact, the subchondral bone may be involved in the pathological process not only primarily, such as in osteochondritis dissecans (OCD), osteonecrosis, and severe trauma, but also secondarily in large degenerative cartilage lesions, and even focal chondral defects, due to the higher mechanical stress on the lesion's edge, may increase in size over time and present with concomitant changes of the underlying subchondral bone plate [10].

This awareness led to the development of a new treatment strategy focusing on the entire osteochondral unit. This approach involves the development of new biphasic products: The bilayer structure allows the entire osteochondral unit to be treated by reproducing the different biological and functional requirements for guiding the growth of both bone and cartilage tissues. Heterogeneous scaffolds have been proposed which combine distinct but integrated layers corresponding to the cartilage and bone regions [11]. These devices aim at fulfilling the different requirements to regenerate cartilage and bone of an osteochondral defect, thus preventing the risk of delamination of different components. Initially, integrated bi-layered osteochondral scaffolds were proposed by using a-hydroxy acid polymers (i.e., poly-lactic acid, poly-lactic-coglycolic acid), combined with a ceramic component (i.e., hydroxyapatite, tricalcium phosphate) in the region corresponding to the subchondral bone, then biphasic but monolithic materials were formed by freeze-drying and chemical cross-linking collagen-based materials (i.e., mineralized or coupled with hyaluronic acid), as well as by ionotropic gelation of alginate-based materials (i.e., containing or not hydroxyapatite ceramic particles), thus allowing specific mechanical properties to be achieved (i.e., elasticity or compression strength) [11–14]. Among the different specific scaffolds developed to reproduce the different biological and functional requirements of bone and cartilage and guide the growth of the two tissues, currently only two osteochondral scaffolds have been commercialized for clinical application.

One is a bilayer porous PLGA-calcium-sulfate biopolymer (TruFit, Smith & Nephew, Andover, MA) [15, 16], which gave controversial results. In fact, whereas some authors have reported a favorable short-term clinical outcome and a slow improvement of the imaging appearance over time [17, 18], others have reported poor results. Barber et al. [19] did not find signs of maturation, osteoconduction, or ossification of the scaffold in any of the nine patients studied with CT scans. Dhollander et al. [20] reported 20% (3 out of 15 patients) of failures at 1-year follow-up and biopsies showing fibrous vascularized repair tissue. Finally, Joshi et al. [21] documented even poorer results at 2 years in 10 patients treated for patellar defects, with all patients except one complaining of pain and swelling, as well as a lack of MRI signs of integration and subchondral bone restoration. The reoperation rate due to implant failure was 70% at final follow-up. In conclusion, the use of this osteochondral bilayer scaffold did not show good results and its use remains questionable.

The second osteochondral scaffold is a three-layered nanostructured biomimetic collagen hydroxyapatite (HA) scaffold. This composite material resembles the composition of the extracellular matrices of cartilage and bone tissue, respectively, and is based on nucleation of HA nanocrystals onto self-assembled collagen fibers [22] to generate a chemically and morphologically graded hybrid biomaterial by stacking a lower mineralized layer, an intermediate layer with reduced amount of mineral (tidemark-like) and an upper layer formed by collagen (reproducing some cartilaginous cues). Equine type I collagen (Coll) was chosen as the organic component, working as a matrix for the mineralization process, due to its good physico-chemical stability and processability and high safety and biocompatibility profile, related to the removal of all potentially immunogenic telopeptides. The mineral phase is represented by magnesium–HA (Mg-HA). Magnesium ions were introduced to increase the physicochemical, structural, and morphological affinities of the composite with newly formed natural bone [23]. The cartilaginous layer, consisting of Type I collagen, has a smooth surface. The intermediate layer consists of a combination of Type I collagen (60% of weight) and Mg-HA

(40% of weight), whereas the lower layer consists of a mineralized blend of Type I collagen (30% of weight) and Mg-HA (70% of weight). Each layer is separately synthesized and the final construct is obtained by physically combining the layers on a Mylar sheet and finally freeze drying and gamma-sterilizing at 25 Kgray [22]. In vitro and animal studies [24, 25] tested this biomaterial and showed good results with cartilage and bone tissue formation. Similar macroscopic, histological, and radiographic results have been obtained by implanting scaffolds loaded with autologous chondrocytes or scaffolds alone: The scaffold was able to induce in situ regeneration through cells coming from the surrounding bone marrow in the animal model. Thus, this scaffold has been introduced into the clinical practice as a cell-free approach (Fig. 13.1).

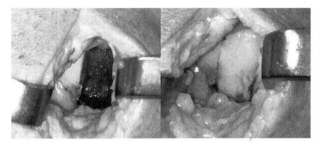

**Figure 13.1** Intraoperative view of an osteochondral lesion of the medial femoral condyle before and after treatment with a biomimetic nanostructured collagen-hydroxyapatite osteochondral scaffold.

## 13.3 Clinical Results in Osteochondral Regeneration

Preliminary results focusing on the surgical technique and intrinsic mechanical stability of implants without any other fixation technique were reported on 13 patients (15 defects) [26]. High-resolution MRI was used for the evaluation of the graft adherence 5–8 weeks after implantation and to evaluate further graft stability and maturation at 6 months. At the earliest follow-up time complete attachment and adherence was found in 13 of the implantation sites. Partial attachment was found in two patients. A possible reason for the early detachment of the implanted biomaterials might be weak mechanical fixation due to inadequate surgical technique with insufficient shoulder coverage of the prepared implantation site. Further analysis at 6 months revealed partial reabsorption of the graft in one case with an incomplete cartilage layer and a complete subchondral structure, whereas in the other case an inhomogeneous tissue filled the entire treated area, probably due to the development of fibrous tissue. Histological analysis, although only performed in two cases, revealed the presence of perfectly formed subchondral bone and complete biomaterial reabsorption. The cartilage repair tissue analyzed 6 months after treatment appeared to be in different degrees of remodeling, but with the presence of two partially differentiated tissues in an ongoing healing process without any presence of "bone step-in."

The first study [27] to report clinical results of this implant involved 30 consecutive patients (9 women, 21 men; mean age, 29.3 years) with chondral or osteochondral knee lesions. Lesion size varied from 1.5 cm$^2$ to 6.0 cm$^2$. Twenty-eight patients were followed for 2 years and were clinically evaluated using the International Knee Documentation Committee (IKDC) and Tegner scores. The Tegner and IKDC objective and subjective scores improved significantly from the baseline evaluation to the 6–, 12–, and 24–month follow-ups. Further analysis showed a slower recovery but the same results for patients who presented with adverse events, older patients, patients who underwent previous surgery, and for those with patellar lesions. Conversely, a faster recovery was observed in active patients. Magnetic resonance imaging evaluation showed complete filling of the cartilage and complete integration of the graft in 70% of the lesions. However, the subchondral lamina and bone were intact in some cases (7% and 47%, respectively). Recently, a 5–year follow-up has been published on 27 patients of the same series [28]. A statistically significant improvement in all clinical scores was obtained from the basal evaluation to the 2– and 5–year follow-ups, and the results were stable over time. The IKDC subjective score improved from 40.0 ± 15.0 to 76.5 ± 14.5 and 77.1 ± 18.0, and the Tegner score from 1.6 ± 1.1 to 4.0 ± 1.8 and 4.1 ± 1.9 at 2 and 5 years, respectively. The MRI evaluation of 23 lesions showed a significant improvement in both MOCART score and subchondral bone status from 2 to 5 years. At 5 years a complete filling of the cartilage was shown in

78.3% of the lesions, complete integration of the graft was detected in 69.6% of cases, the repair tissue surface was intact in 60.9%, and the structure of the repair tissue was homogeneous in 60.9% of cases. The study results highlighted the safety and potential of this procedure, which offered a good clinical outcome with stable results up to a mid-term follow-up. Even though MRI findings improved over time, some abnormalities persisted, but no correlation was found between imaging and clinical results.

One study specifically focusing on OCD lesions was published with clinical and MRI results at short-term follow-up [29]. OCD is an acquired lesion, primarily involving the subchondral bone, which may result in separation and instability of the overlying articular cartilage, thus particularly appropriate for an osteochondral approach. Twenty-seven consecutive patients (19 men, 8 women; age 25.5 ± 7.7 years) affected by symptomatic knee OCD of the femoral condyles (average defect size 3.4 ± 2.2 $cm^2$), grade 3 or 4 on the International Cartilage Repair Society (ICRS) scale were enrolled, treated, and prospectively evaluated by subjective and objective IKDC and Tegner scores preoperatively and at 1- and 2-year follow-up. An MRI was also performed at the two follow-up times. A statistically ignificant improvement in all clinical scores was obtained at 1 year, and a further improvement was found the following year. At the 2-year follow-up, the IKDC subjective score had increased from 48.4 ± 17.8 preoperatively to 82.3 ± 12.2, the IKDC objective evaluation from 40% to 85% of normal knees, and the Tegner score from 2.4 ± 1.7 to 4.5 ± 1.6. The MRI evaluations showed good defect filling and implant integration but also inhomogeneous regenerated tissue and subchondral bone changes in most patients at both follow-up times. No correlation between the MOCART (magnetic resonance observation of cartilage repair tissue) score and clinical outcome was found.

Clinical results have also been published for other complex lesions where the subchondral bone is clearly involved in the aetiopathogenetic process. A case report was published on a 46–year–old athletic patient [30] who, treated with ACL reconstruction on the same knee 10 years earlier, complained of knee pain and presented a deep and extended osteochondral lesion, involving the medial femoral condyle, the trochlea and the patella. A closing–wedge high tibial osteotomy was performed to restore the lower limb normal axis and unload the medial compartment and the biomimetic osteochondral scaffold was implanted through a medial para–patellar approach, to regenerate the damaged articular surface. At 1–year follow-up, the patient was pain–free, had full range of motion, and returned to his pre-operation level of tennis. MRI performed 6 and 12 months after surgery showed stable implants and a hyaline-like signal with good restoration of the articular surface at 6 months. Subchondral edema then progressively decreased over time and at 12 months it was barely evident. Another published case report [31] regards a 50–year–old woman affected by a Schatzker type II tibial plateau fracture of the left knee, who was previously treated with a plate and screws by a lateral approach and cast. Three years after the treatment, the patient complained of pain and instability of the left knee and frequent episodes of effusion, and presented a lateral compartment valgus knee, limited range of motion (ROM), and acute pain at high degrees of flexion. Due to the complexity of the lesion, an integrated approach was applied, restoring the previous anatomic features with both mechanical and biological treatments. The first step was to remove the previous hardware and to perform a tibial lateral plateau open-wedge elevation osteotomy, then implant a homologous bone graft, wedge shaped from a femoral head and fixed with a minimally invasive synthesis (two screws) to correct the tibial plateau depression and the misalignment. Afterwards the joint surface was treated with the osteochondral scaffold. Finally, a hinged dynamic external fixator (EF) was applied to protect the grafts and at the same time allow for early flexion-extension knee movement. At the 1–year follow-up, the patient did not complain of knee pain, had a full range of motion, and returned to her previous activities. The IKDC objective score was normal, the IKDC subjective, EQ VAS and Tegner scores were, respectively 63.2, 83, and 4. At the 24–month follow-up, the activity level was maintained, whereas a further improvement was observed in the IKDC subjective score and EQ VAS evaluation (70.1 and 89, respectively). At the 4 year follow-up the same activity level was observed. The patient was also evaluated using MRI at 12 and 24 months after surgery. The implant remained in site and showed a hyaline-like signal with good restoration of articular surface at both follow-up times. Subchondral edema progressively decreased over time and at 24 months was barely evident in the tibial plateau.

After the promising preliminary results also in the treatment of complex osteochondral lesions, a study specifically focused on the potential of this osteochondral scaffold for the treatment of challenging knee lesions [32]. "Complex cases" were defined according to the presence of at least one of the following inclusion criteria: previous history of intra-articular fracture, tibial plateau lesion, concurrent knee axial realignment procedure, meniscal scaffold, or allograft implantation. The treatment group consisted of 33 patients (24 men, 9 women) who were consecutively treated with the implant of osteochondral scaffold and, when needed, concurrent procedures to address axial misalignment and meniscal resection sequelae. Results were also compared with those of a homogeneous group of 23 patients previously treated and prospectively evaluated after implantation of a chondral scaffold. The IKDC subjective score improved significantly from pre-operative 40.4 ± 14.1 to 12 months' follow-up 69.6 ± 17.0 with a further improvement at the final evaluation at 24 months 75.5 ± 15.0. The same positive trend was confirmed by the VAS and Tegner scores. A comparative analysis showed favorable clinical results for the osteochondral scaffold group. At 12 months of follow-up there was no difference between the treatments, which were comparable; however, at 24 months, the osteochondral scaffold group presented a significantly better performance than the chondral scaffold group. Finally, the osteochondral scaffold was recently used as an alternative to metal resurfacing on unicompartmental osteoarthritis in young patients [33]. This population is particularly challenging, due to a combination of high functional demands and great expectations regarding recovery, but limited treatment options. The indication of unicompartmental knee implants in a young and active population, with great expectations, is not an easy choice for the orthopedic surgeon, especially due to the increased risk of prosthetic revision affecting younger patients. Therefore, a solution to avoid or at least delay metal resurfacing is highly desirable. Forty-three patients affected by unicompartmental OA (Kellegren-Lawrence 3) with full-thickness focal cartilage lesions in stable joints were enrolled and consecutively treated. Mean age at surgery was 40.1 ± 11 years (33 men and 10 women), and mean BMI was 25 ± 3. The lesion size in patients affected by full thickness cartilage lesions was 4.6 ± 2.1 cm$^2$. Thirty-five patients presented an abnormal alignment and were treated by lateral closing-wedge high tibial osteotomy and medial closing-wedge distal femoral osteotomy. In particular, 15 patients were treated with osteotomy and cartilage treatment with an osteochondral biomimetic scaffold implant (3 of them combined with meniscal substitution), 11 with osteotomy and meniscal scaffold implant, 9 with osteotomy and meniscal allograft implant, and 8 with both cartilage and meniscal reconstruction, depending on the main requirements of the specific joint compartment. Only 2 patients were treated surgically for the first time, whereas all other patients had undergone previous surgery, often even multiple treatments. Outcome was prospectively documented before surgery and at 3 years of follow-up using IKDC subjective and objective, and Tegner scores. A significant improvement was observed in terms of clinical scores, both objective and subjective, and activity level from pre-op to the 3 years' follow-up. The analysis performed to determine parameters that might affect the clinical outcome showed that age influenced the final results. In fact, even though a good outcome was obtained at all ages, patients under the age of 40 years presented a higher clinical and subjective improvement thus showing that young patients affected by severe joint unicompartmental degeneration, otherwise doomed to more sacrificing treatments, may benefit from this osteochondral scaffold for the regeneration of the articular surface.

## 13.4  Conclusions

Several regenerative techniques have already shown good results at short and medium-term follow-up but mainly for the treatment of traumatic focal cartilage defects. The subchondral bone is often involved when the articular surface is damaged and needs to be treated in order to have a correct restoration of the most superficial layers of the joint. That is the reason why different osteochondral scaffolds have been developed. Among these, a biomimetic nanostructured osteochondral scaffold, which reproduces the requirements of both bone and cartilage, has been shown to offer good clinical results at mid-term follow-up. This scaffold shows promise even for the treatment of complex lesions, where other procedures are not indicated, and can be considered as a valid option for the treatment of both large chondral or osteochondral lesions. The advantage of these techniques is the possibility of a one-step procedure, on-the-shelf availability of the material, simpler and faster surgical technique, and lower costs. However, some controversial findings have been reported from an imaging point of view, showing the persistence of an altered signal and a slow maturation process of the osteochondral unit. Thus, even if satisfactory results have been already reported, some aspects might be further improved to accelerate the regenerative processes and increase the healing potential, and further clinical investigation with longer-term follow-up and a higher number of patients is required to attest the efficacy and durability of the clinical improvement over time and to understand which patients and lesion types might benefit more from this osteochondral biomimetic scaffold.

## Acknowledgments

B. Di Matteo, F. Perdisa, L. Andriolo, F. Balboni: II Clinic—Biomechanics Laboratory, Rizzoli Orthopaedic Institute, Bologna, Italy. K. Smith: Task Force, Rizzoli Orthopaedic Institute, Bologna, Italy.

## References

1. Kon E, Filardo G, Roffi A, Andriolo L, Marcacci M. New trends for knee cartilage regeneration: From cell-free scaffolds to mesenchymal stem cells. *Curr Rev Musculoskelet Med*, 2012; **5**(3): 236–243.

2. Filardo G, Kon E, Roffi A, Di Martino A, Marcacci M. Scaffold-based repair for cartilage healing: A systematic review and technical note. *Arthroscopy*, January 2013; **29**(1): 174–186.

3. Filardo G, Kon E, Di Martino A, Iacono F, Marcacci M. Arthroscopic second-generation autologous chondrocyte implantation: A prospective 7-year follow-up study. *Am J Sports Med*, October 2011; **39**(10): 2153–2160.

4. Gille J, Schuseil E, Wimmer J, Gellissen J, Schulz AP, Behrens P. Mid-term results of Autologous Matrix-Induced Chondrogenesis for treatment of focal cartilage defects in the knee. *Knee Surg Sports Traumatol Arthrosc*, 2010; **18**(11): 1456–1464.

5. Patrascu JM, Freymann U, Kaps C, Poenaru DV. Repair of a post–traumatic cartilage defect with a cell-free polymer-based cartilage implant: A follow-up at two years by MRI and histological review. *J Bone Joint Surg Br*, 2010; **92**(8): 1160–1163.

6. Dhollander AA, De Neve F, Almqvist KF, et al. Autologous matrix-induced chondrogenesis combined with platelet-rich plasma gel: Technical description and a five pilot patients report. *Knee Surg Sports Traumatol Arthrosc*, 2011; **19**(4): 536–542.

7. Pascarella A, Ciatti R, Pascarella F, et al. Treatment of articular cartilage lesions of the knee joint using a modified AMIC technique. *Knee Surg Sports Traumatol Arthrosc*, 2010; **18**(4): 509–513.

8. Schiavone Panni A, Cerciello S, Vasso M. The management of knee cartilage defects with modified amic technique: Preliminary results. *Int J Immunopathol Pharmacol*, 2011; **24**(1 Suppl 2): 149–152.

9. Kon E, Filardo G, Delcogliano M, Fini M, Salamanna F, Giavaresi G, Martin I, Marcacci M. Platelet autologous growth factors decrease the osteochondral regeneration capability of a collagen-hydroxyapatite scaffold in a sheep model. *BMC Musculoskelet Disord*, September 27, 2010; **11**: 220.

10. Pape D, Filardo G, Kon E, van Dijk CN, Madry H. Disease-specific clinical problems associated with the subchondral bone. *Knee Surg Sports Traumatol Arthrosc*, April 2010; **18**(4): 448–462.

11. Martin I, Miot S, Barbero A, et al. Osteochondral tissue engineering. *J Biomech*, 2007; **40**: 750–765.

12. Scheck RM, Taboas JM, Segvich SJ, Hollister SJ, Krebsbach PH. Engineered osteochondral grafts using biphasic composite solid free-form fabricated scaffolds. *Tissue Eng*, 2004; 1376–1385.

13. Sherwood JK, Riley SL, Palazzolo R, et al. A three-dimensional osteochondral composite scaffold for articular cartilage repair. *Biomaterials*, 2002; **23**: 4739–4751.

14. Gomoll AH, Madry H, Knutsen G, et al. The subchondral bone in articular cartilage repair: Current problems in the surgical management. *Knee Surg Sports Traumatol Arthrosc*, 2010; **18**: 434–447.

15. Melton JT, Wilson AJ, Chapman-Sheath P, Cossey AJ. TruFit CB bone plug: Chondral repair, scaffold design, surgical technique and early experiences. *Expert Rev Med Devices*, 2010; **7**(3): 333–341.

16. Williams RJ, Gamradt SC. Articular cartilage repair using a resorbable matrix scaffold. *Instr Course Lect*, 2008; **57**: 563–571.

17. Bedi AF, LF.; Williams, R.J. III, Potter HG, and the Cartilage Study Group. The maturation of synthetic scaffolds for osteochondral donor sites of the knee: An MRI and T2-mapping analysis. *Cartilage*, 2010; **1**(1): 20–28.

18. Carmont MR, Carey-Smith R, Saithna A, Dhillon M, Thompson P, Spalding T. Delayed incorporation of a TruFit plug: Perseverance is recommended. *Arthroscopy*, 2009; **25**(7): 810–814.

19. Barber FA, Dockery WD. A computed tomography scan assessment of synthetic multiphase polymer scaffolds used for osteochondral defect repair. *Arthroscopy*, 2011; **27**(1): 60–64.

20. Dhollander AA, Liekens K, Almqvist KF, et al. A pilot study of the use of an osteochondral scaffold plug for cartilage repair in the knee and how to deal with early clinical failures. *Arthroscopy*, 2012; **28**(2): 225–233.

21. Joshi N, Reverte-Vinaixa M, Diaz-Ferreiro EW, Dominguez-Oronoz R. Synthetic resorbable scaffolds for the treatment of isolated patellofemoral cartilage defects in young patients: Magnetic resonance imaging and clinical evaluation. *Am J Sports Med*, 2012; **40**(6): 1289–1295.

22. Tampieri A, Sandri M, Landi E, et al. Design of graded biomimetic osteochondral composite scaffolds. *Biomaterials*, 2008; **29**: 3539–3546.

23. Serre CM, Papillard M, Chavassieux P, et al. Influence of magnesium substitution on a collagen-apatite biomaterial on the production of a calcifying matrix by human osteoblasts. *J Biomed Mater Res*, 1998; **42**: 626–633.

24. Kon E, Delcogliano M, Filardo G, et al. Orderly osteochondral regeneration in a sheep model using a novel nano-composite multilayered biomaterial. *J Orthop Res*, 2010; **28**(1): 116–124.

25. Kon E, Mutini A, Arcangeli E, et al. Novel nanostructured scaffold for osteochondral regeneration: Pilot study in horses. *J Tissue Eng Regen Med*, 2010; **4**(4): 300–308.

26. Kon E, Delcogliano M, Filardo G, et al. A novel nano-composite multi-layered biomaterial for treatment of osteochondral lesions: Technique note and an early stability pilot clinical trial. *Injury*, 2010; **41**: 693–701.

27. Kon E, Delcogliano M, Filardo G, Busacca M, Di Martino A, Marcacci M. Novel nano-composite multilayered biomaterial for osteochondral regeneration: A pilot clinical trial. *Am J Sports Med*, June 2011; **39**(6): 1180–1190.

28. Kon E, Filardo G, Di Martino A, Busacca M, Moio A, Perdisa F, Marcacci M. Clinical results and MRI evolution of a nano-composite multilayered biomaterial for osteochondral regeneration at 5 years. *Am J Sports Med*. 2014 Jan; **42**(1): 158–65.

29. Filardo G, Kon E, Di Martino A, Busacca M, Altadonna G, Marcacci M. Treatment of knee osteochondritis dissecans with a cell-free biomimetic osteochondral scaffold: Clinical and imaging evaluation at 2-year follow-up. *Am J Sports Med*, August 2013; **41**(8): 1786–1793.

30. Kon E, Delcogliano M, Filardo G, et al. (2009) Novel nano-composite multi-layered biomaterial for the treatment of multifocal degenerative cartilage lesions. *Knee Surg Sports Traumatol Arthrosc*, **17**: 1312–1315.

31. Filardo G, Di Martino A, Kon E, Delcogliano M, Marcacci M. Midterm results of a combined biological and mechanical approach for the treatment of a complex knee lesion. *Cartilage*, July 2012; **3**(3): 288–292.

32. Filardo G, Kon E, Perdisa F, Di Matteo B, Di Martino A, Iacono F, Zaffagnini S, Balboni F, Vaccari V, Marcacci M. Osteochondral scaffold reconstruction for complex knee lesions: A comparative evaluation. *Knee*, June 27, 2013. pii: S0968-0160(13)00100-2. doi: 10.1016/j.knee.2013.05.007.

33. Marcacci M, Zaffagnini S, Kon E, Marcheggiani Muccioli GM, Di Martino A, Di Matteo B, Bonanzinga T, Iacono F, Filardo G. Unicompartmental osteoarthritis: an integrated biomechanical and biological approach as alternative to metal resurfacing. *Knee Surg Sports Traumatol Arthrosc*. 2013, **21**(11): 2509–17.

# Chapter 14

# Biomimetic Materials in Spinal Surgery: A Clinical Perspective

**Giandomenico Logroscino, Giampiero Salonna, and Carlo Ambrogio Logroscino**

*Catholic Institute of Orthopaedics and Traumatology, Università Cattolica del Sacro Cuore, L.go F. Vito 1, 00168, Rome, Italy*

G.Logroscino@fastwebnet.it

## 14.1 Introduction

The biomaterials designed to replace the bone tissue are indispensible in many medical and surgical fields. Often, spinal surgery requires a large amount of bone tissue for bone fusion so as to obtain a complete and stable correction over time. Autologous grafts are still the gold standard, but their availability is limited. The homologous bone tissue from the bank is a valid alternative, but there are risks related to infectious diseases. The best solution is to have an unlimited amount of "synthetic bone" without the risk of transmissible diseases, but synthetic materials cannot yet replicate the ability of bone tissue to be osteoconductive, osteoinductive, and mechanically resistant. The science of biomaterials is continuously evolving. In the last few years, there

---

*Bio-Inspired Regenerative Medicine: Materials, Processes, and Clinical Applications*
Edited by Simone Sprio and Anna Tampieri
Copyright © 2016 Pan Stanford Publishing Pte. Ltd.
ISBN 978-981-4669-14-6 (Hardcover), 978-981-4669-15-3 (eBook)
www.panstanford.com

has been a progressive improvement of bone substitutes. In the late 1990s, scientists developed some materials designed to reproduce the chemical components of the inorganic matrix of the bone, based using hydroxyapatite. Since then, research has taken major steps forward in the development of artificial materials that are very similar to bone from the biological point of view. The aim was to "deceive" the area around the graft to accept it as its own. This marked the beginning of the era of biomimetic materials, of tissue engineering and of gene therapy.

## 14.2 Historical Background and Indications for Spinal Fusion

Spinal fusion is also referred to as arthrodesis, a word coming from ancient Greek, which indicates the link between two articular surfaces. It has always been one of the most important achievements for vertebral surgery. The history of the treatment of idiopathic scoliosis is emblematic. Initially, this condition was mainly treated by orthopedic doctors with special beds/frames very similar to medieval torture instruments. The spine was pulled along its longitudinal axis and the hump was put under pressure. In more recent times, the correction has been maintained by applying very large casts covering the whole trunk and the pelvis. This treatment induced spectacular corrections, which, however, disappeared and the patients went back to their original situation once the cast was removed. For this reason, some "old generation" orthopedic doctors referred to scoliosis as "orthopedic cancer." In fact, it seemed that this was an incurable and progressive disease, which led to very severe deformities that were incompatible with vital functions. In the most severe cases, this disease led to respiratory distress and death. It was only after the introduction of spinal fusion that the surgical treatment of scoliosis led to hope and life. This exceptional progress was crafted by the American surgeon Hibbs (Fig. 14.1). At the turn of the century, he experimented the efficacy of bone fusion in a series of cases of bone tuberculosis (Pott's disease). He had the brilliant idea of applying this treatment to scoliosis. It was an extraordinary success that marked the beginning of further changes to this technique, with innumerable improvements until today. Hibbs' technique was designed to apply the autologous bone taken for the same patient, generally the iliac bone, to the posterior spine, after dissecting and bleeding the laminae and any part of the posterior arch especially at the level of the concave aspect of the curve. The correction was then maintained with casts until bone fusion was obtained. This entailed a lot of suffering for young women who were obliged to wear the cast for a very long time before and after the procedure. A frequent complication was pseudo-arthrosis (non-union), with the immediate consequence of losing the correction and of creating an imbalance at the level of the coronal and of the sagittal plane. So the patients had to undergo revision surgery with the application of an additional autologous graft and post-operative immobilization. On the one hand, a solution had been found to correct these deformities, but, on the other, this led to an enormous existential sacrifice in subjects at the most sensitive and difficult time of adolescence. Some decades went by before surgery had a major quality jump. The American surgeon P. Harrington [1, 2] (Fig. 14.2) systematically introduced the internal fixation of the spine to correct deformities. The Harrington Instrumentation rapidly spread around the world and immediately attracted the scientific community for its extraordinary potential for young patients suffering from deformities. Harrington had the courage to use steel rods and hooks to fix the spine, which had never been violated with external techniques, being the "custodian" of the noble and delicate structures that allow for motor function (the bone marrow and cauda equina). However, he did not take into consideration the past experience of Hibbs. As a result, the procedure had a high incidence of non-unions and many failures. It was John Howard Moe (Fig. 14.3), the founding member and first president in 1966 of the Scoliosis Research Society, who combined the two methods into a single procedure called "internal fixation and spinal fusion." Paul Harrington said about him, "John Moe was the father of modern-day treatment of scoliosis."

The fundamental role of spinal fusion was once again established. The internal fixation was used to correct deformities and to maintain the correction after the procedure, thus avoiding the hideous constriction of the cast. At the same time, the biological fusion of the spine ensured the long-term result of the treatment. This was a major breakthrough, which literally eliminated non-unions in many studies.

Over the years, the internal instrumentation has been changed, together with the surgical approaches to spine and bone fusion.

The benefits of bone fusion were largely proved in the Far East, precisely in Hong Kong, where in the 1960s, the orthopedic surgeons Hodgson and Stock revolutionized again vertebral surgery with a systematic anterior approach to the spine. It was then possible to reach the spine at 360° both anteriorly and posteriorly. This result was indeed obtained out of the treatment of vertebral tuberculosis (Pott's disease), which was endemic in Hong Kong and claimed many victims among the population living in junks on the water. The damp and unhealthy environment, poor sanitation, and malnutrition triggered severe forms of vertebral tuberculosis. The posterior approach to the spine was not adequate to treat these destructive infections characterized by abscesses and fistulas. The enormous osteolithic destruction of several adjacent vertebral bodies provoked major collapses of the axial skeleton, which could no longer play its supportive role, and paraplegia in the most severe cases. It was only with the anterior, transthoracic, thoracoabdominal, or retroperitoneal lumbar approach that the surgeon could directly reach the septic site to eliminate the cheese-like fluid oozing from the bone, without avoiding distant fistulization and to surgically "debride" the whole septic area. After this major surgical debridement, the spine was weak with many contiguous osteolithic cavities, severely deformed due to the collapse of the axial structure into kyphosis with a major risk of bone marrow lesions. At this point, there was the absolute need to prop up the weakened structure that was bound to progressively collapse into kyphosis. The anterior bone fusion became therefore inevitable and life saving. Bone strut grafts were taken from the fibula, the tibia or from the iliac crest for larger grafts, and were applied mainly to the lumbar spine, when the spine had to be stabilized on one or two levels. Again the postoperative cast was a must. This was the beginning of the era of multiple stage procedures, with an anterior approach to treat the infection and a second posterior approach to stabilize the spine with metal fixation. This allowed for the necessary rigidity to obtain the fusion of the anterior bone graft. Moreover, very soon came further advances in the anterior surgical approach. The Australian surgeon Allan Dwyer, visiting Hong Kong, was impressed by the potential of the surgical anterior approach to the spine and launched the first anterior fixation to stabilize the vertebral bodies [3]. The human invincible spirit went beyond any conceivable limit. The introduction of metal some centimeters away from the aorta and of the iliac vessels seemed science fiction. However, it became a reality. The material was titanium. Titanium screws were applied one after the other into the vertebral bodies. They were then connected by a titanium wire that was locked by a dedicated instrument after the correction (Fig. 14.4). This was certainly the first "segmental instrumentation" for the fixation of the spine. Later these devices were modified by other authors. However, it is worth remembering the first who had the courage to sail beyond the ancient and legendary Pillars of Hercules. As already emphasized, the biological phase is very important to provide a stable and long-lasting result.

Surgery has never stopped and it has consistently advanced with an increasing number of procedures around the world and of surgical indications for all age groups. The introduction of fixation with pedicle screws by the French surgeon Raymond Roy Camille and the successful modifications devised by the American surgeons Steffee and Brantigan (1986) led to an incredible development of lumbar surgery to treat degenerative and traumatic disorders. Even age limits did no longer seemed impossible. The use of pedicle screws provided greater stability with respect to hooks and allowed for a short fixation, without losing so many metamers and preserving motion in the mobile spine. Similarly to other phases of spinal surgery progress, it became evident that, without bone fusion, fixation alone was bound to fail. Screws fractured, especially if the intervertebral disc was "high." Harms and later Brantigan and Steffee had the brilliant idea of using meshes or cages in the intersomatic space (Fig. 14.5). The removal of the intersomatic disc through a posterior approach was eliminated through the insertion of titanium or carbon struts, true biological factors, like autoplastic bone chips taken from the ileus. This made it possible to obtain an intersomatic anterior support (PLIF), which provided immediate stability. At the same time, the bone material inside was introduced into the intersomatic space leading to union and bone continuity between the vertebrae. Sometimes the surgeons utilized a postero-lateral arthrodesis with the iliac bone. With a single surgical approach, it was possible to obtain a 270° fusion, stabilizing the two posterior columns and the anterior one. The evident advantage was the single approach widely used by vertebral surgeons, the very short fixations with less reduction of motion, a more stable implant due to the anterior support and finally the long-term correction deriving from intersomatic and postero-lateral bone fusion. Once again, these technical advances needed some biological factors to obtain long-term results.

Moreover, there are particular situations that necessarily require the right material for the union. For example, the long arthrodeses of the second thoracic vertebra designed to treat multiple curve scoliosis. Sometimes, it is necessary to extend the arthrodesis from the second thoracic vertebra to the fourth lumbar vertebra in adolescents and more rarely in pre-adolescents. Often, these patients do not always have a sufficient bone stock to provide a large amount of graft for bone fusion. In addition, in very young children with congenital scoliosis, it is necessary to perform in situ fusions and, less frequently, to use a homoplastic graft from their mothers or fathers, a great opportunity to use bone substitutes with biomimetic characteristics. Moreover, bone grafts are required to treat deformities in adults, which are often very severe. It is well known that, with advancing age, the quality and quantity of bone decrease, so it is useful to have supplementary biomimetic materials. The same holds true when bone fusion is needed for diseases such as rheumatoid arthritis, which may lead to vertebral collapses or to severe alterations of the cranio-cervical junction and which require fixation for bone fusion. In this case too, the bone tissue is of poor quality. In fact, many surgeons avoid arthrodesis with the risk of having an implant that is short lived and less stable over time.

In more recent times, minimally invasive or even percutaneous techniques have been developed around the world to treat bone fragility-induced vertebral collapses in the fractures young adults and in particular cases when it is necessary to obtain stabilization. Initially, osteoporotic vertebral collapses have been treated with cement (polymethyl methacrylate), but with the spread of this technique and its extension to indications in young subjects, it has increasingly become necessary to use percutaneous cannulas to deliver materials with biomimetic features able to promote bone fusion [4, 5] (Fig. 14.6). Clearly, the introduction of inert materials in young subjects is not supported by surgeons, especially by orthopedic surgeons, who are keen on the biological phases of consolidation, which creates continuity between the fractured components of the bone.

For over 100 years, the efforts of scientists have been designed to improve the results in vertebral fusion. The unstoppable evolution of science towards the future has inevitably led surgery to go beyond the limits of fusion, such as the elimination of motion and the suppression of the articular function between two contiguous segments. The current target is to preserve motion even though the long-term results are still poor. Obstacles like heterotopic ossification and the significant reduction in the range of motion even after some years have not allowed artificial discs to replace bone fusion, which is still the gold standard.

## 14.3 Biomimetic Bone Substitutes

Nature has always been a source of inspiration in the science of materials especially in tissue substitution. In the last few years, research has greatly advanced with the aim to develop materials able to simulate the human extracellular matrix at the chemical and physical level (biomimetism). The concept of "biomimetism" is based on the idea that biological systems are complex systems that produce information at the molecular level through many different chemical, physical, and biological interactions. Biomimetics is therefore the science that studies the biological and biomechanical processes of nature, as a source of inspiration for improving human activities and technologies. Nature is seen as a Model, a Measure and a Guide in the design of technical artifacts.

At present, the biomaterials that are being studied are defined as smart materials or as "biomaterials stimulating a specific cell response at the molecular level" [6]. They are part of a large-scale bone substitution strategy: tissue engineering. It is a multidisciplinary strategy envisaging the use of scaffolds (three-dimensional scaffolds to support tissue growth), cells (especially mesenchymal stem cells), growth factors (Bone Morphogenetic Proteins) and gene therapy. On the basis of this approach, bone substitution strategies can be based on the *matrix-based approaches* (the use of biomimetic bone materials to provide temporary support, which are then resorbed in a predefined period of time), the *cell-based and gene therapy* and the *factor-based therapy* [7].

## 14.4 Tissue Engineering Strategies

### 14.4.1 Smart Materials: Biomimetic Scaffolds

Bone tissue is a specialized connective tissue composed of cells (osteoblasts and osteoclasts) inside a mineralized extracellular matrix. The extracellular matrix has an organic component (35% of dry weight) and an inorganic component (65% of dry weight). The former is made up of Type I collagen fibers (more or less 90%) and of non-collagen proteins (10%), including osteonectin, osteocalcin, and bone sialoprotein [8]. The inorganic component contains more than 98% of tricalcium phosphate, which, in turn, contains about 30% of amorphous calcium phosphate and octocalcium phosphate and the remaining 70% of hydroxyapatite $(Ca_{10}(PO_4)_6-(OH)_2)$. These substances always maintain a dynamic balance, but they change over time and in the same individual according to the bone district examined. The bone extracellular matrix normally contains anionic and cationic substitutes (for example, $Mg^{++}$, $SiO_4$, $Sr^{++}$, $Mn^{++}$), initially interpreted as impurities. Instead they have a specific role in that they interact with the protein, ion and cell matrix [9, 10].

At present, ceramic materials (calcium phosphate ceramics: CPC) are the most extensively investigated and used in the clinical setting since they are extremely similar to the inorganic component [11]. The most frequently used ceramic materials are [12, 13]:

- hydroxyapatite;
- tricalcium phosphate;
- hydroxyapatite and tricalcium phosphate composites in different percentages.

The bone substitutes that are now under investigation are defined as smart materials, since they are able to induce a particular response at the molecular level. The development of these materials is due to a better knowledge of the molecular mechanisms that regulate bone formation and resorption. Some specific molecules (bioligands) or particular three-dimensional structures promote cell adhesion and colonization, as well as resorption. In the last few years, the growing interest in these components and nanotechnologies has resulted in compounds with biological and chemical properties similar to bone. In the past, the synthetic substitutes based on hydroxyapatite were obtained with a simple stoichiometric reaction between the two components (Calcium and Phosphate). The bone tissue is made up of a sophisticated organized structure. The combination of calcium, phosphate, and collagen creates a crystalline structure of hydroxyapatite, arranged into units with a regular orientation of the collagen fibers. The new nanotechnologies, starting from nano-molecular units, have made it possible to derive biologically active and smart macromolecules [14].

Moreover, thanks to these technologies, it has been possible to introduce ions in the compounds (for example, $Mg^{++}$, $SiO_4$, $Sr^{++}$, $Mn^{++}$) that promote specific biological functions in vivo. These ions are able to improve their mechanical functions and promote osteogenesis.

In the development of smart materials, research mainly focuses on

- *doped* ceramic materials;
- improving bioactive properties through nanotechnologies (three-dimensional structure that promote cell adhesion and colonization);
- enhancing mechanical resistance;
- controlling resorption velocity.

## 14.4.2 *"Doped"* Ceramic Substitutes

The inorganic component contains calcium and phosphate but also anion and cation substitutes with different functions. The development of materials that include these ions makes it possible to obtain a material similar to mineralized bone matrix (biomimetic) with peculiar biological activity.

Research mainly focuses on the following:

**Magnesium**: Magnesium is a divalent cation that accounts for 0.1% to 2% of the bone dry weight. Kakei has shown that in the bone of newborn mice, there is a concentration of magnesium ions [15]. Bigi et al. [16, 17] have demonstrated that the immature calcium tissue is rich in magnesium ions that tend to decrease when calcification increases. Moreover, $Mg^{++}$ has important angiogenic functions by inducing the production of nitric oxide through a mechanism similar to the VEGF one [18, 19]. Magnesium and carbonate are present in high concentrations in normal bone tissue in the early osteogenic phase, thus facilitating the invasion of bone cells inside the hydroxyapatite and resorption. However, they tend to disappear when the bone is mature, thus stopping bone growth, reducing the activity of osteoblasts and osteoclasts and causing osteopenia and bone fragility [14, 20–22].

**Calcium carbonate:** Carbonate is the ion most present in the bone (4–8% and it tends to change with age). The levels of carbonate present in the bone mineral are low at birth and they tend to triple in just one week. The cation carbon can be added to HA through A-carbonation, that is the replacement of a hydroxyl group with a carbon ion and B-carbonation, that is the replacement of phosphate with carbon. In many animal species, the A/B carbonation ratio is about 0.7–0.9 [23]. A high A/B ratio was observed in the bone in the elderly. The presence of B-carbonation leads to a lower of degree of crystallinity and to an increase in the solubility in in vitro and in vivo tests. A-CHA shows a low affinity for the adhesion of osteoblastic cells with respect to hydroxyapatite alone and a lower production of collagen in compounds containing A-CHA [24–26].

**Strontium:** Strontium is present in traces in the mineral component of the bone. It stimulates osteogenesis in two ways: by promoting the proliferation, the differentiation and the survival of osteoblasts and by inducing apoptosis in the osteoclasts, thus promoting osteogenesis and inhibiting resorption [27, 28]. Strontium activates the CaSR receptor in the osteoblasts [29, 30] and simultaneously increases the production of OPG (osteoprotegerin) and reduces the expression of RANKL [31]. This ion is assumed to be a key factor in bone degenerative diseases, including osteoporosis [32, 33].

**Manganese:** Manganese is present in traces in the bone tissue. It is believed to have a role in the signaling pathway of PTH [34]. Mn-SOD neutralizes the reacting oxygen species (ROS), which contributes to an increase in osteoclastogenesis and reduction in osteoblastogenesis [35].

**Silicates ($SiO_4$):** They induce angiogenesis probably through an increase production of nitric oxide, which in turn strengthens the production of VEGF [36]. In addition, $SiO_4$ stimulates cell differentiation in an osteoblastic sense and Type 1 collagen synthesis [37]; in animal models, these substitutes stimulate the formation of new bone more than hydroxyapatite alone [38, 39].

**CaP multisubstitutes:** The use of multiple "doped" ions of ceramic calcium phosphate materials is now under investigation (multisubstitute calcium phosphate ceramics). The presence of traces of metals inside these ceramic compounds may change the degradation pattern of these materials, stimulate osteogenesis and inhibit osteoclastogenesis with a combination of effects on the above-mentioned ions [40, 41] with anti-osteoporotic properties [42].

### 14.4.3  Bioactivity of Ceramic Materials

An important characteristic of the biomimetic materials is their ability to adsorb the extracellular matrix (collagen, fibronectin, laminin, etc.) thus promoting cell adhesion and the formation of new tissue [43]. The adsorption of these proteins is a complex phenomenon, guided by chemical, thermodynamic, and kinetic processes that depend upon the properties of the biomaterial surface, on the ionic environment and on the structural/chemical properties of proteins [44]. These properties are

(1) *Roughness of the surface:* Roughness is generally measured in terms of mean quadratic value $(R_a)$, which describes the distance between the peaks (or troughs) of the surface of the material along an arbitrary line. Roughness is largely influenced by the size of the crystal granules of the calcium phosphate ceramics (CPC) particles. Roughness characteristics $(R_a$ and granulometry) less than 100 nm seem to promote a better adsorption of proteins with respect to greater roughness [45].

(2) *Microporosity:* the presence of microporosity extends the surface of the material available for the adsorption of proteins. The high microporosity of CPCs, with pore sizes from 20 to 500 nm, significantly improves protein adsorption. Zhue coll. have shown that hydroxyapatite and the calcium phosphate compounds with high microporosity and/or porosity greater than 20 nm promote a greater adsorption of fibrinogen and insulin with respect to low-porosity materials [46].

(3) *Surface charges, ionic environment, and solubility*: adsorption is affected by the electrostatic charges between the proteins and by the material surface, as well as by the stability of the structural charge of the individual proteins. Crystalline and stable CPCs seem to influence the absorption through

their surface charges, which interact with the protein charges, while amorphous and soluble CPCs influence absorption by provoking changes in the local pH and in ion concentration [47].

### 14.4.4 Fiber-Reinforced Ceramic Materials

Generally, calcium phosphate ceramic cements provide a limited biomechanical support because of their fragility and scarce resistance to traction. This limits their use over time. The development of calcium phosphate ceramic cements with greater resistance would significantly expand the potential field of application. In fact, this would allow for the repair of long bone fractures, for the fixation of cemented joint implants or for the arthrodesis of vertebral bodies [48]. All this has led to the development of materials "reinforced" with fibers that increase their tenacity and resistance to torsion [49]. The fibers used by researchers can be subdivided into two large groups [50]:

- CPCs with non-resorbable fibers: aramide, bioglass, polymers like polyamides, carbon
- CPCs with resorbable fibers: alginate, natural rubber, cellulose, chitosan-polylactide, polycaprolactone

### 14.4.5 Control of the Material Resorption Velocity

Biomimetic materials are similar to the bone extracellular matrix and are subjected to resorption and to gradual remodeling, with the gradual substitution of the developing bone tissue. The resorption velocity has to be adjusted to the regeneration speed of the bone segment.

The bone resorption velocity (solubility) depends on the nature of the calcium phosphate compound and is indicated in Table 14.1 [51–53].

**Table 14.1**  Proprieties of calcium phosphate ceramic materials

| CPCs | Solubility ($K_{sp}$) | Ca/P ratio |
|---|---|---|
| Hydroxyapatite | Low | 1.67 |
| Tricalcium phosphate | Sufficient | 1.7 |
| Tricalcium phosphate phosphate/hydroxyapatite | Variable (it depends on the TCP/HA concentration) | 1.5–1.67 |

## 14.5  Current Research: Future Prospects

As already mentioned, biomimetic materials can be used with a so-called matrix-based approach, that is like simple bone substitutes or combined with cell-based and gene therapies or with factor-based therapy.

## 14.6  Cell-Based and Gene Therapy

Current research is investigating cells that can differentiate in an osteogenic direction and that can produce growth factors in a natural manner. In this way, a reparative response may be activated through the biological stimuli of up and down regulation, according to the local bio-pathological situation. In this connection, two lines of research have been developed: cell-based therapy and gene therapy [41].

In **cell-based therapy**, researchers study adult bone marrow stem cells (BMSC), multipotent cells that are able to differentiate into bone, cartilage, meniscus, tendon, ligament, muscle, and fat tissue [54, 55].

If adequately stimulated by a biological, mechanical and chemical microenvironment, these cells are able to differentiate or to de-differentiate towards a certain type of connective tissue [56].

BMSCs are mainly harvested from the iliac crest. The possible applications of these cells in orthopedics are indicated by Caplan [57]. These applications include tissue engineering, but also cell replacement therapy in genetic diseases such as imperfect osteogenesis or muscular dystrophy. Stem cells like pumps of cytokines/growth factors can be guided towards an osteochondral direction and they can become a source of growth factors or of factors promoting repair or substitutive processes [58].

In the **gene therapy,** cells are programmed to produce osteoinductive molecules through transfection. Many molecules have been studied in animals with significant results:

- growth factors for bone, that are able to induce stem cells to differentiate into osteoblast like cells: bone morphogenetic protein-2 (BMP-2), BMP-4, BMP-7, BMP-9, BMP-12, (LIM mineralization protein-1 (LMP-1) [59, 60], LMP-3 [61–63], RunX-2, OSX;

- growth factors for cartilage: BMPs, transforming growth factor-beta superfamily, IGF-1, FGF, HGF, IL-1 receptor antagonist (IL-1RA), tissue inhibitor of metalloproteinase (TIMP) (these last two are not growth factors, but they are inhibitors of inflammation that destroys cartilage).
- Growth factors for tendons, ligaments, and meniscus: BMP-2, BMP-12, BMP-13, human growth and differentiation factor-5 (GDF-5).

## 14.7 Factor-Based Therapy

The factor-based therapy uses biologically active and protein substances that are able to actively stimulate bone growth (osteoinduction). These factors act through a receptor mechanism by stimulating chemotaxis, osteogenic differentiation, and the production of bone on the part of osteogenic precursor cells. So their action is limited in time and is dose dependent. The study of these factors has led to the introduction in the clinical setting of platelet-derived growth factor (PDGF) of platelet-rich plasma (PRP), of demineralized bone matrix (DBM) and finally of bone morphogenetic proteins (BMPs), including BMP-2,7.

### 14.7.1 Demineralized Bone Matrix

The extracellular DBM (calcium residue <5%) is mainly made up of collagen fibers. On the one hand, it is supposed to mimic the three-dimensional architecture of the bone, thus facilitating and guiding the invasion, the growth and the differentiation of the host cell [64] and, on the other, to have bone growth factors (BMP, IGF, TGF, FGF). These factors are supposed to be able to stimulate the activation and the migration of progenitor stem cells and angiogenesis. DBM does not have mechanical resistance and it is therefore used only as a filler combined to a carrier (glycerol, hyaluronic acid, carboxymethylcellulose).

DBM is safe and effective as a bone graft [bm], but there is still not enough evidence as to the use of this compound as a *stand-alone* substitute [65]. Moreover, there are conflicting data on the concentrations of BMP 2 and BMP 7 on the basis of the methods used to obtain this compound [65, 66].

### 14.7.2 Platelet-Rich Plasma

Platelet gel and PRP are easily obtained from an autologous tissue blood through centrifugation and concentration. These compounds are rich in growth factors, including the platelet-derived growth factor, the insulin-like growth factor and the transforming growth factor [68–70]. PRP has a chemotactic and mitogenic action for osteoblasts and fibroblasts for the synthesis of proteoglycans, that is a prerequisite of the extracellular matrix. Several clinical studies show a failure rate of vertebral surgery with a reduction of vertebral arthrodesis by 15% and 19%, even if used in combination with bone marrow cells [71]. This failure is probably due to the paradoxical inhibition of BMP-2 at high concentrations [72–74].

### 14.7.3 Bone Morphogenetic Proteins

Bone morphogenetic proteins belong to the large and hetero-geneous family of transforming growth factor-a and are deeply involved in the osteogenic process. Of these, BMP-2, BMP-4, BMP-7 (also known as osteonic protein-1) can induce the differentiation of multipotent mesenchymal cells into osteochondrogenic and osteoblastic precursor cell lines [75, 76]. The osteogenic-osteoinductive properties have been observed in many studies. At present, BMP-2 and BMP-7 are authorized by the U.S. FDA and by the European EMA for some applications:

- BMP-2 combined to a collagen carrier is approved for lumbar arthrodesis;
- BMP-7 is approved for tibial bone non-unions in patients with previous failures.

## 14.8 Conclusion

The research in the field of synthetic biomaterials able to reproduce the quality of the bone tissue is continuously evolving. However, it has not reached yet its final target. Nanotechnologies, tissue engineering, and gene therapy are currently the most promising lines of research in the field of biomimetic materials that can become integrated into the bone as if they were bone tissues. From the clinical point of view, there is a growing need for bone substitutes in spinal surgery, because of the increasingly sophisticated technologies and accurate surgical techniques, which cannot do without biology. And today the best bone substitute is bone.

## Acknowledgments

The research leading to these results has received funding from the European Union's Seventh Framework Programme ([FP7/2007-2013]) under grant agreement n° 246373, OPHIS.

## References

1. Harrington PR, Treatment of scoliosis. Correction and internal fixation by spine instrumentation, *J Bone Joint Surg Am*, **44-A**, (1962) pp. 591–610.

2. Harrington PR, The history and development of Harrington instrumentation. By Paul Harrington, 1973, *Clin Orthop Relat Res*, **227**, (1988) pp. 3–5.

3. Dwyer AF, Newton NC, Sherwood AA, An anterior approach to scoliosis. A preliminary report, *Clin Orthop Relat Res*, Jan-Feb; **62**: (1969), 192–202.

4. Logroscino G, Proietti L, Pola E, Spine fusion: Cages, plates and bone substitutes, in *Biomaterials for Spinal Surgery, Part II Spinal Fusion and Intervertebral Discs*. Cambridge, UK: Woodhead Publishing Limited, 2012, pp. 265–294.

5. Logroscino G, Lattanzi W, Bone substitution in spine fusion: The past, the present, and the future, *In Minimally Invasive Surgery of the Lumbar Spine*: Springer, 2014.

6. Hench LL, Polak JM, Third-generation biomedical materials, *Science*, Feb 8, 295(5557), 2002, pp. 1014–1017.

7. Burg KJ, Porter S, Kellam JF, Biomaterial developments for bone tissue engineering, *Biomaterials*, Dec 21(23), pp. 2347–2359, 2000.

8. Landis WJ, Silver FH, Mineral deposition in the extracellular matrices of vertebrate tissues: Identification of possible apatite nucleation sites on type I collagen, *Cells Tissues Organs*, **189**(1–4), pp. 20–24, doi: 10.1159/000151454. Epub 2008 Aug 15, 2009.

9. Fielding GA, Bandyopadhyay A, Bose S, Effects of silica and zinc oxide doping on mechanical and biological properties of 3D printed

tricalcium phosphate tissue engineering scaffolds, *Dent Mater*, **28**(2), 2012, pp. 113–122.

10. Bose S, Fielding G, Tarafder S, Bandyopadhyay A, Understanding of dopant-induced osteogenesis and angiogenesis in calcium phosphate ceramics, *Trends Biotechnol*, **31**(10), 2013, pp. 594–605.

11. Place ES, Evans ND, Stevens MM, Complexity in biomaterials for tissue engineer, *Nat Mater*, **8**(6), 2009, pp. 457–470.

12. LeGeros RZ, Properties of osteoconductive biomaterials: Calcium phosphates, *Clin Orthop Relat Res*, **395**, 2002, pp. 81–98.

13. LeGeros RZ, Lin S, Rohanizadeh R, Mijares D, LeGeros JP, Biphasic calcium phosphate bioceramics: Preparation, properties and applications, *J Mater Sci*, **14**(3), 2003, pp. 201–209.

14. Landi E., Tampieri A., Celotti G., Mattioli Belmonte M., Logroscino G., "Synthetic Biomimetic Nanostructured Hydroxyapatite," in *Bioceramics*. New Orleans USA: Key Engineering Materials, 2005, no. 284–286, pp. 975–8.

15. Kakei M, Nakahara H, Tamura N, Itoh H, Kumegawa M, Behavior of carbonate and magnesium ions in the initial crystallites at the early developmental stages of the rat calvaria, *Ann Anat*, **179**(4), 1997 pp. 311–316.

16. Bigi A, Cojazzi G, Panzavolta S, Ripamonti A, Roveri N, Romanello M, Noris Suarez K, Moro L, Chemical and structural characterization of the mineral phase from cortical and trabecular bone, *J. Inorg Biochem*, **68**(1), 1997, pp. 45–51.

17. Bigi A, Foresti E, Gregorini R, Ripamonti A, Roveri N, Shah JS, The role of magnesium on the structure of biological apatite, *Calcif Tissue Int*, **50**(5), 1992, pp. 439–444.

18. Maier JA, Bernardini D, Rayssiguier Y, Mazur A, High concentrations of magnesium modulate vascular endothelial cell behaviour in vitro, *Biochim Biophys Acta*, May 24, **1689**(1), 2004, pp. 6–12.

19. Cooke JP, Losordo DW, Nitric oxide and angiogenesis, *Circulation*, **105**(18), 2002, pp. 2133–2135.

20. Landi E, Logroscino G, Proietti L, Tampieri A, Sandri M, Sprio S, "Biomimetic Mg-substituted hydroxyapatite: From synthesis to in vivo behaviour, *J Mater Sci Mater Med*, **19**(1), 2008, pp. 239–247.

21. Pola E, Nasto LA, Tampieri A, Lattanzi W, Di Giacomo G, Colangelo D, Ciriello V, Pagano E, Spinelli S, Robbins PD, Logroscino G, Bioplasty

for vertebral fractures: Preliminary results of a pre-clinical study on goats using autologous modified skin fibroblasts, *Int J Immunopathol Pharmacol*, **24**(1 Suppl 2), 2011, pp. 139–142.

22. Sartori M, Giavaresi G, Tschon M, Martini L, Dolcini L, Fiorini M, Pressato D, Fini M, Long-term in vivo experimental investigations on magnesium doped hydroxyapatite bone substitutes, *J Mater Sci Mater Med*, **25**(6), 2014, pp. 1495–1504.

23. Rey C, Collins B, Goehl T, Dickson IR, Glimcher MJ, The carbonate environment in bone mineral: A resolutionenhanced Fourier transform infrared spectroscopy study, *Calcif Tissue Int*, **45**(3), (1989) pp. 157–164.

24. Redey SA, Razzouk S, Rey C, Bernache-Assollant D, Leroy G, Nardin M, Cournot G, Osteoclast adhesion and activity on synthetic hydroxyapatite, carbonated hydroxyapatite and natural calcium carbonate: Relationship to surface energies, *J Biomed Mater Res*, **45**(2), 1999, pp. 140–147.

25. Redey SA, Nardin M, Bernache-Assolant D, Rey C, Dclannoy P, Sedel L, Marie P J, Behavior of human osteoblastic cells on stoichiometric hydroxyapatite and type A carbonate apatite: Role of surface energy, *J Biomed Mater Res*, **50**(3), 2000, pp. 353–364.

26. Landi E, Celotti G, Logroscino G, Tampieri A, Carbonated hydroxyapatite as bone substitute, *J Eur Ceram Soc*, **23**(15), 2003, pp. 2931–2937.

27. Dahl SG, Allain P, Marie PJ, Mauras Y, Boivin G, Ammann P, Tsouderos Y, Delmas PD, Christiansen C, Incorporation and distribuition of strontium in bone, *Bone*, **28**(4), 2001, pp. 446–453.

28. Marie P J, Ammann P, Boivin G, Rey C, Mechanism of action and therapeutic potential of strontium in bone, *Calcif Tissue Int*, **69**(3), 2001, pp. 121–129.

29. Coulombe J, Faure H, Robin B, Ruat M, In vitro effects of strontium ranelate on the extracellular calcium-sensing receptor, *Biochem Biophys Res*, **323**(4), 2004, pp. 1184–1190.

30. Brown E M, Is the calcium receptor a molecular target for the actions of strontium on bone? *Osteoporos Int*, 14 Suppl 3, 2003, pp. 25–34.

31. Tat S K, Pelletier J P, Mineau F, Caron J, Martel-Pelletier J, Strontium ranelate inhibits key factors affecting bone remodeling in human osteoarthritic subchondral bone osteoblasts, *Bone*, **49**(3), (2011) pp. 559–567.

32. Logroscino G, Proietti L, Pola E, Spine fusion: Cages, plates and bone substitute, in *Biomaterials for Spinal Surgery*, (Ambrosio L, Tanner E, ed): Woodhead publishing in materials, 2012.

33. Landi E, Tampieri A, Celotti G, Sprio S, Sandri M, Logroscino G, Sr-substituted hydroxyapatites for osteoporotic bone replacement, *Acta Biomater*, **3**(6), 2007, pp. 961–969.

34. Lewiecki EM, Miller PD, Skeletal effects of primary hyper-parathyroidism: Bone mineral density and fracture risk, *J Clin Densitom*, **16**(1), 2013, pp. 28–32.

35. Wauquier F, Leotoing L, Coxam V, Guicheux J, Wittrant Y, Oxidative stress in bone remodelling and disease, *Trends Mol Med*, **15**(10), 2009, pp. 468–477.

36. Li H, Chang J, Bioactive silicate materials stimulate angiogenesis in fibroblast and endothelial cell co-culture system through paracrine effect, *Acta Biomater*, **9**(6), 2013, pp. 6981–6991.

37. Reffitt DM, Ogston N, Jugdaohsingh R, Cheung HF, Evans BA, Thompson RP, Powell JJ, Hampson G N, Orthosilicic acid stimulates collagen type 1 synthesis and osteoblastic differentiation in human osteoblast-like cells in vitro, *Bone*, **32**(2), 2003, pp. 127–135.

38. Patel N, Brooks R A, Clarke M T, Lee P M, Rushton N, Gibson I R, Best S M, Bonfield W, In vivo assessment of hydroxyapatite and silicate-substituted hydroxyapatite granules using an ovine defect model, *Mater Sci*, **16**(5), 2005, pp. 429–440.

39. Sprio S, Tampieri A, Landi E, Sandri M, Martorana S, Celotti G, Logroscino G, Physico-chemical properties and solubility behaviour of multi-substituted hydroxyapatite powders containing silicon, *Mater Sci Eng C*, **c-28**, 2008, pp. 179–187.

40. Bose S, Tarafder S, Banerjee SS, Davies NM, Bandyopadhyay A, Understanding in vivo response and mechanical property variation in MgO, SrO and $SiO_2$ doped b-TCP, *Bone*, **48**(6), 2011, pp. 1282–1290.

41. Khan SN, Cammisa FP Jr, Sandhu HS, Diwan AD, Girardi FP, Lane JM, The biology of bone grafting, *J Am Acad Orthop Surg*, **13**(1), 2005, pp. 77–86.

42. Iafisco M, Ruffini A, Adamiano A, Sprio S, Tampieri A, Biomimetic magnesium-carbonate-apatite nanocrystals endowed with strontium ions as anti-osteoporotic trigger, *Mater Sci Eng C Mater Biol Appl*, **35**, 2014, pp. 212–219.

43. Keselowsky BG, Collard DM, García AJ, Surface chemistry modulates fibronectin conformation and directs integrin binding and specificity to control adhesion, *J Biomed Mater Res Part A*, **66**(2), 2003, pp. 247–259.

44. Fujii E, Ohkubo M, Tsuru K, Hayakawa S, Osaka A, Kawabata K, Bonhomme C, Babonneau F, Selective protein adsorption property

and characterization of nano-crystalline zinc-containing hydroxyapatite, *Acta Biomater*, **2**(1), 2006, pp. 69–74.

45. Li B, Liao X, Zheng L, Zhu X, Wang Z, Fan H, Zhang X, Effect of nanostructure on osteoinduction of porus biphasic calcium phosphate ceramics, *Acta Biomater*, **8**(10), 2012, pp. 3794–3804.

46. Zhu XD, Zhang HJ, Fan HS, Li W, Zhang XD, Effect of phase composition and microstructure of calcium phosphate ceramic particles on protein adsorption, *Acta Biomater*, **6**(4), 2010, pp. 1536–1541.

47. Zhu XD, Fan HS, Xiao YM, Li DX, Zhang HJ, Luxbacher T, Zhang XD, Effect of surface structure on protein adsorption to biphasic calcium-phosphate ceramics in vitro and in vivo, *Acta Biomater*, **5**(4), 2009, pp. 1211–1218.

48. Dos Santos LA, de Oliveira LC, da Silva Rigo EC, Carrodéguas RG, Boschi AO, Fonseca de Arruda AC, Fibre reinforced calcium phospathe cement, *Artif Organs*, **24**(3), 2000, pp. 212–216.

49. Beaudoin JJ, *Handbook of Fibre-Reinforced Concrete*. New Jersey: Noyes Publication, 1990.

50. Canal C, Ginebra M P, Fibre-reinforced calcium phosphate cements: A review, *J Mech Behav Biomed Mater*, **4**(8), 2011, pp. 1658–1671.

51. Klein CP, de Blieck-Hogervorst JM, Wolke JG, de Groot K, Studies of the solubility of different calcium phosphate ceramic particles in vitro, *Biomaterials*, **11**(7), 1990, pp. 509–512.

52. Barrère F, van Blitterswijk CA, de Groot K, Bone regeneration: Molecular and cellular interactions with calcium phosphate ceramics, *Int J Nanomed*, **1**(3), 2006, pp. 317–332.

53. Bell LC, Mika H, Kruger BJ, Synthetic hydroxyapatite-solubility product and stechiometry of dissolution, *Arch Oral Biol*, **23**(5), 1978 pp. 329–336.

54. Barba M, Cicione C, Bernardini C, Campana V, Pagano E, Michetti F, Logroscino G, Lattanzi W, Spinal fusion in the next generation: Gene and cell therapy approaches, *Sci World J*, 2014; 406159. doi: 10.1155/2014/406159. eCollection 2014.

55. Campana V, Milano G, Pagano E, Barba M, Cicione C, Salonna G, Lattanzi W, Logroscino G, Bone substitutes in orthopaedic surgery: from basic science to clinical practice, *J Mater Sci Mater Med*, vol. (Epub ahead of print), May 28, 2014.

56. Khan SN, Tomin E, Lane JM, Clinical applications of bone graft substitutes, *Orthop Clin North Am*, **31**(3), 389–398, 2000.

57. Murphy MB, Moncivais K, Caplan AI, Mesenchymal stem cells: Environmentally responsive therapeutics for regenerative medicine, *Exp Mol Med*, **15**, 2013, pp. 45–54.

58. Caplan AI, Review: Mesenchymal stem cells: Cell-based reconstructive therapy in orthopedics, *Tissue Eng*, **11**, 2005, pp. 7–8.

59. Boden SD, Titus L, Hair G, Liu Y, Viggeswarapu M, Nanes MS, Baranowski C, Lumbar spine fusion by local gene therapy with a cDNA encoding a novel osteoinductive protein (LMP-1), *Spine*, **23**(23), 1998, pp. 2486–2492.

60. Viggeswarapu M, Boden SD, Liu Y, Hair GA, Louis-Ugbo J, Murakami H, Kim HS, Mayr MT, Hutton WC, Titus L, Adenoviral delivery of LIM mineralization protein-1 induces new-bone formation in vitro and in vivo, *J Bone Joint Surg Am*, Mar; **83-A**(3), 2001, pp. 364–376.

61. Pola E, Gao W, Zhou Y, Pola R, Lattanzi W, Sfeir C, Gambotto A, Robbins PD, Efficient bone formation by gene transfer of human LIM mineralization protein-3, **11**(8), 2004, pp. 683–693.

62. Lattanzi W, Parrilla C, Fetoni A, Logroscino G, Straface G, Pecorini G, Stigliano E, Tampieri A, Bedini R, Pecci R, Michetti F, Gambotto A, Robbins PD, Pola E, "Ex vivo-transduced autologous skin fibroblasts expressing human Lim mineralization protein-3 efficiently form new bone in animal models", *Gene Ther*, vol. 15, no. 19, pp. 1330–1343, Oct 2008.

63. Barba M, Pirozzi F, Saulnier N, Vitali T, Natale MT, Logroscino G, Robbins PD, Gambotto A, Neri G, Michetti F, Pola E, Lattanzi W, Lim Mineralization Protein 3 induces the osteogenic differentiation of Human Amniotic Fluid Stromal Cells through Kruppel-like Factor-4 down-regulation and further bone-specific gene expression, *J Biomed Biotechnol*, 2012: 813894. doi: 10.1155/2012/813894. Epub 2012 Oct 2.2012.

64. Lane JM, Bone morphogenic protein science and studies, *J Orthop Trauma*, **19**(10 Suppl), 2005, pp. S17–S22.

65. Mahantesha, Shobha KS, Mani R, Deshpande A, Seshan H, Kranti K, Clinical and radiographic evaluation of demineralized bone matrix (grafton) as a bone graft material in the treatment of human periodontal intraosseous defects, *J Indian Soc Periodontol*, **17**(4), 2013, pp. 495–502.

66. Kinney RC, Ziran BH, Hirshorn K, Schlatterer D, Ganey T, Demineralized bone matrix for fracture healing: Fact or fiction?, *J Orthop Trauma*, 2010, **24**(Suppl 1), pp. S52–S55, 2010.

67. Grabowski G, Cornett CA, Bone graft and bone graft substitutes in spine surgery: Current concepts and controversies, *J Am Acad*, **21**(1), pp. 51–60, 2013.

68. Witte LD, Kaplan KL, Nossel HL, Lages BA, Weiss HJ, Goodman DS, Studies of the release from human platelets of thegrowth factor for cultured human arterial smooth muscle cells, *Circ Res*, **42**(3), 1978, pp. 402–409.

69. Kaplan KL, Broekman MJ, Chernoff A, Lesznik GR, Drillings M, Platelet alpha-granule proteins: Studies on release and subcellularlocalization, *Blood*, **53**(4), 1979, pp. 604–618.

70. Ross R, Vogel A, The platelet-derived growth factor, *Cell*, **14**(2), 1978, pp. 203–210.

71. Kitoh H, Kawasumi M, Kaneko H, Ishiguro N, Differential effects of culture-expanded bone marrow cells on the regeneration of bone between the femoral and the tibial lengthenings, *J Pediatr Orthop*, **29**(6), 2009, pp. 643–649.

72. Tsai CH, Hsu HC, Chen YJ, Lin MJ, Chen HT, Using the growth factors-enriched platelet glue in spinal fusion and its efficiency, *J Spinal Disord Tech*, **22**(4), 2009, pp. 246–250.

73. Castro FP Jr, Role of activated growth factors in lumbar spinal fusions, *J Spinal Disord Tech*, **17**(5), 2004, pp. 380–384.

74. Weiner BK, Walker M, Efficacy of autologous growth factors in lumbar intertransverse fusions, *Spine*, **28**(17), 2003, pp. 1968–1970.

75. Miyazono K, Maeda S, Imamura T, BMP receptor signaling: Transcriptional targets, regulation of signals, and signaling crosstalk", *Cytokine Growth Factor Rev*, **6**(3), 2005, pp. 251–263.

76. Wu X, Shi W, Cao X, Multiplicity of BMP signaling in skeletal development, *Ann N Y Acad Sci*, **1116**, 2007, pp. 29–49.

# Chapter 15

# Bioartificial Endocrine Organs: At the Cutting Edge of Translational Research in Endocrinology*

Roberto Toni,[a,b,k] Elena Bassi,[a] Fulvio Barbaro,[a] Nicoletta Zini,[c] Alessandra Zamparelli,[a] Marco Alfieri,[a] Davide Dallatana,[a] Salvatore Mosca,[a] Claudia della Casa,[a] Cecilia Gnocchi,[d] Giuseppe Lippi,[e] Giulia Spaletta,[f] Elena Bassoli,[g] Lucia Denti,[g] Andrea Gatto,[g] Francesca Ricci,[h] Pier Luigi Tazzari,[h] Annapaola Parrilli,[i] Milena Fini,[i] Monica Sandri,[j] Simone Sprio,[j] and Anna Tampieri[j]

[a]*Department of Biomedical, Biotechnological and Translational Sciences (S.Bi.Bi.T), Laboratory of Regenerative Morphology and Bioartificial Structures/S.Bi.Bi.T. Museum, Section of Human Anatomy, University of Parma School of Medicine, Parma, Italy*
[b]*Unit of Anthropometry and Constitutional Medicine, Center for Sport and Exercise Medicine, University of Parma School of Medicine, Parma, Italy*
[c]*CNR—National Research Council of Italy, IGM, IOR, Bologna, Italy*
[d]*Laboratory of Hematochemistry, Maggiore Hospital—Parma, Italy*
[e]*Clinical Biochemistry Section, Department of Biomedical and Motor Neurological Sciences, University of Verona, Verona, Italy*
[f]*Department of Mathematics, University of Bologna, Bologna, Italy*
[g]*Department of Engineering "Enzo Ferrari" (DIEF), University of Modena and Reggio Emilia, Modena, Italy*
[h]*Blood Transfusion Medicine, Saint Orsola—Malpighi Hospital, Bologna, Italy*
[i]*Laboratories of Preclinical and Surgical Studies, and Biocompatibility, Innovative Technologies, and Advanced Therapies (BITTA), Rizzoli Research Innovation Technology (RIT), IOR, Bologna, Italy*
[j]*ISTEC—CNR, Faenza, Italy*
[k]*Department of Medicine, Division of Endocrinology, Diabetes and Metabolism, Tufts Medical Center—Tufts University School of Medicine, Boston, MA, USA*

roberto.toni@unipr.it, roberto.toni@unibo.it, roberto.toni@tufts.edu

---

*This work is dedicated to the memory of Giorgio Toni, on occasion of the 12th anniversary of his demise, in recognition of his pioneering studies on mammalian morphogenesis that provided innovative perspectives on the role played by the stromal and vascular structures in addressing cell fate and activity during embryonic and adult life. His work has been of great inspiration to the concept of organomorphic bioengineering introduced here.

*Bio-Inspired Regenerative Medicine: Materials, Processes, and Clinical Applications*
Edited by Simone Sprio and Anna Tampieri
Copyright © 2016 Pan Stanford Publishing Pte. Ltd.
ISBN 978-981-4669-14-6 (Hardcover), 978-981-4669-15-3 (eBook)
www.panstanford.com

**358** | *Bioartificial Endocrine Organs*

## 15.1 Introduction

Bioartificial endocrine organs comprise classical endocrine glands, and soft (parenchyma) and hard (mineralized) tissue organs involved in endocrine-metabolic regulation. These bioconstructs are one of the newest promises of regenerative medicine, but their bioengineering "on the laboratory bench" and thus, outside the living body (i.e. ex situ) remains a substantial challenge [1, 2]. Based on current concepts [3–5], bioartificial endocrine organs can be engineered ex situ using macroscopic, three-dimensional (3D) scaffolds that mimic the 3D architecture of the native, organ stromal support (here coined *organomorphism*) reproduced with either natural or synthetic biomaterials. Once pluripotent stem cells, tissue-committed progenitors, and differentiated primary cells are seeded and co-cultured with the organomorphic scaffold, their self-assembly is expected up to the formation of a 3D macroscopic, functional and immuno-tolerant organ, replicating the native one. However, 3D systems exhibiting appropriate flow and trophic performance (bioreactor) are required to maximize homing, survival, growth, and differentiation/transdifferentiation of seeded elements [3, 6, 7]. Embryonic stem cells (ESCs) and induced pluripotent stem cells are also raising hopes as valuable sources to bioengineer human bioartificial viscera [8, 9]; thus, in the near future they may become another option to reconstruct ex situ bioartificial endocrine organs.

### 15.1.1 Basic Principles for ex situ Growth and Differentiation of Endocrine Cells to Engineer Complex, 3D Organomorphic Bioconstructs

In the first step, source cells (ideally adult, autologous stem cells/ progenitors) are isolated from native organs, and in vitro seeded, grown, and expanded using bidimensional (2D) plates. This process may also take place in suspension without adhesion, or inside a 3D gel environment (collagen, basal membrane extract—Matrigel), depending on the type of progenitor elements. Cells, then, are moved to a dynamic bioreactor system that includes either a 3D biocompatible scaffold or a 3D acellular natural matrix as a support. The geometry of these supports can either be random or similar to that of the native organ (i.e. be organomorphic);

in addition, the scaffolds can either be physical or virtual, and specifically: (1) *physical scaffolds*, whose (a) natural supports, like acellular organomorphic matrixes, are obtained by decellularization of a congener organ and, (b) synthetic supports, made of either bioerodible polymers (e.g. esters of $\alpha$-hydroxy acids including the polylactic or PLLA and polyglycolic and/or their blends, and lactone polyesters like poly-$\varepsilon$-caprolactone or PCL) or organic products like collagen, proteoglycans, agarose, alginate, gelatin, chitosan, hyaluronic acid, and fibronectin among others, are assembled using a number of reverse engineering techniques, to provide a 3D substrate for growth of seeded cells [10, 11]; (2) *virtual scaffolds*, are initially "drawn" under guidance of a software, to address cells into a pre-shaped context (e.g. bio-printing and bio-plotting) [12, 13] and, later transformed as either 3D holographic, electromagnetic, magnetic, or two-phase liquid fields using photons, electric charges, paramagnetic nanoparticles, and solutions of compounds at different viscosity, to push cells into pre-ordered growth trajectories [14–17]. As a result, these "templates" obligate the seeded elements to organize into ordered, 3D architectures like cylinders, spheres, cords, prismatic spaces, folded layers, angled planes, nets and lattice. Thus, it is clear that to bioengineer ex situ a desired 3D cell assembly it must be present a 3D "scaffold", either physical or virtual. Figure 15.1 summarizes the biophysical and geometrical principles supporting the self-assembly of cells growing onto 3D scaffolds.

In a further step, an adequate cell-scaffold interface can be provided through extracellular proteins/ramified sugars able to act as a sort of "glue" for seeded cells, and cells are stimulated to proliferate by appropriate growth factors and specific physical stimuli (e.g. perfusion/perifusion flow of culture media, constant $O_2$ supply, metabolic waste removal, shear stress, mechanical stretching) [22–24]. In a last step, the bioartificial organ is transplanted into a host living organism, and its vascular supply provided by local vessels, i.e. by natural in situ re-vascularization, especially whether it is implanted inside tissue highly conductive for vessel formation (subepidermal layer, serosa, kidney capsule) [25–27]. In this manner, it should not be necessary to reproduce ex situ the intrinsic vascularization of the bioengineered organ. However, offering to the extrinsic vessels elective pathways for penetration into the bioconstruct, possibly recapitulating the

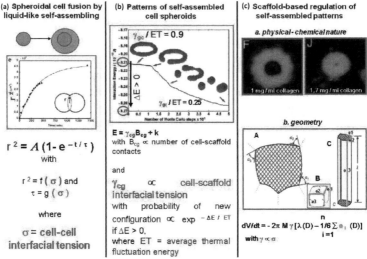

**Figure 15.1** (A) Developing cells may behave like water droplets. Their fusion into a higher degree spheroid occurs as function of cell–cell interfacial tension $\sigma$, through change in the circular interfacial area $A$ having instantaneous squared radius $r^2$; as a result, the higher is $\sigma$, the wider is $A$ and the larger is $r^2$; (B) spontaneously formed, multicellular spheroids may 3D arrange in metastable (i.e. stable at weak equilibrium) geometrical structures (e.g. toroidal-like patterns) depending on the energy of interaction between the spheroids and the surrounding environment (scaffold/matrix). The cell–environment interfacial tension $\gamma_{cg}$ is a critical parameter, with the highest probability to keep a metastable pattern in the presence of maximal $\gamma_{cg}$ and minimal fluctuations in average biological thermal energy ET; (C) The physical-chemical properties of the scaffold/matrix are key factors for changes in cell–environment interfacial tension, with metastable (ring-like) patterns occurring at low environmental content in collagen (F); in contrast, collapse to a multi-spheroidal bulk occurs at higher environmental content in collagen (J). In addition, changes in the volume of assembling spheroids also depend on the 3D geometry of the environment (scaffold/matrix). Indeed, the interposition of scaffold branches between adjacent cell domains reduces the available triplets of contact edges ($\alpha_1$–$\alpha_3$ angles in $A \equiv e_1$–$e_3$ edges in B, C) between microstructures (term $e_i$ on the right-hand-side of the equation being the length of the i-th triple edge), limiting their volume increase (term $dV/dt$ on the left-hand-side of the equation) [from 2, 18–21, partly modified].

original vascular trajectories present in the natural, end-stage structure could improve the process of revascularization. Indeed, by assuming the ex situ regeneration as a process occurring in a developing structure [28], it is expected that the vascular geometry may play per se a morphogenetic influence, especially in endocrine viscera [29–31]. Thus, the presence of a scaffold geometrically reproducing the vascular arborisation of the natural organ might ensure a physiological endothelial/epithelial interface during the process of in vivo revascularization. To this end, we have initiated a research program focussed on the development of innovative reverse engineering technologies to prototype with biomaterials ramified, vascular-like scaffolds reproducing the intrinsic arterial tree of human and rat, parenchymal and endocrine organs [32–35]. This with the intent to overcome the limitations in structural resolution of current additive layer manufacturing techniques.

## 15.1.2 Lessons from Embryonic Development for an ex situ Developmental Bioengineering of Endocrine Organs: The Organomorphic Principle

The evidence that to reconstruct "on the laboratory bench" a 3D organ requires a 3D substrate for seeded cells, either physical (acellular organomorphic matrix, scaffold of biocompatible material) or virtual (machine-driven deposition of cells) is the reflection of a general biological property of embryonic development, including that of endocrine glands. In fact, during in vivo organogenesis stem cells and precursor elements (i.e. progenitors, and transient amplifying cells) acquire different phenotypes (immunotolerance included) depending upon the geometry of their host environment or "niche" [36], a phenomenon proved to occur also in bioengineered contexts [37, 38]. In particular, factors related to the 3D geometry of the system, like elasticity and stiffness of the extracellular matrix strongly contribute to address cell fate [39, 40]. Therefore, the 3D architecture of cell assembly and its inherent physical-chemical properties are fundamental to regulate expansion and functional differentiation of the resident cells.

In addition, the need of a pre-defined environmental "geometry" for ex situ growth of cells towards a specific 3D morphology is in agreement with the experimental evidence that the 3D architecture of the cell seeding context is highly influential to their phenotype fate [41, 42]. In particular, as predicted by the morphoregulatory theory of topobiology, the tissue environmental geometry provides a mechano-chemical regulation on cell growth and differentiation [43]. Specifically, the morphoregulatory input induces histodifferentiation and, thus, brings about organ functional activity. As a result, organ physical topology becomes coincidental with organ signal topology (Fig. 15.2) [44].

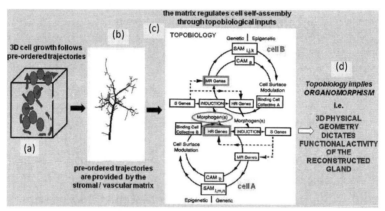

**Figure 15.2** (a) In a 3D environment, the geometry of the vectors representing the average mechanical/elastic forces naturally involved during growth and differentiation of seeded cells tends to coincide with (b) the geometry of the natural stromal/vascular scaffold (SVS) of the forming organ. As such, growing cells are expected to receive a key mechano-chemical input from the geometry of the SVS per se. Indeed, based on the topobiology theory (c) the scaffold-based signal is transmitted to the growing cells (cell A) through interaction with cell-(CAM) and substrate-(SAM) adhesion molecules, resulting in induction of historegulatory (HR) genes (i.e. tissue-specific), and release of specific morphogens. The morphogens induce selector (S) genes (e.g. homeotics) in adjacent cell clusters (cell B), giving rise to simultaneous activation of both morphoregulatory (MR) and new HR genes, eventually leading to a chain reaction that "guides" cellular self-assembly to a specific organ shape (provided by morphoregulatory molecules) and function (provided by historegulatory molecules). This mechanism (d) leads to a coincidence between physical topology of cell aggregates and signal topology of growing and differentiating cells, making changes in 3D organ shape critical to the maturation of organ physiological performance [from 2, 43, partly modified].

To this purpose, recent studies in mouse models have shown that in endoderm-derived endocrine organs, like the liver and pancreatic islets, specific morphogens are released by the cardiac and diaphragmatic mesoderm surrounding the ventral multipotent endoderm at a very early embryonic age (six somites), to induce competence and specification of domains destined to become the liver, whereas inhibiting those for ventral pancreas. Thus, it is clear that the embryonic source of the forthcoming connective and vascular tissue (i.e. the mesoderm) regulates the commitment of those endodermal cells destined to give rise to the 3D liver parenchyma. Indeed, in the post-specification step mesoderm-derived, fibroblasts and endothelial cells invade the primitive, endodermal hepatic bud to favour a peculiar 3D laminar organization of hepatoblasts (hepatic cords) into the liver parenchyma, simultaneously inducing selective enzymatic activities in dependence on cell position within the hepatic cords [31]. In a very similar manner, during the post-specification step of pancreas mesoderm-derived, fibroblasts from the notochord and endothelial cells from the dorsal aorta migrate into both dorsal and ventral pancreatic buds, favouring the 3D and functional "patterning" of endocrine islets [29]. Finally, knock-out studies have shown that pharyngeal mesoderm-dependent genes (like Sonic Hedgehog, Hoxa5, and Tbx1), as well as neural-crest derived ectomesenchyma (i.e. primitive connective tissue of neuroectodermal origin) may regulate thyroid size and vascularisation, suggesting a permissive role of mesoderm in mammalian thyroid morphogenesis [45–47] (Fig. 15.3).

Therefore, in endoderm-derived endocrine organs like the liver, pancreatic islets, and thyroid the inner stromal/vascular scaffold (SVS), i.e. the natural organomorphic matrix, may act as a pivotal mechano-chemical information for growth and differentiation of stem and progenitor cells during morphogenesis. As a result, endocrine bioconstructs engineered ex situ are expected to become biologically similar to the native endocrine organ as much as accurate provision of structural and functional factors involved in the natural development and physiological maturation come into play. In particular, the presence of a 3D context reproducing ex situ the geometrical, physical and biochemical properties of the inner SVS seems to be a key factor to elicit the morphogenetic potential of cultured cells, and establish a reconstruction procedure retracing their developmental steps. In conclusion, a generic 3D architecture of the scaffold/matrix seems not sufficient to bioengineer ex situ an entire and functional 3D organ. In fact, the 3D growing architecture dictates the functional differentiation of the resident cells. Consequently, only a 3D geometry of the scaffold recapitulating that of the supporting and trophic system in the parent organ may fulfil the scale requirements necessary to guide ex situ cell auto-assembly up to the formation of a viable and physiologically competent, macroscopic endocrine organ.

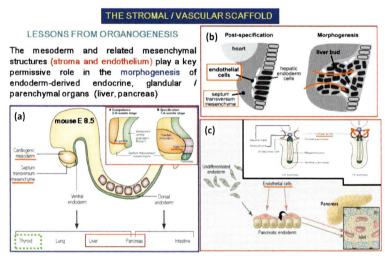

**Figure 15.3** Early embryonic development of endoderm-derived, endocrine organs (liver and pancreatic islets) in the mouse. (a) Sagittal schematics of the six-somite age, mouse embryo. The mesoderm (light orange) adjacent to the primitive endodermal tube (green) regulates commitment of liver and pancreatic buds (and also that of thyroid and lungs); (b) early post-specification step of liver morphogenesis. Mesoderm-derived cells (stromal and endothelial) enter the multipotent endodermal cell groups of the liver, to laminate the future hepatic parenchyma; (c) early post-specification step of pancreas morphogenesis. Mesoderm-derived cells (stromal and endothelial) from the notochord and dorsal aorta (orange arrows in the upper inset) invade the multipotent endodermal cell groups of the dorsal and ventral pancreas, to induce 3D organization of endocrine pancreatic islets (lower inset) [from 29, 31, partly modified].

### 15.1.3 Current Results on ex situ Bioengineering of Bioartificial Endocrine Organs

In the case of endocrine organs, a primary problem is the lack of a general model of 3D organomorphic scaffolding onto which grow the seeded cells, up to the formation of different tissues and their self-assembly in entire 3D organs. In addition, no adequate artificial device (i.e. bioreactor) has yet been identified to homogeneously irrigate the seeded cells throughout the thickness of the solid regenerating parenchyma, although recent hollow fibre systems have provided encouraging results with the liver [48, 49]. In particular, it is well known that in the presence of cell layers thicker than 0.2–0.5 mm, oxygen ($O_2$) and culture media cannot adequately penetrate the depth of the growing endocrine mass, and cell necrosis ensues [50, 51]. This is the reason why we believe that the technique (called "cell-sheets") to in vitro seed cells in a sandwich-like context where layers of developing tissue alternate with layers of biocompatible "matrix" (corresponding to a geometrically amorphous support) is not suitable to ex situ bioengineer entire 3D endocrine glands, but only parts of their tissues.

A number of attempts have been made to partially reconstruct endocrine tissues using the cell-sheet technology, amorphous gels, reticular matrices, and 3D biocompatible scaffolds without any organomorphic geometry. In rodents, both ESCs and dissociated pancreatic cells have been induced in vitro to re-organize as groups of insulin-producing cells, and single functional islets [26, 52, 53]; isolated secondary ovarian follicles have been grown up to multilayer follicles, and successfully used for in vitro fertilization [54]; both ESCs overexpressing thyroid transcription factors, and differentiated thyrocytes after mechanical dispersion have been observed to in vitro self-organize into uni- and multicellular follicles, especially when cultured in a 3D system, and to form layers of functional thyroid tissue [55–57]; parathyroid cells have been assembled in functional organoids [58]; and an embryonic anterior pituitary bud has been reconstructed from ESCs committed by forced gene expression to multipotent pituitary cells, eventually differentiated to secretory phenotypes [59]. Preliminary data have also been published on the use of biocompatible templates mimicking the 3D macroscopic morphology of the rat testis and human ovary. In the case of the testis, Sertoli cells seeded on this support have been able to differentiate into testicular cords [60]. In the case of the ovary, human theca interna cells colonizing the honeycomb-like spaces of an ovarian matrix phantom made of agarose were observed to promote self-assembling of cumulus granulosa-oocyte complexes up to the formation of mature oocytes with polar bodies and theca layers [61]. Finally, it has been recently shown that the decellularized natural stroma of pig adrenals may allows for cell proliferation and cortisol production by in vitro seeded human embryonic adrenocortical cells [62]. All these results suggests that the application of the organomorphic principle to the construction of the scaffold/matrix may become a key factor for successfully bioengineer ex situ entire 3D endocrine organs.

## 15.2 The New Concept of the Organomorphic Scaffold-Bioreactor Unit for Endocrine Organ Bioengineering

Based on the above-mentioned premises, in 2007 we have proposed an innovative concept for the ex situ bioengineering of endocrine organs, and we have applied it to the bioengineering of an anatomically simple gland, the thyroid. We have designed with biocompatible material a scaffold–bioreactor unit that reproduces both the 3D native morphology of the human thyroid SVS and the natural thyrocyte/vascular flow interface [63]. We have reasoned that the thyroid contains only two secretory cell types, whose thyrocytes are the main component. Thyrocytes are organized into a highly regular 3D microstructure, the spherical follicles that, to a higher degree of architecture are arranged into irregular polyhedrons, called lobules. At a higher geometrical level, the lobules are packed together into conic-like or oval-like 3D volumes, called lobes. We have observed that the 3D macro-microscopic geometry of the natural, SVS of the lobes replicates the macro-microscopic follicular and lobular anatomy in a fractal-like manner [34, 64], i.e. is organomorphic (Fig. 15.4). In simple words, the SVS can be considered the equivalent of a "photographic negative"

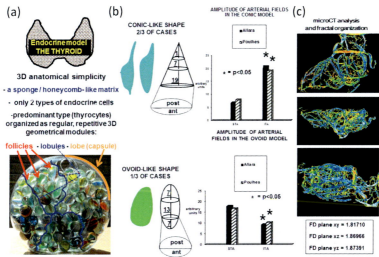

**Figure 15.4** (a) Structural organization of the mammalian, thyroid gland. The thyroid architecture is based on a sponge-like matrix made of stromal (connective) bundles, blood vessels and nerves (or stromal/vascular scaffold—SVS), the latter two components coursing inside the fibrous trusses of the SVS. A single predominant cell type occurs (thyrocytes), allocated in spherical structures (follicles), further organized in prismatic- and/or pyramidal-like modules (lobules), collectively gathered inside large volumes (lobes), surrounded by a stromal "wrapping" (capsule); (b) through retrospective analysis of published anatomical data (Allara E., 1936; Pouhels et al., 1952) we have determined that the amplitude of the intralobar thyroid vascularisation (superior thyroid artery or STA and inferior thyroid artery or ITA) is influenced by the macroscopic 3D geometry (either conic-like or ovoidal) of the thyroid lobes. Volumes for arterial arborisation corresponding to thirds of a regular cone and ovoid are depicted inside each geometrical figure. This has suggested that each lobe is organized as a topological space, where the SVS components are strictly interrelated, including thyrocytes [63, 65]; (c) indeed, through prospective studies based microCT, and computer analysis of vascular casts from cadaveric glands, we have found a consistent degree of auto-similarity (fractal dimension or FD) in the anatomy of the SVS, suggesting that the lobe is a space phase where growing thyrocytes may self-assemble guided by the rules of the chaotic attractor inherent the SVS geometry [34, 64].

of the lobe architecture [2, 65]. Finally, we have analyzed whether this assumption fulfils the theoretical and experimental requirements to guide 3D growth and differentiation of thyrocyte stem/progenitor cells and, possibly, also that of vascular endothelial precursor cells [2, 66–68].

### 15.2.1 Design of a Thyromorphic, Scaffold-Bioreactor Unit for ex situ Bioengineering, and Its Application to Patient-Tailored Bioconstructs

The basic concepts supporting the design of our thyromorphic, scaffold-bioreactor unit are shown in Fig. 15.5. The modelling significantly differs from current and popular ideas how to regenerate/reconstruct both endocrine and non-endocrine soft tissue organs, and take inspiration from the morphogenetic role exerted by the SVS. It is based on a microporous, biodegradable replica of the adult thyroid SVS, serving as a conductive pathway for trophic solutions and colonizing cells. It is equipped with a double media supply driven by peristaltic pumps, consisting of a high pressure perfusion through the microporous channels, mimicking the natural intraglandular vessels, and a low pressure perifusion bathing a highly hydrophilic, amorphous field of low/intermediate viscosity material (e.g. polysaccharides, collagen) constituting the seeding space. In this manner, the perfusate can percolate throughout this viscous volume down to the length of the SVS, where it can both re-enter the channel system of the scaffold, and be filtered through a membrane, where tissue catabolic wastes accumulates. The membrane can be changed at specific time intervals to avoid increase of toxins and cellular debris at the base of the scaffold.

Alternatively, the perifusate can continuously bath the surface of the viscous seeding space, thus its peripheral convective flow would be expected to drain cellular waste at the limits of the reactor through an external circuit. Computational fluid dynamic assessment is introduced, to accommodate and maximize performance to cell growth. A minimal shear stress of growing cells is expected, due to the organ-specific geometry of the scaffold, favouring morphogenesis. This system is believed to exhibit a high tissue convection of $O_2$, due to (1) increase in extravascular medium re-circulation, (2) increase in $O_2$ flow to the external surface of clustered cells and (3) increase in $O_2$ diffusion to the internal cell mass. Flow-through $O_2$ sensor foils are integrated into the growing space to monitor cell-related $O_2$ changes. In this manner, the bioengineered SVS may provide a 3D replica of the natural vascular pathways, capable of conducting continuously culture media and $O_2$ inside the growing tissue mass, up to its finest levels [2, 63, 65]. A theoretical modelling of ex situ self-assembly of thyroid cells grown in a thyromorphic, scaffold-bioreactor unit is shown in Fig. 15.6.

In addition, since each individual has his own organ size and shape, and thus his own specific organ functional performance, the design of the unit is flexible enough to accommodate 3D geometrical constraints adequate to restrain the proliferation of the self-assembling cells within the physical limits of the

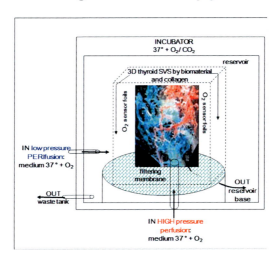

**Figure 15.5** Schematic view of our prototype of organomorphic scaffold-bioreactor unit for ex situ reconstruction of a bioartificial, human thyroid gland. The 3D microporous channels replicate the natural thyroid stromal/vascular scaffold, i.e. are organomorphic, and are believed to play a morphogenetic permissive role for seeded cells (either stem cells/progenitor, and differentiated elements). Based on their vessel-like geometry, they are expected to ensure a high culture medium and $O_2$ flow to the internal cell mass of the growing endocrine tissue [from 2, partly modified].

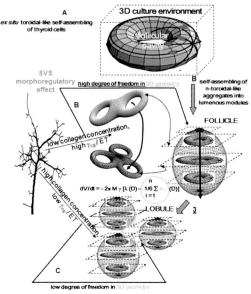

**Figure 15.6** Theoretical modelling of ex situ self-assembling of thyroid cells, including stem cells/progenitors and differentiated elements, when grown in a thyromorphic scaffold-bioreactor unit (for basic principles see Fig. 15.1). (A) in a 3D space at constant temperature (culture environment), single or few cells (red short arrow heads) spontaneously tend to give rise to metastable patterns (e.g. ring-like structures or toroids); (B) by initially interacting with sparse stromal bundles of the engineered SVS, cells experiment a high cell-scaffold interfacial tension, and low geometrical constraints. Although this condition may favour maintenance of the native metastable organization, the perfusion/perifusion dynamics of culture media increase the thermal energy of the environment, and self-aggregation of metastable patterns into luminous modules (follicle-like structures) is expected to occur. However, those patterns experimenting the lowest interfacial tension may lose stability, allowing for single cell replication (primarily stem cells/progenitors) and expansion of the cells mass; (C) the increase in the cell population favours interactions with progressively denser stromal bundles of the SVS. As a result, low cell-scaffold interfacial tension and high geometrical constraints occur. Thus, progressive reduction in accumulation of self-assembling follicles ensues, leading to a higher order of architecture (lobular structure). Supposedly, the entire process should take place via a feedback autoregulation, and a self-controlled inflation of the growing tissue should result.

organomorphic bioreactor. Such a condition can be satisfied by reproducing with fidelity the size and shape of the SVS of the specific subject at the time of clinical request. Although this may be a practical problem when anatomical and structural changes occur to the organ as a result of an underlying disorder (e.g. hyperplasia, inflammatory infiltration, cancer), thus distorting large part of its SVS, nevertheless general geometrical properties of the SVS may help to overcome this limit. In fact, in a normal soft tissue organ including the thyroid, the SVS is constituted by repetitive 3D ramified units that entangle the 3D macroscopic perimeter of the entire parenchymal mass. Therefore, knowing the geometrical/mathematical rules and variables governing the architecture of the repetitive units and their volume expansion within the 3D limits of the organ, it might be possible to predict the final shape and size of a specific patient-tailored SVS starting from any still unaffected, random area of the target organ.

To reach this aim, we have developed a computational algorithm (whose implementation is currently under study) able to reproduce both a fractal-like growth of the SVS, and the volume and shape of the organ, whose output is exportable in STL format adequate for reverse engineering [2, 33, 34, 63]. In particular, we have applied this procedure to the virtual simulation of a normal human thyroid SVS inside the volume of an adult thyroid lobe. In this manner, a complete 3D ramification of the SVS was obtained and its expansion restrained inside the natural limits of the mature parenchyma. To achieve this result, we have used mean vascular and lobar anatomical parameters, focussing our reconstruction to the vascular arborisation of second, third and fourth-order, intraglandular arteries. The origin of second-order branches onto the surface of the lobe was fixed to a number representing the average of normal anatomical combinations stemming from the superior and inferior thyroid arteries, and in a pattern reproducing that observable in the course of a standard selective angiography (Fig. 15.7). On these bases, a digital model of a patient-tailored, thyroid SVS can be obtained, and hopefully reproduced with a rapid prototyping technology [32, 33], eventually to be used as an organomorphic scaffold in a patient-tailored, thyromorphic bioreactor. On a broader perspective, we believe that with this methodology it will be possible to generate patient-tailored, simulations of complete SVS for a number of other endocrine glands and soft tissue organs at clinical request.

## 372 | Bioartificial Endocrine Organs

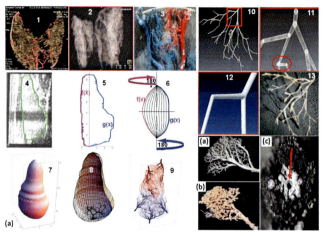

**Figure 15.7** Computational reconstruction of the intraglandular arterial matrix of the human thyroid lobe, and rapid prototyping of an isolated arterial branch. In a first step, a number of morphometric parameters including the mean intravascular calibers in relations to the order of arterial ramification, the numerosity of arterial branches, their binary splitting, and the putative fractal dimension were calculated from both in vivo angiotomographic images, and polyvinylic corrosion casts of the arterial distribution on the isolated, cadaveric gland (phases 1–3). In a second step, an in vivo 2D ultrasonographic image of the thyroid lobe (phase 4) was used to provide a 3D reconstruction of the lobar shape and volume (phases 5–7), the latter representing a fixed space for growth of an averaged 3D simulation (STL language) of the vascular matrix (phases 8–9). In a final step, the STL simulation of a single arterial branch was chosen (phase 10), its computational modelling corrected for edge radii, missing triangles, and inverted normals (phases 11–12), and physically reproduced with test resin, using additive layer manufacturing (Multi Jet Modelling, ProJetTM HD 3000, 3D Systems Inc.). Note the geometrical consistency between the digital and physical models (phase 13); (a) injection/corrosion cast of human kidney arteries made with polyvinylic resin, after spray-gun painting with colloidal silver paste (master); (b) copper shell mould produced by electroforming on the resin master; (c) inlet/outlet hole of a metallized, vascular branch after thermal dissolution of the master. The hole provides access for filling under vacuum the vascular spaces with biomaterials, thus allowing for faithful reproduction of the original 3D, vascular geometry [from 2, 32, 33, 65, partly modified].

## 15.2.2 Studies on the Role of the Native Stroma in Addressing the Morphogenesis of the Embryonic Human Thyroid Gland

To substantiate our concept of the morphoregulatory role played by the geometry of the native SVS, we conducted a series of morphological studies aimed at investigating the anatomical organization of the inner stromal scaffold in the early developing human thyroid, and the possible contribution of neural-crest derived elements to it [1]. This has been possible by profiting of the large collection of perfectly-preserved, human embryos at different Carnegie stages (CS) of development kept at the S.Bi.Bi.T. Museum in Parma, Italy. Using embryos at CS13 (first month from conception), we observed a close association of the thyroid bud with the mesodermic aortic sac. As a consequence, endodermal multipotent stem cells resulted organized in parallel, pseudostratified cords separated by linear spaces filled with fibrillary, stromal-like material. However, at CS19 (second month from conception) this structural arrangement was replaced by radial epithelial cords containing neural-crest derived, neuroendocrine cells immunopositive for chromogranin A. In addition, primitive follicular lumina were apparent, indicating initial steps of functional secretory differentiation of thyroblasts.

Based on these results, we have proposed a primary role for the embryonic stroma in addressing the post-specification morphogenesis of the human thyroid bud. Specifically, stromal cells from the surrounding mesoderm are believed to penetrate the mass of endodermal thyroid progenitors, and to deposit a mesodermal fibrillary component to induce their 3D lamination. This process would provide a mechano-chemical signal to favour differentiation of endodermal, multipotent stem cells into committed progenitor cells, like thyroblasts. Endothelial penetration/differentiation might subsequently induce thyroblasts proliferation, and decline in multipotent stem cells, as previously suggested to occur in humans at this developmental step [1]. In conclusion, it seems very likely that the 3D geometry of the natural stromal matrix acts per se in the developing thyroid to release a morphoregulatory input. This supports our proposal that the SVS plays a key role in addressing proliferation and fate of growing endocrine cells.

### 15.2.3 Studies on the Growth and Differentiation of Adult Rat Thyroid Cells in 3D Culture Systems

Our concepts of developmental bioengineering have received additional support from in vitro studies on adult rat thyroid cells grown in 3D culture. As opposed to adult thyrocytes grown on standard, 2D plastic plate where they spread randomically in a pavement-like pattern, thyrocytes seeded in a 3D Matrigel (12.5–50%) system depict stable growth trajectories. This behaviour is likely due to similarly-oriented vectors of mechanical/elastic forces, coming into play as a result of the 3D environment. In a 3D space, in fact, cell membrane adhesions and superficial tensions are expected to act on the entire cell surface, giving rise to an optimal shear stress. Thus, cells initially self-assemble into metastable (i.e. at weak equilibrium) high energy 3D patterns, like rings and morula-like spheres [2, 67, 68]. Shortly after, these spheres disappear and cells may either exhibit an epithelial-mesenchymal transition, or give rise to conventional follicles, suggesting mature phenotypes [58]. Therefore, it is clear that the 3D environment is a basic requirement to promote growth and differentiation of thyroid progenitor cells into functionally active thyrocytes [66–68].

In addition, when primary rat thyroid cells are cultured on a decellularized, 3D natural matrix of the rat thyroid lobe, and in the absence of any differentiating factor like TSH, they tend to spontaneously recellularize the decellularized, native follicular spaces. Consistently, thyroid hormones are released in the culture medium up to 7 days. Since we have shown that both differentiated cells, and stem cells/progenitors coexist in primary thyroid culture [16], these results suggest that the 3D geometry of the lobe matrix may guide both mature and immature elements to self-assemble into functional follicular units [66–68] (Fig. 15.8). In summary, all these evidences point to the concept that a thyromorphic (i.e. organomorphic to the thyroid) scaffold-bioreactor unit could act as an ideal device to promote the ex situ reconstruction of an entire, immuno-tolerant thyroid gland suitable for clinical transplantation.

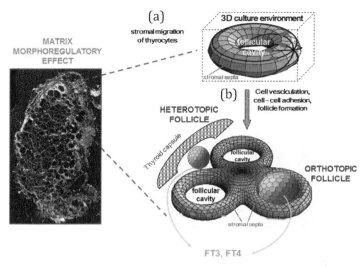

**Figure 15.8** Modelling of short-term, ex situ recellularization of the decellularized, rat thyroid lobe matrix in static culture, as reconstructed by recent experimental evidence of our group [1, 63, 66–69]. (a) The 3D geometry of the stromal septa of the matrix is believed to guide seeded thyroid cells including stem cells/progenitors and differentiated thyrocytes, ideally expected to self-assemble into functional follicular units, even in the absence of dynamic, bioreactor-based culture media flows, and differentiation factors like TSH; (b) cells self-assemble on the matrix via epithelial–mesenchymal transitions, migration through septa, cell vesciculation, cell–cell adhesion, and formation of single- and multiple-cell, follicle-like structures; (c) follicle-like structures may be generated either inside empty follicular spaces of the matrix (orthotopic follicles) or outside the original follicular cavities, like under the thyroid capsule (heterotopic follicles), and are able to release in the culture medium free thyroid hormones (FT3, FT4).

The robustness of our reasoning is currently confirmed by the evidence that recellularization of decellularized stromal matrixes of mammalian soft tissue organs including kidney, liver, pancreas and lungs has been obtained following injection of congener endothelial and parenchymal cells through the patent matrix

**376** | *Bioartificial Endocrine Organs*

vessels [70–74]. Unfortunately, immuno-tolerance of allogenic decellularized stromal matrices is virtually unknown [75] and, due to the presence of unremoved cell contaminants host-versus-graft reactions represent a risk upon transplantation [76], even if using autologous cells for recellularization. In contrast, in the presence of bioartificial structures based on biocompatible thermoplastic materials like PLLA and PCL, or natural compounds like collagen, chitosan, and alginate immunogenic reactions are expected to be minimal, or even absent. To conclude, also current literature data highlights the paramount importance of the relation between the 3D microanatomy of the intrinsic vascular tree and the adjacent parenchymal cells for ex situ bioengineering a thick mass of viable tissue, in particular endocrine organs.

## 15.2.4 Studies on the ex situ Bioengineering of the Rat Anterior Pituitary Gland, Adrenal Cortex, Thymus and Cerebral Neocortex

In an effort to extend the morphoregulatory role of the SVS to the ex situ bioengineering of other endocrine and soft tissue organs as a proof of concept, we have undertaken a number of experimental programs aimed at reconstructing on the laboratory bench the anterior pituitary, adrenal cortex, thymus and parts of the central nervous system, specifically the frontal neocortex.

Using as an experimental model the rat, observations have been made on the feasibility of decellularizing the natural SVS of the anterior pituitary gland, adrenal cortex, thymus and cerebral neocortex after surgical removal of the entire organs, and their processing with variable sequences of liquid N2 freezing at −80°C/ thawing at 4°C, followed by alternate washings with trypsin, Triton X-100, and deoxycholic acid for several days, or similar procedures. In this manner, we were able to detach the resident cells in the adenohypophysis, adrenal cortex and thymus, while preserving the 3D macro- and microscopic architecture of their SVS [1]. In contrast, cellular debris were found throughout the neocortex, although many areas remained devoid of neuronal and glial cell bodies, revealing the dense fibrillary textures (i.e. the cerebral "matrix") believed to serve as a natural SVS for 3D guidance of neural cell processes (Fig. 15.9) [77]. This last finding is in agreement with recent observations on the porcine brain [78].

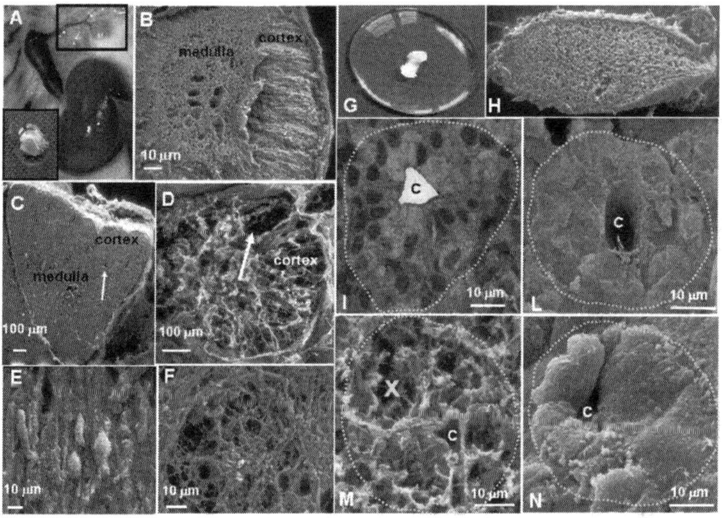

**Figure 15.9** (A) Rat adrenal gland in situ, and after surgical excision (inset); (B) scanning electron microscopy (SEM) image of the decellularized adrenal gland, including cortex and medulla; (C) SEM image of the rat thymic lobe. Arrow points to a vessel; (D) SEM image of the decellularized cortex (i.e. cortex matrix) of the rat thymus. Arrow points to a vessel; (E) SEM image of the rat frontal neocortex, layers 3–4. Note neuronal and glial perikarya; (F) SEM image of the decellularized rat frontal neocortex, layers 3–4. Note empty neuronal and glial spaces, and the dense fibrillary network of the cerebral matrix; (G) rat anterior pituitary gland after surgical excision, floating in a drop of buffer; (H) SEM image of the decellularized matrix of the rat anterior pituitary; (I) light microscopic appearance of rat anterior pituitary tissue (toluidine blue staining). Note the typical "rosette" (dotted line) of adenohypophysial cells (asterisk) around a blood capillary (c); (L) SEM image of a typical rat pituitary "rosette" (dotted line) around a capillary (c); (M) SEM image of the decellularized rat pituitary matrix. Note the empty cellular spaces (X) at the level of a typical "rosette"(dotted line) with central capillary (c); (N) SEM image of the rat pituitary matrix, recellularized for 7 days with primary pituitary cells in static culture. Note that cells in the engineered tissue attempt to re-organize a typical "rosette" (dotted line) around a capillary (c) space.

In a second step, primary rat anterior pituitary cells were used to recellularize the decellularized adenohypophysial SVS. Using the same technique applied with the rat thyroid SVS, primary pituitary elements were seen to colonize the empty niches of the pituitary SVS by assuming a "rosette" configuration around an empty vascular channel, in a way that replicates the normal pattern of anterior pituitary cells in vivo (Fig. 15.9). Since we preserved the marginal zone of the anterior pituitary during cell seeding preparation [79], we assume that adult pituitary stem cells contributed to the SVS recellularization. Therefore, these results suggests that the anterior pituitary SVS may act as a morphoregulatory guidance for growth and self-assembly of both differentiated and progenitor adenohypophysial cells. In conclusion, all these data confirm that the organomorphic principle is fundamental for a successful ex situ bioengineering of endocrine glands and soft tissue organs, and urge to develop free form fabrication technologies as much sensitive as possible to faithfully replicate with synthetic and/or natural biomaterials the 3D geometry of the SVS of the native organs to be reconstructed.

## 15.3 Conclusions

We have proposed an innovative concept for ex situ bioengineering of soft tissue, endocrine organs based on the organomorphic principle. To prove this hypothesis, we have designed an organomorphic scaffold-bioreactor unit reproducing the 3D macro-microscopic architecture of the SVS of the adult human thyroid gland, chosen as a suitable and simplified model of parenchymal endocrine viscera. Numerous experimental data have been collected to support this approach, including in vivo and in vitro studies with computational microanatomy of the intraglandular thyroid vessels coupled to reverse engineering techniques and synthetic biomaterials, immunocytochemical studies on early embryological steps of thyroid development, culture of primary thyroid cells in 3D systems, and recellularization of the decellularized, natural thyroid SVS. We have concluded that the organomorphism of the scaffold and bioreactor has the potential to guide self-assembly of seeded cells ex situ, up to the reconstruction of a macroscopic, functional and immune-tolerant human thyroid gland.

In an effort to confirm these assumptions, we have extended our studies to the isolation of the SVS of other endocrine and soft tissue viscera like the pituitary gland, adrenals, thymus, and parts of the cerebral cortex. We have obtained preliminary results supporting the organomorphic principle for engineering all these organs. On a broader perspective, we believe this approach may accelerate the field of regenerative medicine into a phase of radical solution for a number of challenging or incurable, endocrine-metabolic disorders. Specifically, conditions like diabetes mellitus, permanent hypoparathyroidism and/or hypothyroidism following total thyroidectomy for cancer, adrenal insufficiency and congenital adrenal hyperplasia, primitive male hypogonadism and infertility, female infertility with hyperandrogenism and obesity (e.g. the polycystic ovary syndrome), pituitary insufficiency, and rare conditions of the immune-endocrine and metabolic regulation including branchial arch disorders (DiGeorge syndrome), congenital lysosomal storage defects (e.g. Gaucher disease), and bone abnormalities (e.g. osteogenesis imperfecta, Paget disease of the youth, skeletal dysplasia) might be definitively cured by substituting the affected organ with a bioartificial one. In addition, this strategy might offer an alternative source of soft tissue organs, currently available only from cadaveric donors, and provide patient-tailored bioconstructs.

The transformative impact of this view is believed to open also to the reconstruction of nervous structures, still believed impossible to be assembled outside the living body, and potentially usable in the treatment of spinal trauma, stroke, neurodegenerative disorders, and brain cancer. Finally, we think that a program based on organomorphic scaffold–bioreactor systems could have a major impact on the bioengineering, biomaterial and pharmaceutical industry giving rise to patents for bioartificial organ prototypes, new functionalized molecules for scaffold fabrication, and commercial kits to test drugs at cellular level in 3D, organomorphic environments.

## Acknowledgements

The authors are grateful to Drs. Prisco Mirandola and Daniela Galli, and to the PhD students Valentina Strusi and Simone Mastrogiacomo, Section of Human Anatomy, S.Bi.Bi.T., University of Parma, Italy for technical and scientific support during the preparation of the experimental protocols, to Dr. Michele Iafisco, ISTEC-CNR, Faenza, Italy for suggestions on biomaterial handling and applications, to Prof. Nadir Mario Maraldi, Laboratory of Musculoskeletal Cell Biology, IOR and University of Bologna, Italy, for insights on acellular matrixes and generous provision of laboratory equipment, and to Prof. Francesco Antonio Manzoli, Scientific Direction IOR, Bologna, Italy for constant financial support to the research activities. We are also indebted to Ronald M. Lechan, Endocrine Division, Tufts University—Tufts Medical Center, Boston, MA, USA for sound criticism on various aspects of the research program. Supported by Grants MIUR FIRB RBAP10MLK7_004, and ACPR12_00312.

## References

1. Sprio, S., Sandri, M., Iafisco, M., Panseri, I., Cunha, C., Ruffini, A., Zini, N., Toni, R., Tampieri, A. (2013). Biomimetic biomaterials in regenerative medicine. In: *Biomimetic biomaterials, Structure and applications*, ed. Ruys, A. J., Chapter 1, (Whoodhead Publishing, Cambride, U.K.) pp. 3–45.

2. Toni, R., Tampieri, A., Zini, N., Strusi, V., Sandri, M., Dallatana, D., Spaletta, G., Bassoli, E., Gatto, A., Ferrari, A., Martin, I. (2011). Ex situ bioengineering of bioartificial endocrine glands: A new frontier in regenerative medicine of soft tissue organs. *Ann. Anat.*, **193**, pp. 381–394.

3. Atala, A. (2009). Engineering organs. *Curr. Opin. Biotechnol.*, **20**, 575–592.

4. Furth, M. E., Atala, A. (2008). Producing organs in the laboratory. *Curr. Urol. Rep.*, **9**, 433–436.

5. Koh, C., Atala, A. (2004). Tissue engineering, stem cells, and cloning: Opportunities for rigenerative medicine. *J. Am. Soc. Nephrol.*, **15**, pp. 1113–1125.

6. Parenteau, N., Rosenberg, L., Hardin-Young, J. (2004). The engineering of tissues using progenitor cells. *Curr. Top. Develop. Biol.*, **64**, pp. 101–139.

7. Perl, S., Kushner, J., Buchholz, B. A., Meeker, A. K., Stein, G. M., Hsieh, M. Kirby, M., Pechhold, S., Liu, E. H., Harlan, D., Tisdale. (2010). Significant human-cell turnover is limited to the first three decades of life as determined by in vivo thymidine analog incorporation and radiocarbon dating. *J. Clin. Endocrinol. Metab.*, **95**, pp. E234–E239.

8. Okita, K., Ichisaka, T., Yamanaka, S. (2007). Generation of germline competent induced pluripotent stem cells. *Nature*, **448**, pp. 313–317.

9. Warren, L., Manos, P., Ahfeldt, T., Loh, Y.-H., Li, H., Lau, F., Ebina, W., Mandal, P. K., Smith, Z. D., Meissner, A., Daley, G. Q., Brack, A. S., Collins, J. J., Cowan, C., Schlaeger, T. M., Rossi, D. J. (2010). Highly efficient reprogramming to pluripotency and directed differentiation of human cells with synthetic modified mRNA. *Cell Stem Cell*, **7**, pp. 1–13.

10. Kim, B. S., Baez, C. E., Atala, A. (2000). Biomaterials for tissue engineering. *World J. Urol.*, **18**, pp. 2–9.

11. Lee, J., Cuddihy, M. J., Kotov, N. A. (2008). Three-dimensional cell culture matrices: State of the art. *Tissue Eng. Part B Rev.*, **14**, pp. 61–86.

12. Boland, T., Mironov, V., Gutowska, A., Roth, E. A., Markwald, R. R. (2003). Cell and organ printing 2: Fusion of cell aggregates in three-dimensional gels. *Anat. Rec. A Discov. Mol. Cell Evol. Biol.*, **272**, pp. 497–502.

13. Mironov, V., Boland, T., Trusk, T., Forgacs, G., Markwald, R. R. (2003). Organ printing: Computer-aided jet-based 3D tissue engineering. *Trends Biotechnol.*, **21**, pp. 157–161.

14. Albrecht, D. R., Underhill, G. H., Wassermann, T. B., Sah, R. L., Bhatia, S. N. (2006). Probing the role of multicellular organization in three-dimensional microenvironments. *Nat. Methods*, **3**, pp. 369–375.

15. Landers, R., Hubnerb, U., Schmelzeisenb, R., Mulhaupt, R. (2002). Rapid prototyping of scaffolds derived from thermoreversible hydrogels and tailored for applications in tissue engineering. *Biomaterials*, **23**, pp. 4437–4447.

16. Nguyen, K. T., West, J. L. (2000). Photopolymerizable hydrogels for tissue engineering applications. *Biomaterials*, **23**, pp. 4307–4314.

17. Panseri, S., Russo, A., Giavaresi, G., Sartori, M., Veronesi, F., Fini, M., Salter, D. M., Ortolani, A., Strazzari, A., Visani, A., Dionigi, C., Bock, N., Sandri, M., Tampieri, A., Marcacci, M. (2012). Innovative magnetic scaffolds for orthopedic tissue engineering. *J. Biomed. Mater. Res. Part A*, **100A**, pp. 2278–2286.

18. Jakab, K., Neagu, A., Mironov, V., Markwald, R. R., Forgacs, G. (2004). Engineering biological structures of prescribed shape using self-assembling multicellular systems. *Proc. Natl. Acad. Sci. U. S. A.*, **101**, pp. 2864–2869.

19. Jakab, K., Norotte, C., Damon, B., Marga, F., Neagu, A., Besch-Williford, C. L., Kachurin, A., Church, K. H., Park, H., Mironov, V., Markwald, R., Vunjak-Novakovic, G., Forgacs, G. (2008). Tissue engineering by self-assembly of cells printed into topologically defined structures. *Tissue Eng. Part A*, **14**, pp. 413–421.

20. MacPherson, R. D., Srolovitz, D. J. (2007). The von Neumann relation generalized to coarsening of three-dimensional microstructures. *Nature*, **446**, pp. 1053–1055.

21. Marga, F., Neagu, A., Kosztin, I., Forgacs, G. (2007). Developmental biology and tissue engineering. *Birth Defects Res. (Part C)*, **81**, pp. 320–328.

22. Badylak, F. (2002). The extracellular matrix as a scaffold for tissue reconstruction. *Cell. Dev. Biol.*, **13**, pp. 377–383.

23. Langer, R., Vacanti, J. P. (1993). Tissue engineering. *Science*, **260**, pp. 920–926.

24. Song, J. J., Ott, H. C. (2011). Organ engineering based on decellularized matrix scaffolds. *Trends Mol. Med.*, **17**, pp. 424–432.

25. Grikscheit, T., Ochoa, E. R., Srinivasan, A., Gaissert, H., Vacanti, J. P. (2003). Tissue-engineered esophagus: Experimental substitution by onlay patch or interposition. *J. Thorac. Cardiovasc. Surg.*, **126**, pp. 537–544.

26. Kodama, S., Kojima, K., Furuta, S., Chambers, M., Paz, A. C., Vacanti, C. A. (2009). Engineering functional islets from cultured cells. *Tissue Eng. Part A.*, **15**, pp. 3321–3329.

27. Oberpenning, F., Meng, J., Yoo, J. J., Atala, A. (1999). De novo reconstitution of a functional mammalian urinary bladder by tissue engineering. *Nat. Biothec.*, **17**, pp. 149–155.

28. Martin, Y., Vermette, P. (2005). Bioreactors for tissue mass culture: Design, characterization, and recent advances. *Biomaterials*, **26**, pp. 7481–7503.

29. Edlund, H. (2002). Pancreatic organogenesis. Developmental mechanisms and implications for therapy. *Nat. Rev. Gen.*, **3**, pp. 524–532.

30. Fagman, H., Nilsson, M. (2011). Morphogenetics of early thyroid development. *J. Mol. Endocrinol.*, **46**, R33–R42.

31. Zaret, K. S. (2002). Regulatory phases of early liver development: Pradigms of organogenesis. *Nat. Rev. Gen.*, **3**, pp. 499–512.

32. Bassoli, E., Denti, L., Gatto, A., Paderno, A., Spaletta, G., Zini, N., Strusi, V., Dallatana, D., Toni, R. (2011). New approaches to prototype 3D vascular-like structures by additive layer manufacturing, in High Value *Manufacturing. Advanced Research in Virtual and Rapid Prototyping* (eds. Bartolo, P. J., et al.), *Proc. 5th Int. Conf. Adv. Res. & Rapid Protot.*, CRC Press, Taylor & Francis, London, pp. 35–42.

33. Bassoli, E., Denti, L., Gatto, A., Spaletta, G., Paderno, A., Zini, N., Parrilli, A., Giardino, R., Strusi, V., Dallatana, D., Mastrogiacomo, S.,

Zamparelli, A., Iafisco, M., Toni, R. (2012). A combined additive layer manufacturing (ALM)/indirect replication method to prototype 3D vascular-like structures of soft tissue and endocrine organs, *Virt. Phys. Protot.*, **7**, pp. 3–11.

34. Bassoli, E., Denti, L., Gatto, A., Spaletta, G., Sofroniou, M., Parrilli, A., Fini M., Giardino, R., Zamparelli, A., Zini, N., Barbaro F., Bassi, E., Mosca, S., Dallatana, D., Toni. R. (2014). A planar fractal analysis of the arterial tree of the human thyroid gland: Implications for additive manufacturing of 3D ramified scaffolds. In: High Value Manufacturing. *Advanced Research in Virtual and Rapid Prototyping*, eds. Bartolo, P. J. et al., Proc. 5th Int. Conf. Adv. Res. & Rapid Protot. CRC Press, Taylor & Francis, London, pp. 423–429.

35. Mastrogiacomo, S., Strusi, V., Dallatana D., Barbaro F., Zini N., Zamparelli A., Iafisco, M., Parrilli A., Giardino R., Lippi G., Spaletta, G., Bassoli, E., Gatto. A., Sandri, M., Sprio, S.,Tampieri, A., Toni, R. (2012). Poly-L-lactic acid and poly-$\varepsilon$-caprolactone as biomaterials for ex-situ bioengineering of the rat thyroid tissue, *I.J.A.E.*, **117** (suppl to 2), p. 120.

36. Scadden, D. T. (2006). The stem-cell niche as an entity of action. *Nature*, **44**, pp. 1075–1079.

37. Burdick, J. A., Vunjak-Novakovic, G. (2009). Engineered microenvironments for controlled stem cell differentiation. *Tissue Eng. Part A.*, **15**, pp. 205–219.

38. Lund, A. W., Yener, B., Stegemann, J. P., Plopper, G. E. (2009). The natural and engineered 3D microenvironment as a regulatory cue during stem cell fate determination. *Tissue Eng. Part B Rev.*, **15**, pp. 371–380.

39. Discher, D. E., Mooney, D. J., Zandstra, P. W. (2009). Growth factors, matrices, and forces combine and control stem cells. *Science*, **324**, pp. 1673–1677.

40. Engler, A. J., Sen, S., Sweeney, H. L., Discher, D. E. (2006). Matrix elasticity directs stem cell lineage specification. *Cell*, **126**, pp. 677–689.

41. Freytes, D. O., Wan, L. Q., Vunjak-Novakovic, G. (2009). Geometry and force control of cell function. *J. Cell Biochem.*, **108**, 1047–1058.

42. Vogel, V., Sheetz, M. (2006). Local force and geometry sensing regulate cell functions. *Nat. Rev. Mol. Cell Biol.*, **7**, pp. 265–275.

43. Edelman, G. M. (1988). *Topobiology, an Introduction to Molecular Embryology*, Basic Book Inc, New York.

44. Engler, A. J., Humbert, P. O., Wehrle-Haller, B., Weaver, V. M. (2009). Multiscale modeling of form and function. *Science*, **324**, 208–212.

45. Fagman, H., Grande, M., Gritli-Linde, A., Nilsson, M. (2004). Genetic deletion of sonic hedgehog causes hemiagenesis and ectopic development of the thyroid in mouse. *Am. J. Pathol.*, **164**, 1865–1872.

46. Lania, G., Zhang, S., Huynh, T, Caprio, C., Moon, A. M., Vitelli, F., Baldini, A. (2009). Early thyroid development requires a Tbx1–Fgf8 pathway. *Dev. Biol.*, **328**, pp. 109–117.

47. Meunier, D., Aubin, J., Jeannotte, L. (2003). Perturbed thyroid morphology and transient hypothyroidism symptoms in Hoxa5 mutant mice. *Dev. Dyn.*, **227**, pp. 367–378.

48. Schmelzer, E., Triolo, F., Turner, M. E., Thompson, R. L., Zeilinger, K., Reid, L. M., Gridelli, B., Gerlach, J. C. (2010). Three-dimensional perfusion bioreactor culture supports differentiation of human fetal liver cells. *Tissue Eng. A*, **16**, pp. 2007–2016.

49. Zeilinger, K., Schreiter, T., Darnell, M., Söderdahl, T., Lübberstedt, M., Dillner, B., Knobeloch, D., Nüssler, A. K., Gerlach, J. C., Andersson, T. B. (2011). Scaling down of a clinical three-dimensional perfusion multicompartment hollow fiber liver bioreactor developed for extracorporeal liver support to an analytical scale device useful for hepatic pharmacological in vitro studies. *Tissue Eng. C Methods*, **17**, pp. 549–556.

50. Kaihara, S., Borenstein, J., Koka, R., Lalan, S., Ochoa, E. R., Ravens, M., Pien, H., Cunningham, B., Vacanti, J. P. (2000). Silicon micromachining to tissue engineer branched vascular channels for liver fabrication. *Tissue Eng.*, **6**, pp. 105–117.

51. McClelland, R. E., Coger, R. N. (2000). Use of micropathways to improve oxygen transport in a hepatic system. *J. Biomech. Eng.*, **122**, pp. 268–273.

52. Lee, J. I., Nishimura, R., Sakai, H., Sasaki, N., Kenmochi, T. (2008). A newly developed immunoisolated bioartificial pancreas with cell sheet engineering. *Cell Transplant.*, **17**, pp. 51–59.

53. Wang, X., Ye, K. (2009). Three-dimensional differentiation of embryonic stem cells into islet-like insulin-producing clusters. Tissue Eng. *Part A*, **15**, pp. 1941–1952.

54. Xu, M., Kreeger, P. K., Shea, L. D., Woodruff, T. K. (2006). Tissue-engineered follicles produce live, fertile offspring. *Tissue Eng.*, **12**, pp. 2739–2746.

55. Antonica, F., Kasprzyk, D. F., Opitz, R., Iacovino, M., Liao, X. H., Dumitrescu, A. M., Refetoff, S., Peremans, K., Manto, M., Kyba, M., Costagliola, S. (2012). Generation of functional thyroid from embryonic stem cells. *Nature*, **491**, pp. 66–71.

56. Arauchi, A., Shimizu, T., Yamato, M., Obara, T., Okano, T. (2009). Tissue-engineered thyroid cell sheet rescued hypothyroidism in rat models after receiving total thyroidectomy comparing with nontransplantation models. *Tissue Eng. Part A.*, **15**, pp. 3943–3949.

57. Toda, S., Sugihara, H. (1990). Reconstruction of thyroid follicles from isolated porcine follicle cells in three-dimensional collagen gel culture. *Endocrinology*, **126**, pp. 2027–2034.

58. Ritter, C. S., Slatopolsky, E., Santoro, S., Brown, A. J. (2004). Parathyroid cells cultured in collagen matrix retain calcium responsiveness: Importance of three-dimensional tissue architecture. *J. Bone Min. Res.*, **19**, pp. 491–498.

59. Suga, H., Kadoshima, T., Minaguchi, M., Ohgushi, M., Soen, M., Nakano, T., Takata, N., Wataya, T., Muguruma, K., Miyoshi, H., Yonemura, S., Oiso, Y., Sasai, Y. (2011). Self-formation of functional adenohypophysis in three-dimensional culture. *Nature*, **480**, pp. 57–63.

60. Gassei, K., Schlatt, S. (2007). Testicular morphogenesis: Comparison of in vivo and in vitro models to study male gonadal development. *Ann. N. Y. Acad. Sci.*, **1120**, 152–167.

61. Krotz, S. P., Robins, J. C., Ferruccio, T. M., Moore, R., Steinhoff, M. M., Morgan, J. R., Carson, S. (2010). In vitro maturation of oocytes via the pre-fabricated self-assembled artificial human ovary. *J. Assist. Reprod. Genet.*, **27**, pp. 743–750.

62. Allen, R. A., Seltz, L. M., Jiang, H., Kasick, R. T., Sellaro, T. L., Badylak, S. F., Ogilvie, J. B. (2010). Adrenal extracellular matrix scaffolds support adrenocortical cell proliferation and function in vitro. *Tissue Eng. Part A.*, **16**, pp. 3363–3337.

63. Toni, R., Casa, C. D., Spaletta, G., Marchetti, G., Mazzoni, P., Bodria, M., Ravera, S., Dallatana, D., Castorina, S., Riccioli, V., Castorina, E. G., Antoci, S., Campanile, E., Raise, G., Rossi, R., Ugolotti, G., Martorella, A., Roti, E., Sgallari, F., Pinchera, A. (2007). The bioartificial thyroid: A biotechnological perspective in endocrine organ engineering for transplantation replacement. *Acta Biomed.*, **78**(1), pp. 129–155.

64. Parrilli, A., Zini, N., Spaletta, G., Bassoli, E., Gatto, A., Toni, R., Ceglia, L., Fini, M. (2013). Micro-CT of 3D vascular structure: Clues for innovative scaffolds in organ engineering. *Proc. Bruker MicroCT User Meeting*, 2013, pp. 135–139.

65. Toni, R., Casa, C. D., Bodria, M., Spaletta, G., Vella, R., Castorina, S., Gatto, A., Teti, G., Falconi, M., Rago, T., Vitti, P., Sgallari, F. (2008). A study on the relationship between intraglandular arterial distribution and thyroid lobe shape: Implications for biotechnology of a bioartificial thyroid. *Ann. Anat.*, **190**, pp. 432–441.

66. Strusi, V., Zini, N., Dallatana, D., Parrilli, A., Giardino, R., Lippi, G., Spaletta, G., Bassoli, E., Gatto, A., Iafisco, M., Sandri, M., Tampieri, A., Toni, R., (2011). Ex situ bioengineering of the rat thyroid using as a scaffold the three-dimensional (3D) decellularized matrix of the glandular lobe: Clues to the organomorphic principle. *I.J.A.E.*, **116** (supp to 1), p. 180.

67. Strusi, V., Zini, N., Dallatana, D., Mastrogiacomo, S., Parrilli, A., Giardino, R., Lippi, G., Spaletta, G., Bassoli, E., Gatto, A., Iafisco, M., Sandri, M., Tampieri, A., Toni, R. (2012). Endocrine bioengineering: Reconstruction of a bioartificial thyroid lobe using its three-dimensional (3D) stromal/vascular matrix as a scaffold. *End. Abst.*, **29**, p. 1586.

68. Toni, R., Strusi, V., Zini, N., Dallatana, D., Mastrogiacomo, S., Parrilli, A., Giardino, R., Lippi, G., Spaletta, G., Bassoli, E., Gatto, A., Iafisco, M., Sandri, M., Tampieri, A., (2012). Bioengineering of the thyroid lobe: Use of its stromal/vascular matrix as a scaffold for ex situ reconstruction. *Endocr. Rev.*, **33**, (03_Meeting Abstracts), OR26–3.

69. Barbaro, F., Zamparelli, A., Zini, N., Dallatana, D., Bassi, E., Mosca, S., Parrilli, A., Fini, M., Giardino, R., Toni, R. (2013). Adult stem/progenitor cells of the rat thyroid: side population distribution, intermediate filament expression, and long-term in vitro expansion. *I.J.A.E*, **118**, (supplement to 2), p.19.

70. Baptista, P. M., Orlando, G., Mirmalek-Sani, S. H., Siddiqui, M., Atala, A., Soker, S. (2009). Whole organ decellularization-a tool for bioscaffold fabrication and organ bioengineering. *Proc. Conf. IEEE Eng. Med. Biol. Soc.*, pp. 6526–6529.

71. Goh, S.-K., Bertera, S., Olsen, P., Candiello, J. E., Halfter, W., Uechi, G., Balasubramani, M., Johnson, S. A., Sicari, B. M., Kollar, E., Badylak, S. F., Banerjee, I. (2013). Perfusion-decellularized pancreas as a natural 3D scaffold for pancreatic tissue and whole organ engineering. *Biomaterials*, **34**, 6760–6772.

72. Mirmalek-Sani, S.-H., Orlando, G., McQuilling, J. P., Pareta, R., Mack, D. L., Salvatori, M., Farney A. C., Stratta R. J., Atala, A., Opara, E. C., Sokera, S. (2013). Porcine pancreas extracellular matrix as a platform for endocrine pancreas bioengineering. *Biomaterials*, **34**, pp. 5488–5495.

73. Ott, H. C., Clippinger, B., Conrad, C., Schuetz, C., Pomerantseva, I., Ikonomou, L., Kotton, D., Vacanti, J. P. (2010). Regeneration and orthotopic transplantation of a bioartificial lung. *Nat. Med.*, **16**, pp. 927–933.

74. Uygun, B. E., Soto-Gutierrez, A., Yagi, H., Izamis, M. L., Guzzardi, M. A., Shulman, C., Milwid, J., Kobayashi, N., Tilles, A., Berthiaume, F., Hertl,

M., Nahmias, Y., Yarmush, M. L., Uygun, K. (2010). Organ reengineering through development of a transplantable recellularized liver graft using decellularized liver matrix. *Nat. Med.*, **16**, pp. 814–820.

75. Badylak, S. F., Gilbert, T. W. (2008). Immune response to biologic scaffold materials. *Sem. Immunol.*, **20**, pp. 109–116.

76. Keane, T. J., Londono, R., Turner, N. J., Badylak, S. F. Consequences of ineffective decellularization of biologic scaffolds on the host response. (2012). *Biomaterials*, **33**, pp. 1771–1181.

77. Dityatev, A., Seidenbecher, C. I., Schachner, M. (2010). Compartmentalization from the outside: The extracellular matrix and functional microdomains in the brain. *Trends Neurosci.*, **33**, pp. 503–512.

78. DeQuach, J. A., Yuan, S. H., Goldstein, L. S., Christman, K. L. (2011). Decellularized porcine brain matrix for cell culture and tissue engineering scaffolds. *Tissue Eng Part A.*, **17**, pp. 2583–2592.

79. Vankelecom, H. (2006). Pituitary stem/progenitor cells: Embryonic players in the adult gland? *Eu. J. Neurosci.*, **32**, pp. 2063–2081.

# Index

ACL, *see* anterior cruciate ligament
AFM, *see* atomic force microscope
anterior cruciate ligament (ACL) 309, 315
anterior pituitary 376–378
apatite crystals 7, 53, 131, 135
apatite formation, in vitro 120, 124–125, 127, 129, 131, 133, 135
apatite nanocrystals 47, 49, 59–60, 65–66
apatite nanoparticles 49, 62, 65, 69–70
apatites 47–50, 61–66, 107, 123–124, 126–127, 137, 195
articular cartilage 146, 163, 283–285, 287
atomic force microscope (AFM) 51, 53, 57
autologous bone grafts 182
axons 212–217, 223, 226, 228

bacterial nano-cellulose (BNC) 159–166, 168, 170
bioactive materials 110, 122
bioartificial endocrine organs 357–378
biochemical gradients 30–31, 33, 35

biocompatible nanobiomaterials 11
biological apatites 47, 57–59, 61, 63, 120–121, 131
biological systems 3, 48–49, 51, 53, 55, 57, 119, 189, 287, 341
biomaterial delivery systems 292
biomaterial design strategies 29
biomaterial functionalization 25
biomaterial handling 379
biomaterial implantation 28
biomaterial matrix 227
biomaterial nanotopography 289
biomaterial reabsorption, complete 326
biomaterials
  bone-implantable 68
  ceramic 99
  implanted 28, 66, 224
  innovative bone substitute 66
  load-bearing 64
  nanostructured 65
  natural 24, 378
  protein-based 285
  regenerative 110
  smart 307, 313
  specialized 247
  stiff 286

biomimetic apatite 120–122,
  124, 129, 131–137,
  195, 290
biomimetic apatite
  nanocrystals 60
biomimetic bone
  substitutes 341
biomimetic materials 250,
  307, 315, 336, 345–347,
  349
 smart 307, 315
biomimetics 2–3, 5, 11–12,
  15, 64, 228, 230, 290,
  306–307, 315, 325, 330,
  341, 343
biomorphic
  transformations 99
bionanocomposites 2–3
biopolymers 2, 23, 149, 152,
  158, 161, 170
bisphosphonates 66–67, 102
blood vessels 54, 57, 68, 91,
  93, 146, 180, 215, 218,
  223, 227, 367
BMPs, *see* bone
  morphogenetic proteins
BMSCs, *see* bone marrow stem
  cells
BNC, *see* bacterial
  nano-cellulose
bone
 alveolar 9, 55
 autologous 337
 cancellous 23, 54, 151, 181
 iliac 337, 339
 mammalian 64, 132
 mineral 11, 103
 osteoporotic 105, 109
bone allografts 182
bone apatite 52, 121–122, 137
 biological 120, 137
bone augmentation 64, 105

bone cells 4, 33, 89, 344
 immature 33
bone cements 104–105
bone defects 13, 64, 100,
  182, 187, 191, 313–314
bone distraction 91, 313
bone grafts 91, 182, 340, 348
 homologous 91, 328
bone graft substitutes 65, 180
bone growth 110, 344
bone loss 4, 101
bone marrow 14, 146, 228,
  312, 325, 337
bone marrow cells 349
bone marrow stem cells
  (BMSCs) 94, 184, 287,
  347
bone mineral 6, 344
bone mineral crystals 59
bone mineralization 103
bone morphogenetic proteins
  (BMPs) 50, 66–67,
  92, 213, 243, 290, 341,
  347–349
bone regeneration 4, 47–48,
  50, 52, 54, 56, 58, 60,
  62–70, 89–91, 137, 152,
  180, 182, 184
bone remodeling 66, 87
bone repair 11, 89, 179, 182,
  295
bone replacement 286, 291
bone resorption 10, 102
bone scaffolding 98, 110
bone scaffolds 4, 93
 ceramic 12
 regenerative 4
bone sialoprotein 50, 342
bone substitutes 288, 336, 342,
  347
bone tissue 4–5, 32, 86–87,
  120–121, 147, 154,

181–185, 195, 288, 290,
313, 335, 340, 342–344,
349
developing 346
homologous 335
in-growing 188
bone tissue biomimesis 290
bone tissue engineering 181,
183, 185
bone tissue formation 8, 325
bone tissue growth 199
bone tissue in-growth 188
bone tissue regeneration 10,
47, 92, 179, 199
controlled 294
bone trabeculae 86

calcifications 48–49,
57–58, 343
pathological 49, 57–58
calcium 9, 11, 52, 58, 97–98,
109, 121, 129, 152, 159,
181, 286, 343
calcium phosphate cements
(CPCs) 105–107,
109–110, 342, 345–346
calcium phosphates 48, 98,
107, 120–121, 124–127,
183, 346
CAMs, see cell adhesion
molecules
CaP biomaterials 66–67
CaP nanoparticles 70–71
carbonated hydroxy apatite
(CHA) 120, 122, 126, 132
cardiac hypertrophy 261,
267, 273
cardiomyocytes 261–262,
267, 272

cartilage 1, 6, 9, 12, 145–147,
149, 151, 180–181,
285–287, 306, 313, 315,
323–326, 330, 347–348
cell adhesion 25, 93, 99, 109,
186, 198–199, 285–286,
292, 294, 342–343, 345
cell adhesion molecules (CAMs)
25, 213, 227, 362
cell–biomaterial
communication 291
cell–material interactions 24,
288
cells
anterior pituitary 377–378
bone-related 65
bone tumor 65
glial 213
osteoblast 6, 8, 86, 195
parathyroid 365
cellular–biomaterial
interaction 292
ceramic materials 94, 165,
183, 342–343, 345
CG, see collagen-GAG
CHA, see carbonated hydroxy
apatite
chondrocytes 8, 146, 163,
165, 186, 243
collagen 5–7, 9–10, 12, 50–51,
158–166, 168–169,
184–185, 224–226,
285–286, 289, 312,
314–316, 324–325,
343–345, 358–360
mineralized 51, 54
collagen fibers 5–7, 9, 135,
342–343, 348
collagen fibrils 50, 52, 121,
163, 287
collagen-GAG (CG) 250

## Index

cortical bone 54, 181–182
CPCs, *see* calcium phosphate cements
cytocompatibility 163–164, 166–167, 291
cytokines 28, 30, 292

DBM, *see* demineralized bone matrix
DEJ, *see* dentin-enamel junction
demineralized bone matrix (DBM) 348
dentin 9, 54–56
dentine 2, 9, 48–49
dentin-enamel junction (DEJ) 55–56
DMEM, *see* Dulbecco's modified Eagle's medium
dorsal root ganglia (DRG) 225–226
DRG, *see* dorsal root ganglia
Dulbecco's modified Eagle's medium (DMEM) 154, 163–166, 168–169

ECM, *see* extra cellular matrix
ECM proteins 26, 225–226, 245, 288
EGF, *see* epidermal growth factor
electrospinning 242, 244, 246–247
  coaxial 229, 244–245
embryonic development 213–214, 361
embryonic stem cells (ESCs) 26, 358, 365

endocrine organs 358, 361, 364–366, 378
endoneurial tubes 216–217, 223–224
endoneurium 215–216, 223
endothelial cells 212–213, 215, 217, 226, 251, 363
endothelial outgrowth cells (EOCs) 189
EOCs, *see* endothelial outgrowth cells
epidermal growth factor (EGF) 292
ESCs, *see* embryonic stem cells
extra cellular matrix (ECM) 22–24, 27–28, 147, 180–181, 213, 225, 243, 284, 288, 308

FGF, *see* fibroblast growth factor
fibrils 23, 52, 54, 158, 160, 162–163, 170, 288
  mineralized 52–53
fibroblast growth factor (FGF) 213, 292, 348
fibroblasts 28, 186, 212–213, 215, 217, 349, 363
fibrosis 261–262
fractures 55, 91, 101, 103–105, 121, 246, 313, 340
  vertebral compression 102, 104

gelling agents 148, 152–153
genes 71, 187, 362
gene therapy 15, 336, 341, 347, 349

GFs, *see* growth factors
giant cells  29, 309
graphene  274
growth factors (GFs)  23,
    25–27, 30–32, 34, 36,
    66–67, 186, 213–214,
    229–230, 241–242,
    244, 246–248, 250, 292,
    347–349

hard tissue regeneration  14,
    295
heart  180, 260–262, 266,
    268–273
heart failure  259–260, 262
human blood plasma  120,
    122–123, 125, 127, 135,
    137, 186
human bone morphogenetic
    proteins  242
hyaluronic acid  7, 27, 151,
    153–154, 159, 164–165,
    168, 170, 246, 287,
    322–323, 348, 359
hydrogels  7, 27, 152, 158, 167,
    170, 246, 250–251
hydrolyses  107–109
hydroxyapatite  8, 10, 56, 70,
    94, 147, 150, 153, 157,
    165, 170, 286, 323, 336,
    342–346
hydroxyapatite crystals  56
hydroxyapatite nanocrystals
    182, 185, 290

ionotropic gelation  147–148,
    150–152, 155–157, 167,
    323

lesions  284, 312, 322, 326–328
leukocytes  28, 34
liver  11, 295, 363–365, 375

macrophage phenotype  29
macrophages  28–29, 109, 226
magnesium  6, 129, 314–315,
    343
magnetic nanoparticles  13–14,
    187–190, 192, 194, 198,
    293
magnetic resonance imaging
    (MRI)  11, 293–294,
    322, 326–328
magnetic scaffolds  12, 159,
    179–180, 187, 190–191,
    193, 198–199, 294–295
  nanocomposite  192, 198
magnetism  13, 180, 187,
    189, 191
magnetite  11, 194–195, 295
mechanotransduction  182
meniscal tissue regeneration
    311, 315
mesenchymal stem cells
    (MSCs)  14, 65, 146–147,
    155–156, 165, 169–170,
    184, 194, 228, 289, 322
mesoporous silica
    nanoparticles (MSNs)
    36, 248
metalloproteinase  28, 348
microRNA  260, 263–265, 267,
    269, 273
MicroRNA-based therapy
    259–260, 262, 264, 266,
    268–270, 272, 274
mimicking  9, 33, 223–224, 291,
    294, 366, 368

mimicry 22–23, 25, 27, 29, 225, 246–247, 249
miRNA 264–269
MRI, *see* magnetic resonance imaging
mRNA 265, 268–269
MSCs, *see* mesenchymal stem cells
MSNs, *see* mesoporous silica nanoparticles
multi-functional hard tissues 5, 7, 9
myelination 214–215, 226, 228
myocardium 261–262, 271–272
myofibroblasts 262–263, 272

nano-apatites 47–48, 50, 52, 54, 56, 58, 60, 62, 64, 66, 68, 70
nanobiomagnetism 1–2, 4, 6, 8, 10–14
nanocomposites 2, 186, 197
nanocrystalline apatites 48–49, 58–61, 63–64, 66
nanopores 272–273
nanosized apatites 62, 65
natural biochemical gradients 246–247, 249
natural bone 3, 159, 185, 314
NCPs, *see* non-collagenous proteins
nerve growth factor (NGF) 213, 226–227, 229
nerve regeneration 149, 211–212, 215, 218–219, 223–225, 228–230
nerve regenerative templates 222–223, 225, 227, 229

neural guides 220–224
neurons 212–215, 217
neurotmesis 216–219, 221
   surgical approaches to 217–219
NGF, *see* nerve growth factor
niomaterials, apatite-based 64
non-collagenous proteins (NCPs) 50

organic polymers 295
organomorphic principle 361, 366, 378–379
organomorphic scaffold-bioreactor unit 366, 378
osteoarthritis 146, 283, 309
osteoblasts 50, 54, 57, 65, 87, 102–103, 108, 137, 182, 185–186, 294, 342, 344, 347, 349
osteochondral defects 145–147, 151, 170–171, 199, 242, 311, 323
osteochondral regeneration 7, 283, 312, 325, 327, 329
osteochondral scaffolds 3, 312, 324, 328–330
   nanostructured collagen-hydroxyapatite 325
osteoclasts 50, 54, 86–87, 102, 109, 182, 342, 344
osteogenesis 92, 184, 343–344
osteoinductive materials 314–315
osteointegration 64–66
osteons 51, 54
osteoporosis 10, 90, 101–103, 108, 344
osteoporosis-related fractures 101, 103, 105, 107

osteotomy 91, 313, 330

pancreatic islets 363–364
PDGF, *see* platelet-derived
 growth factor
perineurium 215–216,
 218, 223
peripheral nerve
 regeneration 230
peripheral nerves 212–217,
 223, 227, 230
peripheral nervous
 system 211–213
platelet-derived growth
 factor (PDGF) 229,
 348–349
platelet-rich-plasma (PRP) 92,
 242, 348–349
PLGA 31–32, 35, 183, 249, 286
PLGA microspheres 31
PLGA-pSi 35–36, 248–249
pri-miRNAs 264–265
progenitor cells 1, 250, 322,
 363
protein adsorption 29, 345
protein-biomaterial systems
 244
proteins
 non-collagenous 50
 non-collagenous bone 50
 reporter 249
protein stability 32
PRP, *see* platelet-rich-plasma
pSi particles 32–33
pulsed electromagnetic fields
 12

recellularization 375–376, 378
red blood cells 33–34

SBF, *see* simulated body fluid
SBF solutions 122, 125, 127,
 130–135, 137
scaffold architecture 288–289,
 294
scaffold bioactivity 184, 197
scaffold design 288
scaffold fabrication 159, 379
scaffold fixation 192
scaffolds
 biomimetic 5, 9–11, 247, 250,
 286–287, 316, 342
 biphasic 147–148, 150,
 157–158, 160, 163,
 166–168, 287
 bilayered 199, 287
 bio-inspired 5, 7, 9
 bioactive 64, 243
 biocompatible 358, 365
 biological 308
 bioresorbable 181
 collagen biomaterial 250
 fiber-deposited 193–194
 fibre-reinforced 163, 167
 fibrous 225
 hybrid 12, 64
 monolithic 147, 151, 157,
 170
 monophasic 151, 163–164
 nerve scaffolds 229–230
 organomorphic 358, 367,
 369, 371, 373, 375, 377
 osteoconductive 11
 polycaprolactone 244
 polyurethane 311, 315
 synthetic 90, 308
 three-dimensional 247, 341
 tissue-engineered 192, 246
 tubular 190
Schwann cells 212–217, 224,
 226–228
 exogenous 227–228

immature 213–215
mature 214
migrating 226, 228
nonmyelinating 214
Schwann precursor cells 213
signaling molecules 27,
246–247
simulated body fluid (SBF)
120, 122–125, 127, 129,
131–132, 134–135, 186
smart biomimetic
biomaterials 306
SMFs, *see* static magnetic field
spinal fusion 12, 293,
336–337, 339
spinal surgery 64, 314, 316,
335–336, 338, 340, 342,
344, 346, 348, 350
spine 102, 336–339
spongy bone 87, 96, 181, 290
static magnetic field (SMFs) 13,
189, 293–294
stem cells 147, 228, 312, 347
adult bone marrow 347
cultured bone marrow 94
embryonic 358
human mesenchymal
155–156, 170, 194
mesenchymal 14, 65,
146–147, 289
multipotent 373
neural crest 216
stromal cells, human bone
marrow 189
stromal/vascular scaffold
(SVS) 362–363, 366–368,
370–371, 373, 376, 378
strontium 108–109, 344
SVS, *see* stromal/vascular
scaffold
synthetic biomaterials 25, 29,
220, 349, 358, 378

tendons 87, 145, 184, 306,
308, 313, 315, 347–348
therapeutic agents 66,
227–228, 274
thymus 376, 378
thyrocytes 366–367, 374
thyroid 363–364, 366, 371,
374
thyroid cells 369–370, 374
tissue
cardiac 273
cartilage 146, 154, 157, 159,
163, 284, 323
cartilage repair 288, 326–327
human bone 135
ligament 88
musculoskeletal 305–306
natural bone 98
nerve 220, 229
skeletal 57
stromal 219, 223
vascular 13, 190, 363
tissue engineering strategies
342–343, 345
tissue regeneration 4, 10, 22,
30, 147, 181, 221, 243,
246, 284, 288, 293–295
tissue repair 213, 216, 315
tissue transplantation
305–306
titanium 65, 128–129, 131,
339
tooth 1, 55–57
trabecular bone 98, 193, 287
tumors 68–70, 180, 187–188,
198

vascular endothelial growth
factor (VEGF) 67, 180,

215, 227, 229, 244, 251, 292, 343–344

vascularization 181, 183, 219, 222–223, 227–228, 286, 307

VEGF, *see* vascular endothelial growth factor

vertebroplasty 104–105

Wallerian degeneration 216–217, 219

wound healing 23, 28, 30, 245

X-ray diffraction (XRD) 51, 53, 62, 109

XRD, *see* X-ray diffraction